Ocular
Inflammatory Disease

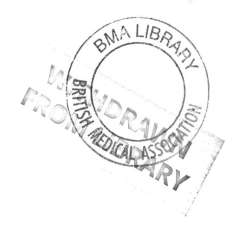

Commissioning Editor: Paul Fam
Project Development Manager: Helen Sofio
Editorial Assistant: Sven Pinczewski
Project Manager: Glenys Norquay
Designer: Andy Chapman
Illustration Manager: Mick Ruddy
New Illustrations: Richard Prime
Marketing Manager (UK): Gaynor Jones
Marketing Manager (USA): Lisa Damico

Ocular
Inflammatory Disease

Jack J Kanski MD MS FRCS FRCOphth

Honorary Consultant Ophthalmic Surgeon
Prince Charles Eye Unit
King Edward VII Hospital
Windsor, UK

Carlos E Pavésio MD FRCOphth

Consultant Ophthalmic Surgeon
Moorfields Eye Hospital
London, UK

Stephen J Tuft MA MChir MD FRCOphth

Consultant Ophthalmic Surgeon
Moorfields Eye Hospital
London, UK

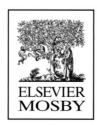

ELSEVIER
MOSBY

MOSBY An Affiliate of Elsevier Limited

First published 2004
  Reprinted 2004, 2005, 2007

ISBN 0 323 03737 2

British Library Cataloguing in Publication Data
A catalogue record for this book is available from the British Library

Library of Congress Cataloguing in Publication Data
A catalogue record for this book is available from the Library of Congress

Notice
Medical knowledge is constantly changing. As new information becomes available, changes in treatment, procedures, equipment and the use of drugs become necessary. The author, contributor and the publishers have, as far as it is possible, taken care to ensure that the information given in this text is accurate and up to date. However, readers are strongly advised to confirm that the information, especially with regard to drug usage, complies with the latest legislation and standards of practice.

The Publisher

your source for books,
journals and multimedia
in the health sciences
www.elsevierhealth.com

Working together to grow
libraries in developing countries

www.elsevier.com | www.bookaid.org | www.sabre.org

ELSEVIER   BOOK AID
             International   Sabre Foundation

The
publisher's
policy is to use
**paper manufactured
from sustainable forests**

Printed in China
Last digit is the print number: 9   8   7   6   5   4   3   2

Contents

Preface

Inflammation is the central mechanism of the majority of acquired ocular diseases. Its importance has been highlighted by the recognition that even conditions such as diabetes and macular degeneration have an inflammatory basis. While some inflammatory processes are limited to the eye and others are associated with systemic disorder, all are potentially treatable.

Effective management of inflammatory eye disease rests on the correct identification of the clinical picture. Distinguishing infectious from non-infectious disease is of paramount importance since therapy will be radically different. Familiarity with the clinical features of the many different manifestations of inflammation is essential.

It has been our intention to create a book that would provide a succinct and practical guide with clear descriptions of the important clinical presentations. The text has been richly illustrated with clinical details and examples. A description of the diagnostic features, the recommended investigations, differential diagnosis, and management of each condition is presented.

We have prepared a practical guide rather than a comprehensive review of each subject. However, key references for further study are provided. We trust that trainees at all levels will find this book an excellent companion.

JJK
CEP
SJT

Chapter 1

Blepharitis

ANATOMY

The eyelids provide a mechanical and functional component essential to the health of the ocular surface.

1. **The grey line** divides the eyelids into an anterior and posterior lamella (Fig. 1.1).

- The anterior lamella is composed of skin containing the bases of the eyelashes and the orbicularis oculi muscle.

- The posterior lamella consists of conjunctival mucous membrane and the meibomian glands within the tarsal plate.

- The grey line helps contain the anterior margin of the tear meniscus.

2. **The glands** in the lid margin are of the following three types:

a. *Meibomian glands* are modified sebaceous glands that empty through a single row of about 30 openings on each lid; double rows of openings are a rare normal anatomical variant.

- The structure of the glands can be visualised by transillumination of the everted lid. The glands and their openings may be congenitally absent in ectodermal dysplasia and their numbers reduced following chronic inflammation (gland dropout).

- Each gland consists of a central duct with multiple acini, the cells of which synthesise lipids (meibum) that pass into the duct when the cells degenerate (holocrine gland function).

- The meibum consists of polar and non-polar lipids. The latter link the surface polar lipids to lipocalins in the aqueous layer and thus help maintain a stable tear film. Oleic acid is the most abundant lipid.

- The rate of lipid production is under neuronal, hormonal and vascular control. Androgen, oestrogen and progesterone receptors have been identified. The meibomian lipids normally have a melting point below 32°C and this temperature can increase in the presence of disease.

b. *The glands of Zeis* are modified sebaceous glands that are associated with lash follicles.

c. *The glands of Moll* are modified sweat glands, the ducts of which open either into a lash follicle or directly onto the anterior lid margin between the lashes.

3. **The lashes** are slightly more numerous in the upper lid than in the lower lid.

- The lash roots lie against the anterior surface of the tarsus, between the pretarsal orbicularis oculi muscle and the muscle of Riolan.

- The cilia pass between the orbicularis oculi and the muscle of Riolan and exit the skin at the anterior lid margin and curve away from the globe (Fig. 1.2).

- Scarring of the tarsal plate and conjunctiva can alter lash position and direction. Following intense inflammation, abnormal lashes can grow from meibomian gland openings (distichiasis).

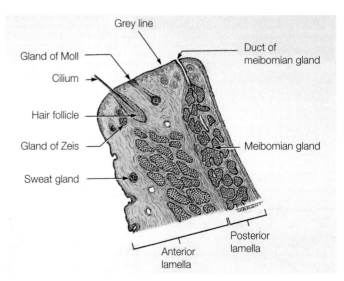

Fig. 1.1 Cross-section of the lower lid

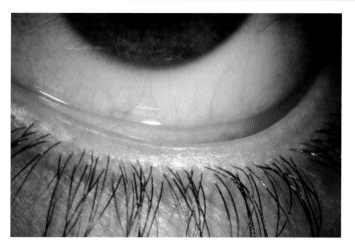

Fig. 1.2 Normal lower lid

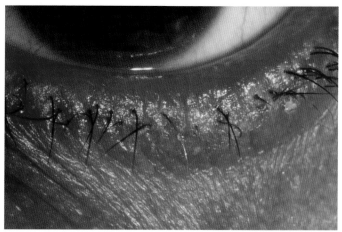

Fig. 1.3 Hard scales around the bases of lashes (collarettes) and madarosis in staphylococcal blepharitis

CHRONIC MARGINAL BLEPHARITIS

Chronic marginal blepharitis is a very common cause of ocular discomfort and irritation. It may be subdivided into anterior and posterior, although there is often considerable overlap in symptoms and features of both are often present. Patients with anterior disease tend to be younger than those with posterior blepharitis, but both types can result in conjunctivitis, keratitis, exacerbation of ocular allergy and dry eye. The poor correlation between symptoms and signs, uncertain aetiology and mechanisms of the disease process, conspire to make management difficult.

NB: Some signs of blepharitis (e.g. lid margin telangiectasis, pouting of meibomian gland orifices) may occur as a part of the normal ageing process in asymptomatic individuals.

Anterior blepharitis

Pathogenesis

Anterior blepharitis affects the area surrounding the bases of the eyelashes and may be staphylococcal or seborrhoeic.

Staph. epidermidis and *P. acnes* are normal skin flora, but *Staph. aureus* is more common in patients with staphylococcal blepharitis than in unaffected individuals. The inflammatory capacity of components of the cell wall of Gram-positive bacteria is well documented and it is possible that there is also an abnormal cell-mediated response to some components of the cell wall of *Staph. aureus*. This response may also be responsible for the red eye reaction and the peripheral corneal infiltrates seen in some patients. Seborrhoeic blepharitis is often associated with generalised seborrhoeic dermatitis that may involve the scalp, nasolabial folds, behind the ears, and the sternum.

NB: Because of the intimate relationship between the lids and ocular surface, chronic blepharitis may cause secondary inflammatory and mechanical changes in the conjunctiva and cornea.

Diagnosis

1. **Symptoms** do not provide a reliable clue to the type of blepharitis.

- Burning, grittiness, mild photophobia, and crusting and redness of the lid margins with remissions and exacerbations are characteristic.

- Symptoms are usually worse in the mornings, although in patients with associated dry eye they may increase during the day.

NB: Because of poor correlation between the severity of symptoms and clinical signs, it can be difficult to objectively assess the benefit of treatment.

2. **Signs**

a. Staphylococcal blepharitis

- Hard scales and crusting mainly located around the bases of the lashes (collarettes) (Figs 1.3 and 1.4).

- Mild papillary conjunctivitis (Fig. 1.5) and chronic conjunctival hyperaemia are common (Fig. 1.6).

- Acute folliculitis and external hordeola (styes) may develop by spread of infection to the lash follicles (Fig. 1.7).

- Lid margin ulceration in severe disease.

- Scarring and notching (tylosis) of the lid margin in long-standing cases (Fig. 1.8).

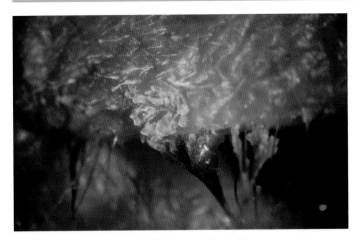

Fig. 1.4 Severe scaling in staphylococcal blepharitis

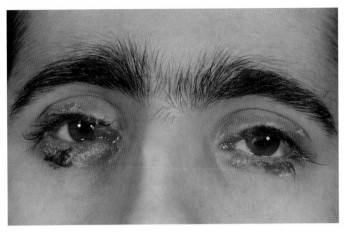

Fig. 1.7 Severe staphylococcal blepharitis with a stye in the right lower lid

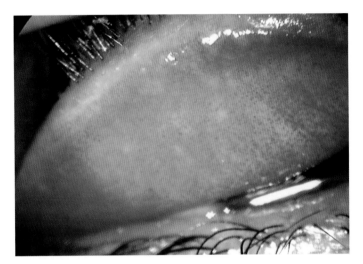

Fig. 1.5 Papillary conjunctivitis in staphylococcal blepharitis

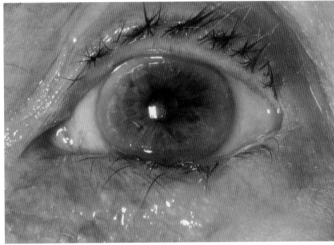

Fig. 1.8 Scarring and notching of the lower lid margin in longstanding staphylococcal blepharitis

- The lashes in longstanding cases may become white (poliosis) (Fig. 1.9), thin and fewer in number (madarosis) (Fig. 1.10), and misdirected inwards (trichiasis) (Fig. 1.11).

- Secondary corneal changes include superficial punctate corneal erosions involving the inferior third of the cornea, marginal keratitis (Fig. 1.12), phlyctenulosis (Fig. 1.13) and vascularisation (Fig. 1.14).

- Associated tear film instability and dry eye are common.

b. Seborrhoeic blepharitis

- Hyperaemic and greasy anterior lid margins with sticking together of lashes (Fig. 1.15).

- The scales are soft and located anywhere on the lid margin and lashes (Fig. 1.16).

- The majority of patients have seborrhoeic dermatitis elsewhere (Fig. 1.17).

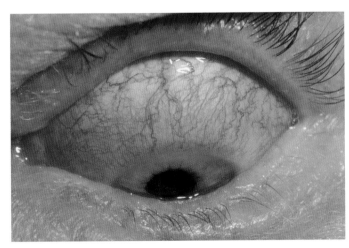

Fig. 1.6 Bulbar conjunctival hyperaemia in staphylococcal blepharitis

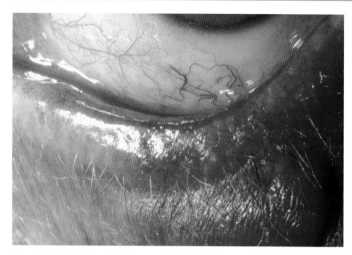

Fig. 1.9 Poliosis in staphylococcal blepharitis

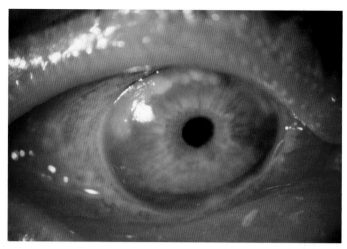

Fig. 1.12 Marginal keratitis in staphylococcal blepharitis

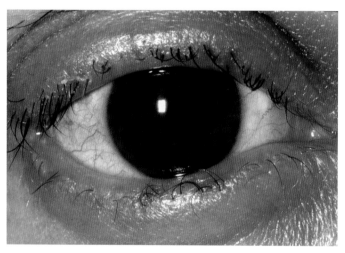

Fig. 1.10 Madarosis and misdirection of lashes, particularly in the lower lid, in staphylococcal blepharitis

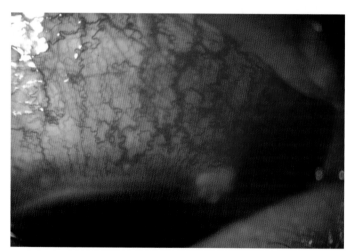

Fig. 1.13 Limbal phlycten in staphylococcal blepharitis

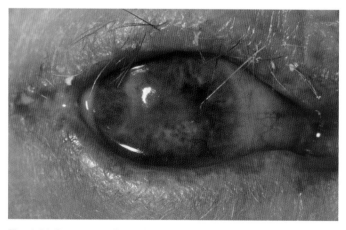

Fig. 1.11 Severe madarosis, trichiasis and keratopathy in staphylococcal blepharitis

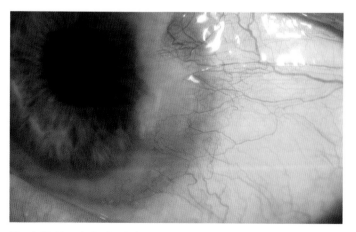

Fig. 1.14 Vascularisation in longstanding staphylococcal blepharitis

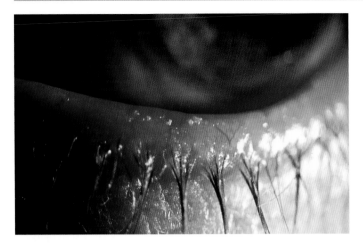

Fig. 1.15 Mild seborrhoeic blepharitis

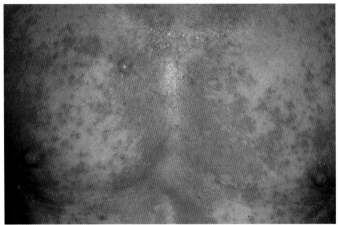

Fig. 1.17 Seborrhoeic dermatitis on the chest

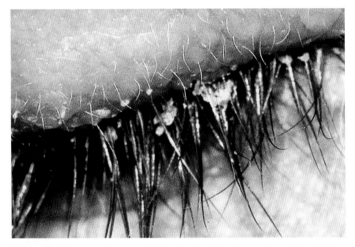

Fig. 1.16 Severe seborrhoeic blepharitis (Courtesy of J Silbert, from *Anterior Segment Complications of Contact Lens Wear*, Butterworth-Heinemann, 1999)

3. Investigations

a. ***Cultures*** may be taken in severe cases, but this is not otherwise indicated. *Staph. epidermidis* and *Staph. aureus* are the most common isolates. However, there is a poor correlation between the isolate, antibiotic sensitivity spectrum and clinical response to antibiotic treatment.

b. ***Biopsy*** should be performed if tumour is suspected.

Treatment

There is little evidence to support any particular treatment protocol for anterior blepharitis. Patients should be advised that lifelong treatment may be necessary, that a permanent cure is unlikely, but that control of symptoms is usually possible. In longstanding cases, several weeks of intensive treatment may be needed to achieve improvement.

1. Lid hygiene

- A warm compress applied for several minutes to soften crusts at the bases of the lashes.

- Lid cleaning to mechanically remove crusts involves scrubbing the lid margins once or twice daily with a cotton bud dipped in a dilute solution of baby shampoo or sodium bicarbonate.

- Commercially produced soap/alcohol impregnated pads for lid scrubs are available, but care should be taken not to induce mechanical irritation.

- The eyelids can also be cleaned with diluted shampoo when washing the hair.

- Gradually, lid hygiene can be performed less frequently as the condition is brought under control, but blepharitis often recurs if it is stopped completely.

2. Antibiotics

a. ***Topical*** sodium fusidic acid, bacitracin or chloramphenicol is used to treat acute folliculitis but is of limited value in longstanding cases. Following lid hygiene, the ointment should be rubbed onto the anterior lid margin with a cotton bud or clean finger.

b. ***Oral*** azithromycin (500 mg daily for 3 days) may be helpful to control ulcerative lid margin disease.

3. Weak topical steroids such as fluorometholone 0.1% q.i.d. for 1 week is useful in patients with severe papillary conjunctivitis, marginal keratitis and phlyctenulosis, although repeated courses may be required.

4. Tear substitutes are required for associated tear film instability and dry eye.

Posterior blepharitis

Pathogenesis

Posterior blepharitis is caused by meibomian gland dysfunction with keratinisation of the meibomian gland orifices and gland dropout, although it is unclear if these are primary or secondary phenomena. Alterations in meibomian gland secretions cause relative loss of non-polar lipids and an

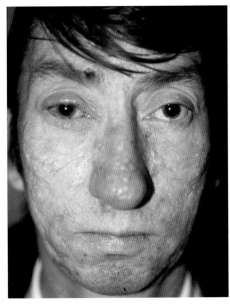

Fig. 1.18 Severe acne rosacea and chalazion involving the right lower lid associated with posterior blepharitis

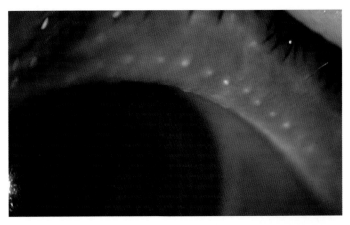

Fig. 1.20 Plugging of meibomian gland orifices in posterior blepharitis

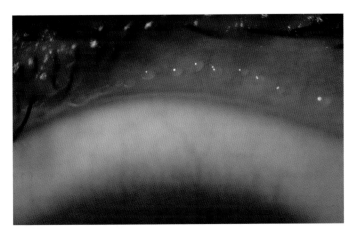

Fig. 1.19 Capping of meibomian gland orifices with oil in posterior blepharitis

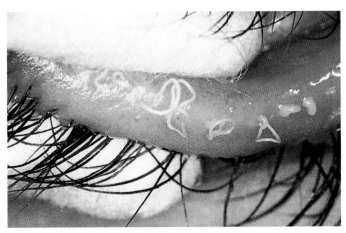

Fig. 1.21 Toothpaste-like plaques expressed from the meibomian glands in posterior blepharitis (Courtesy of J Silbert, from *Anterior Segment Complications of Contact Lens Wear*, Butterworth-Heinemann, 1999)

increase in cholesterol esters, waxes and unsaturated fatty acids.

Bacterial lipases may give rise to the formation of free fatty acids. This results in an increase in the melting point of the meibum, preventing expression from the glands, so contributing to ocular surface irritation and possibly enabling growth of *Staph. aureus*. Loss of the tear film phospholipids that act as surfactants results in increased tear evaporation and osmolarity, and an unstable tear film. There is a strong association between meibomian gland dysfunction and acne rosacea (Fig. 1.18).

Diagnosis

There is a poor correlation between the severity of symptoms and the clinical signs.

1. **Symptoms** are similar to anterior blepharitis.

2. **Signs** of meibomian gland dysfunction

- Excessive and abnormal meibomian gland secretion which may manifest as capping of meibomian gland orifices with oil globules (Fig. 1.19).

- Pouting, recession, or plugging of the meibomian gland orifices (Fig. 1.20).

- Pressure on the lid margin results in expression of meibomian fluid that may be turbid or appear like toothpaste (Fig. 1.21); in severe cases the secretions become so inspissated that expression is impossible.

- The posterior lid margin shows hyperaemia and telangiectasia (Fig. 1.22).

- Lid transillumination may show gland loss and cystic dilatation of meibomian ducts.

- Meibomian cysts are common and may be multiple and recurrent (Fig. 1.23).

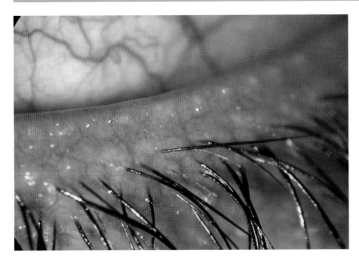

Fig. 1.22 Hyperaemia and telangiectasia of the posterior lid margin in posterior blepharitis

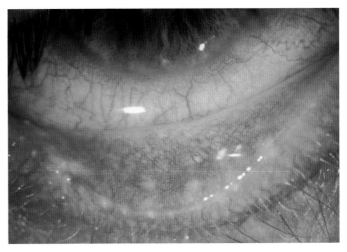

Fig. 1.25 Conjunctival concretions in posterior blepharitis

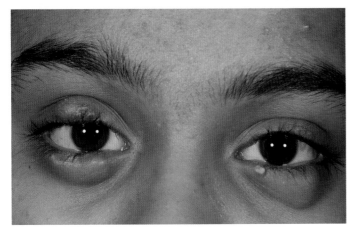

Fig. 1.23 Multiple meibomian cysts in posterior blepharitis

- The tear film is oily and foamy, and froth may accumulate on the lid margins or inner canthi (Fig. 1.24). The tear film break-up time may be reduced; about 40% of patients have associated aqueous tear film deficiency.

- Conjunctival changes include papillary conjunctivitis, inclusion cysts and concretions (Fig. 1.25). Subconjunctival scarring associated with shortening of the fornices may occur in chronic disease.

- Inferior corneal punctate epithelial erosions are common.

Treatment

It is very important to inform the patient that cure is unlikely. Although remission may be achieved, recurrence is common, particularly if treatment is stopped.

1. Lid hygiene

- Warm compresses and hygiene are performed as for anterior blepharitis except the emphasis is on massaging the lid to express accumulated meibum.

- Massaging toward the lid margin edge to 'milk' meibum and physical expression of the glands by the physician is of uncertain benefit (see Fig. 1.21).

2. Systemic tetracyclines are the mainstay of treatment.

- The rationale for the use of tetracyclines is their ability to block staphylococcal lipase production at concentrations well below the minimum inhibitory concentration. They also inhibit the action of tear matrix metalloproteinase.

- Tetracyclines are particularly indicated in patients with recurrent phlyctenulosis and marginal keratitis, although repeated courses of treatment may be needed.

- Gastrointestinal upset is the most common side effect.

- Tetracyclines inhibit absorption of oral contraceptives.

- Photosensitisation and pigmentation of the skin and mucous membranes can occur.

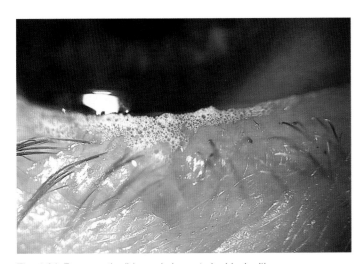

Fig. 1.24 Foam on the lid margin in posterior blepharitis

NB: Tetracyclines should not be used in children under the age of 12 years (erythromycin is an alternative) or in pregnant or breastfeeding women, because they are deposited in growing bone and teeth, and may cause staining of teeth and dental hypoplasia.

a. **Oxytetracycline** 250 mg b.d. for 6–12 weeks; tetracycline probably has a similar effect although evidence is lacking.

b. **Doxycycline** 100 mg b.d. for 1 week and then daily for 6–12 weeks.

c. **Minocycline** 100 mg daily for 6–12 weeks; skin pigmentation may develop after prolonged use (Fig. 1.26).

d. **Erythromycin** 250 mg b.d. may be used in children.

3. **Topical therapy** involves antibiotics, steroids and tear substitutes for evaporative dry eye.

Associated conditions

1. **Tear film instability and dry eye** is found in 30–50% of patients, probably as a result of imbalance between the aqueous and lipid components of the tear film allowing increased evaporation. Tear film break-up time is typically reduced.

2. **Chalazion formation**, which may be multiple and recurrent, is common, particularly in patients with posterior blepharitis.

3. **Epithelial basement membrane disease** and recurrent epithelial erosion may be exacerbated by posterior blepharitis.

4. **Cutaneous**

a. **Acne rosacea** is often associated with meibomian gland dysfunction (see Fig. 1.18).

b. **Seborrhoeic dermatitis** is present in >90% of patients with seborrhoeic blepharitis (see Fig. 1.17).

c. **Acne vulgaris** treatment with isotretinoin is associated with the development of blepharitis in about 25% of patients; it subsides when the treatment is stopped.

5. **Bacterial keratitis** is associated with ocular surface disease secondary to chronic blepharitis.

6. **Atopic keratoconjunctivitis** is often associated with staphylococcal blepharitis. Treatment of the blepharitis

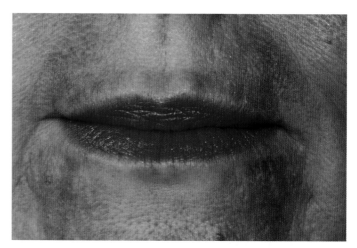

Fig. 1.26 Skin pigmentation due to prolonged use of minocycline

Table 1.1 Summary of characteristics of chronic blepharitis

	Feature	Anterior blepharitis		Posterior blepharitis
		Staphylococcal	Seborrhoeic	
Lashes	Deposit	Hard	Soft	
	Loss	++	+	
	Distorted or trichiasis	++	+	
Lid margin	Ulceration	+		
	Notching	+		++
Cyst	Hordeolum	++		
	Meibomian			+
Conjunctiva	Phlyctenule	+		+
Tear film	Foaming			++
	Dry eye	+	+	++
Cornea	Punctate erosions	+	+	++
	Vascularisation	+	+	++
	Infiltrates	+	+	++
Associated dermatitis		Atopic	Seborrhoeic	Acne rosacea

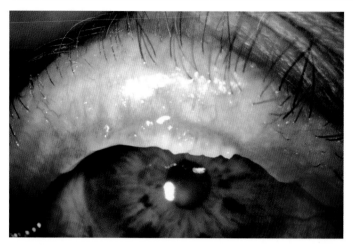

Fig. 1.27 Sebaceous cell carcinoma causing localised thickening of the lid margin and madarosis

Ficker L, Ramakrishnan M, Seal D, et al. Role of cell-mediated immunity to staphylococci in blepharitis. *Am J Ophthalmol* 1991;111:473–479.

McCulley JP, Dougherty JM, Deneau DG. Classification of chronic blepharitis. *Ophthalmology* 1982;89:1173–1180.

McCulley JP, Shine WE. Changing concepts in the diagnosis and management of blepharitis. *Cornea* 2000;19:650–658.

Mathers WD. Ocular evaporation in meibomian gland dysfunction and dry eye. *Ophthalmology* 1993;100:347–351.

Mathers WD, Shields, WJ, Sachdev MS, et al. Meibomian gland dysfunction and chronic blepharitis. *Cornea* 1991;10:277–285.

Seal D, Ficker L, Ramakrishnan M, et al. Role of staphylococcal toxin production in blepharitis. *Ophthalmology* 1990;97:1684–1688.

Shimazaki J, Goto E, Ono M, et al. Meibomian gland dysfunction in patients with Sjögren syndrome. *Ophthalmology* 1998;105:1485–1488.

MISCELLANEOUS BLEPHARITIS

Phthiriasis palpebrarum

Pathogenesis

The crab louse *Phthirus pubis* is adapted to living in pubic hair (Fig. 1.28). An infested person may transfer the lice to another hairy area such as the chest, axillae or eyelids. Phthiriasis palpebrarum is an infestation of lashes.

Diagnosis

1. **Symptoms** consist of chronic irritation and itching of the lids.

2. **Signs**

- The lice are anchored to the lashes by their claws (Fig. 1.29).

- The ova and their empty shells appear as oval, brownish, opalescent pearls adherent to the base of the cilia (Fig. 1.30).

- Conjunctivitis is uncommon.

often helps the symptoms of allergic conjunctivitis and vice versa.

7. **Contact lens intolerance.** Long-term contact lens wear is associated with posterior lid margin disease. Inhibition of lid movement and the normal expression of meibomian oil may be the cause. There may also be associated giant papillary conjunctivitis, making comfortable lens wear difficult. Blepharitis is also a risk factor for contact lens-associated bacterial keratitis.

Differential diagnosis

A number of conditions may masquerade as chronic blepharitis. Misdiagnosis may delay initiation of appropriate treatment and can be life threatening.

1. **Infiltrating lid tumours** should be suspected in patients with apparently asymmetric or unilateral chronic blepharitis, particularly when associated with loss of lashes (Fig. 1.27).

2. **Ocular cicatricial pemphigoid** and other mucocutaneous disorders.

3. **Dermatoses** with lid margin involvement, most notably, discoid lupus erythematosus, psoriasis and ichthyosis.

4. **Factitious** blepharitis, especially in patients with chronic unilateral conjunctivitis.

FURTHER READING

Bron AJ, Benjamin L, Snibson GR. Meibomian gland disease. Classification and grading of lid changes. *Eye* 1991;5:395–411.

Doherty JM, McCulley JP, Silvany RE, et al. The role of tetracycline in chronic blepharitis: inhibition of lipase production in staphylococci. *Invest Ophthalmol Vis Sci* 1991;32:2970–2975.

Driver PJ, Lemp MA. Meibomian gland dysfunction. *Surv Ophthalmol* 1996;40:343–367.

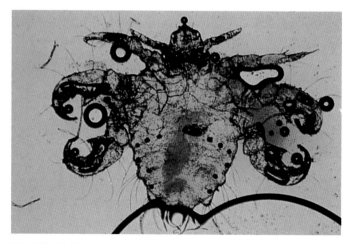

Fig. 1.28 *Phthirus pubis* (crab or pubic louse) (Courtesy of Hart and Shears, from *Color Atlas of Medical Microbiology*, Mosby, 2004)

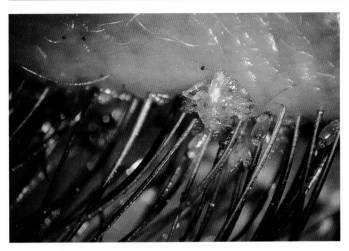

Fig. 1.29 Lice in phthiriasis palpebrarum

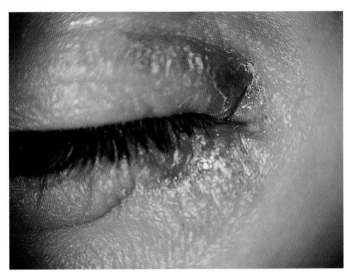

Fig. 1.31 Angular blepharitis

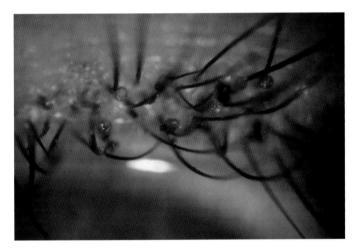

Fig. 1.30 Ova and shells in phthiriasis palpebrarum

Treatment

1. **Mechanical removal** of the lice and their attached lashes with fine forceps.

2. **Topical** yellow mercuric oxide 1% or petroleum jelly applied to the lashes and lids twice a day for 10 days.

3. **Delousing** of the patient, family members, clothing and bedding is important to prevent recurrences.

> **NB:** One-third of patients with pubic lice have a sexually transmitted disease.

Angular blepharitis

Angular blepharitis involves the lateral and median canthus. Similar changes may be seen in patients with severe allergic conjunctivitis.

1. **Pathogenesis.** The infection is usually caused by *Moraxella lacunata* or *Staph. aureus*, although other bacteria, and rarely herpes simplex, have also been implicated.

2. **Signs**

- Often unilateral, red, scaly, macerated skin at the canthus (Fig. 1.31).

- Associated papillary and follicular conjunctivitis may occur.

3. **Treatment** involves topical chloramphenicol, bacitracin or erythromycin cream.

Childhood blepharokeratoconjunctivitis

Childhood blepharokeratoconjunctivitis is a poorly defined condition which tends to be more severe in Asian and Middle Eastern populations.

Diagnosis

1. **Presentation** is usually at about 6 years of age with chronic redness and irritation that results in constant eye rubbing and photophobia which may be misdiagnosed as allergic eye disease.

2. **Signs**

- Chronic anterior or posterior blepharitis which may be associated with recurrent styes or meibomian cysts.

- Conjunctival changes include diffuse hyperaemia, bulbar phlyctens, and follicular or papillary hyperplasia.

- Superficial punctate keratopathy, marginal keratitis, peripheral vascularisation (Fig. 1.32) and axial subepithelial haze.

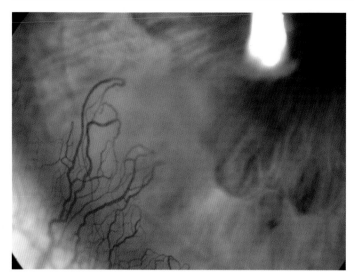

Fig. 1.32 Peripheral corneal vascularisation in childhood blepharokerato-conjunctivitis

Treatment

* Treatment of blepharitis with lid hygiene and topical antibiotic ointment at bedtime.

* Topical low-dose steroid (prednisolone 0.1% or fluoro-metholone 0.1%).

* Oral erythromycin syrup 125 mg daily for 4–6 weeks.

FURTHER READING

Farpour B, McClellan KA. Diagnosis and management of chronic blepharoconjunctivitis in children. *J Paediatr Ophthalmol Strabismus* 2001;38:204–212.

Rundle PA, Hughes DS. Phthirus pubis infestation of the eyelids. *Br J Ophthalmol* 1993;77:815–816.

Viswalingam M, Rauz S, Morlet N, et al. Blepharokeratoconjunctivitis in children: diagnosis and treatment. *Br J Ophthalmol* 2005;89:400–403.

Chapter 2

Dry eye disorders

INTRODUCTION

Dry eye occurs when there is inadequate tear volume or function resulting in an unstable tear film and ocular surface disease. However, the tear film should not be considered in isolation, but as part of a functional unit also comprising the corneal and conjunctival epithelium, the lacrimal glands and the lids. A stimulus to any part of this unit can elicit a unified response. Using the term 'ocular surface and tear disorders' to describe the resultant spectrum of diseases reflects the interrelationship between these contributing factors. Different disorders in this group share some common features: (a) characteristic symptoms; (b) tear film instability, (c) tear hyperosmolarity and (d) signs of ocular surface damage.

Epidemiology

Dry eye is a common condition with a prevalence of self-reported symptoms of about 11–33% of the population over 45 years. Depending on the diagnostic criteria used, about 2.2% have symptoms of dry eye and reduced Schirmer test; however, only 0.4–0.5% of the population receive treatment. Risk factors are age, female gender, arthritis, and oestrogen hormonal replacement. Symptoms of dry eye are more common in people who use VDUs or wear contact lenses.

Physiology

Aqueous tear secretion

- The main lacrimal glands produce about 95% of the aqueous component of tears, and the accessory lacrimal glands of Krause and Wolfring produce the remainder.

- Secretion of tears has basic (resting) and much greater reflex components. Reflex secretion occurs in response to corneal and conjunctival sensory stimulation, tear break up, and ocular inflammation mediated via the fifth cranial nerve. It is reduced by topical anaesthesia and during sleep. Secretion can increase 500% in response to injury.

- Inadequate tear function results in symptoms of irritation and damage to the ocular surface that constitutes keratoconjunctivitis sicca (KCS). Dry eye and KCS are synonymous and it is now evident that inflammation is also an important component.

Spread of the tear film

- The tear film is mechanically spread over the ocular surface through a neuronally controlled blinking mechanism and is cleared through the nasolacrimal drainage system.

- Three factors are required for effective resurfacing of the tear film: (a) normal blink reflex, (b) contact between the external ocular surface and eyelids, and (c) a normal corneal epithelium.

- Considerable force is applied to the epithelium during blinking, producing about 1 mm of retropulsion. The tear film must be able to disperse the associated shearing force on the epithelium.

- In addition to the specialised functions described below, the tear film provides a smooth optical surface to the cornea and freely transmits oxygen and carbon dioxide.

Tear film constituents

The tear film has three layers:

- Lipid layer secreted by the meibomian glands.

- Aqueous layer secreted by the lacrimal glands.

- Mucin layer secreted principally by conjunctival goblet cells and also the lacrimal glands.

However, it is now clear that this is an oversimplification and there are gradients of constituents from the ocular surface to the lipid layer. Each layer has separate functions, disease of which can lead to functional changes resulting in symptoms of dry eye.

OUTER LIPID LAYER

1. Composition

- The outer lipid layer is composed of two phases: a polar surfactant phase containing phospholipids adjacent to the aqueous–mucin phase, and an outer surface non-polar phase containing waxes, cholesterol esters and triglycerides.

- The polar lipids are bound to lipocalins within the aqueous layer which are small secreted proteins that have the ability to bind hydrophobic molecules and may also contribute to tear viscosity.

- Lid movement during blinking is important in releasing lipids from the glands. The thickness of the layer can be increased by forced blinking and conversely reduced by infrequent blinking during periods of visual concentration.

2. Functions

- To prevent evaporation of the aqueous layer of the tear film and maintain tear film thickness.

- To act as a surfactant, allowing spread of the tear film.

- Deficiency results in evaporative dry eye.

MIDDLE AQUEOUS LAYER

1. Composition

- Water, electrolytes, dissolved mucins and proteins.

- Growth factors derived from the lacrimal gland, production of which increases in response to injury.

- Pro-inflammatory interleukin cytokines, which accumulate during sleep, when tear production is reduced.

2. Functions

- Antibacterial due to the presence of proteins such as IgA, lysozyme and lactoferrin.

- To wash away debris and noxious stimuli and allow the passage of leucocytes after injury.

- The aqueous phase is anchored to the apical glycocalyx of the external epithelial cells. In deficiency states it becomes hyperosmolar and epithelial cell damage occurs.

INNER MUCIN LAYER

1. Composition

- Mucins which are high-molecular-weight glycoproteins that may be transmembrane or secretory. The latter are further classified as gel-forming or soluble.

- The secretory ocular mucins are principally produced by the conjunctival goblet cells and also by the lacrimal glands. The superficial epithelial cells of the cornea and conjunctiva produce transmembrane mucins that form the glycocalyx.

- Epithelial staining with rose bengal indicates that the transmembrane and gel mucin layer is absent and the cell surface exposed. Damage to the epithelial cells will prevent normal tear film adherence.

2. Functions

- To permit wetting by converting the corneal epithelium from a hydrophobic to a hydrophilic surface.

- Lubrication.

NB: Deficiency of the mucin layer may be a feature of both aqueous deficiency and evaporative states. Goblet cell loss is associated with cicatrising conjunctivitis, vitamin A deficiency, chemical burns and toxicity to medications.

Regulation of tear film components

1. Hormonal

- Androgens are the prime hormones that regulate lipid production.

- Oestrogen and progesterone receptors have been identified in conjunctiva and lacrimal gland tissue, and appear to be essential for normal function of these tissues.

- Postmenopausal women and the elderly may be relatively androgen-deficient and this may account for some of the observed involutional changes. Androgen may also be a natural suppressor of inflammation.

2. Neural fibres adjacent to the lacrimal gland and goblet cells result in aqueous and mucus secretion.

Mechanism of disease

- Inflammation in the conjunctiva and accessory glands is present in 80% of patients with KCS.

- There is increased expression of HLA class II antigens and expression of markers of apoptosis and inflammatory cytokines in the epithelium, resulting in apoptosis, squamous metaplasia, and loss of goblet cells.

- Inflammation may thus be the cause and consequence of dry eye, amplifying and perpetuating disease. The presence of inflammation is the rationale for steroid therapy.

- Hyperosmolarity of tears is also a key mechanism of disease, and may be the major pathway for epithelial cell damage.

Classification

The classification outlined in Table 2.1 is usually applied, although most individuals have considerable overlap between mechanisms.

Table 2.1 Classification of keratoconjunctivitis sicca

1. **Aqueous layer deficiency**
   - Sjögren syndrome
   - Non-Sjögren
2. **Evaporative**
   - Meibomian gland disease
   - Exposure
   - Defective blinking
   - Contact lens associated
   - Environmental factors

rheumatoid arthritis, systemic lupus erythematosus, scleroderma, dermatomyositis and polymyositis, mixed connective disease, relapsing polychondritis and primary biliary cirrhosis (see Ch. 8). Detection of these conditions is important. Diagnostic criteria require confirmation of disease and two other objective criteria.

NB: Exclusion criteria for Sjögren syndrome include head or neck irradiation, hepatitis C infection, AIDS, lymphoma, sarcoidosis, graft-versus-host disease and the use of anticholinergic drugs.

Sjögren syndrome

Sjögren syndrome is a systemic autoimmune condition characterised by lymphocytic infiltration of the exocrine glands and mucous membranes, resulting in a secondary reduction in secretion leading to abnormalities in the tear film and ocular surface disease. The primary features are a dry eye with dry mouth. It affects approximately 0.4% of the population and it is more common in women.

NB: Detection of associated disease is important because patients are also at risk of developing ocular inflammation (keratitis, scleritis and uveitis) or a life-threatening systemic vasculitis.

1. **Diagnostic criteria**

a. Symptomatic

- Ocular symptoms or the use of artificial tear substitutes.
- Oral symptoms of dry mouth, swollen salivary glands or the need for frequent drinks.

b. Objective

- Objective evidence of dry eyes (see below).
- Positive involvement of minor salivary gland on labial biopsy.
- Salivary involvement demonstrated by sialography or scintilography.
- Laboratory evaluation for extractable nuclear antigens (anti-Ro and anti-La, antinuclear antigen or rheumatoid factor).

2. **Primary** Sjögren syndrome may have systemic symptoms (arthralgia, myalgia and fatigue) that do not constitute a readily classifiable disease (see Ch. 8). Diagnostic criteria require histology or serology to be positive with a total of four criteria fulfilled, or three of the four objective criteria.

3. **Secondary** Sjögren syndrome is associated with an underlying distinct autoimmune disease. Examples include

Causes of non-Sjögren dry eye

1. **Primary** age-related hyposecretion is the most common.

2. **Lacrimal tissue destruction**

- Tumour.
- Inflammation (e.g. pseudotumour or sarcoidosis).

3. **Absence or reduction of lacrimal gland tissue**

- Surgical removal.
- Rarely congenital.

4. **Conjunctival scarring with obstruction of lacrimal gland ductules**

- Chemical burns.
- Cicatricial pemphigoid.
- Stevens–Johnson syndrome.
- Old trachoma.

5. **Neurological lesions with sensory or motor reflex loss**

- Familial dysautonomia (Riley–Day syndrome).
- Parkinson's disease.
- Reduced sensation may also contribute to dry eye after laser in-situ keratomileusis (LASIK) and contact lens wear.

6. **Vitamin A deficiency.**

Evaporative dry eye

1. **Meibomian gland dysfunction**

- Posterior blepharitis.
- Rosacea.
- Atopic keratoconjunctivitis.
- Congenital meibomian gland absence.

2. Exposure and defective blinking

- Severe proptosis.
- Facial nerve palsy.
- Eyelid scarring.
- Following blepharoplasty.

3. Miscellaneous

- Contact lens wear.
- Environmental, such as air conditioning.

FURTHER READING

Baudouin C. The pathology of dry eye. *Surv Ophthalmol* 2001;45:S211–S220.

Brewitt H, Sistani F. Dry eye disease: the scale of the problem. *Surv Ophthalmol* 2001;45:S199–S202.

Lin PY, Tsai SY, Cheng CY, et al. Prevalence of dry eye among an elderly Chinese population in Taiwan: the Shihpai Eye Study. *Ophthalmology* 2003;110:1096–1101.

Moss SE, Klein R, Klein BE. Prevalence of and risk factors for dry eye syndrome. *Arch Ophthalmol* 2000;118:1264–1268.

Rolando M, Zierhut M. The ocular surface and tear film and their dysfunction in dry eye disease. *Surv Ophthalmol* 2001;45:S203–S210.

Schein OD, Munoz B, Tielsch JM, et al. Prevalence of dry eye among the elderly. *Am J Ophthalmol* 1997;124:723–728.

Shimazaki J, Goto E, Ono M, et al. Meibomian gland dysfunction in patients with Sjögren syndrome. *Ophthalmology* 1998;105:1485–1488.

Stern ME, Beuerman RW, Fox RI, et al. The pathology of dry eye: the interaction between the ocular surface and lacrimal glands. *Cornea* 1998;17:584–589.

Tiffany JM. Tears in health and disease. *Eye* 2003;17:923–926.

Tseng SC, Tsubota K. Important concepts for treating ocular surface and tear disorders. *Am J Ophthalmol* 1997;124:825–835.

Vitali C, Bombardieri S, Jonsson R, et al. Classification criteria for Sjögren's syndrome: a revised version of the European criteria proposed by the American-European Consensus Group. *Ann Rheum Dis* 2002; 61:554–558.

Watanabe H. Significance of mucin on the ocular surface. *Cornea* 2002;21:S17–S22.

DIAGNOSIS

Clinical features

Symptoms

- The major symptoms are feelings of dryness, grittiness and burning that characteristically worsen during the day.
- Stringy discharge, transient blurring of vision, redness and crusting of the lids are also common.
- Less frequent symptoms include itching, photophobia and a tired or heavy feeling.
- Lack of emotional or reflex tearing is uncommon.

> **NB:** The symptoms of KCS are frequently exacerbated on exposure to conditions associated with increased tear evaporation (e.g. air-conditioning, wind, and central heating) or prolonged reading, when blink frequency is reduced.

Signs

1. Lid margin

- Meibomian gland dysfunction may be present.
- Eyelid malposition or trichiasis.

2. Conjunctiva

- Mild keratinisation and redness.
- Scarring over the upper tarsal plate may occur in Sjögren syndrome.

3. Tear film

- In the normal eye, as the tear film breaks down, the mucin layer becomes contaminated with lipid but is washed away. In the dry eye, the lipid-contaminated mucin accumulates in the tear film as particles and debris that move with each blink (Figs 2.1 and 2.2).
- The marginal tear meniscus is a crude measure of the volume of aqueous in the tear film. In the normal eye, the

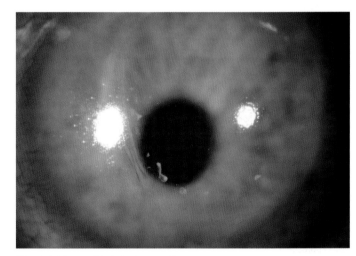

Fig. 2.1 Mucus debris in the tear film

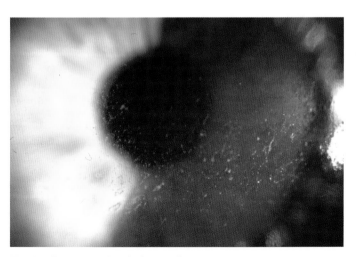

Fig. 2.2 Extensive debris in the tear film

meniscus is about 1 mm in height, while in the dry eye, the tear meniscus becomes thin (Fig. 2.3) or absent.

- Froth in the tear film or along the eyelid margin occurs in meibomian gland dysfunction (see Fig. 1.24).

4. Cornea

- Punctate epithelial erosions that stain with fluorescein involving the interpalpebral zone and inferior cornea (see Fig. 2.3).

- Filaments consist of mucus strands lined with epithelium, attached at one end to the corneal surface (Fig. 2.4); the unattached end moves with each blink.

- Mucus plaques consist of semi-transparent, white-to-grey, slightly elevated lesions of various sizes (Fig. 2.5). They are composed of mucus, epithelial cells and proteinaceous and lipoidal material and are usually seen in association with corneal filaments; both stain with rose bengal (Fig. 2.6).

- Complications in very severe cases include peripheral superficial corneal neovascularisation, epithelial breakdown, melting (Fig. 2.7) and perforation (Fig. 2.8), bacterial keratitis and toxicity from medications.

Special investigations

The aim of investigation is to confirm and quantify the diagnosis of dry eye. Unfortunately, although the repeatability of symptoms is good, that of clinical tests is poor, as is the correlation between symptoms and tests. The reliability of tests improves as the severity of dry eye increases. The tests measure the following parameters:

- Stability of the tear film (break-up time).

- Tear production (Schirmer, fluorescein clearance and tear osmolarity).

- Ocular surface disease (corneal stains and impression cytology).

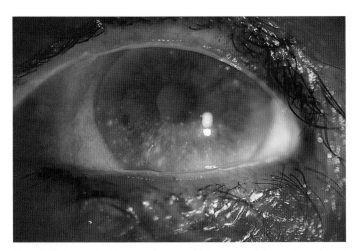

Fig. 2.3 Thin marginal tear meniscus and inferior punctate erosions stained with fluorescein

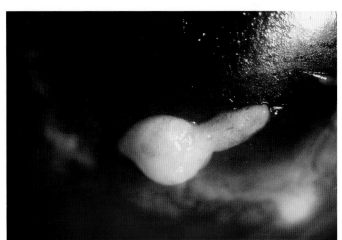

Fig. 2.5 Very large mucus plaque and a very dry cornea (Courtesy of Watson, Hazleman, Pavèsio and Green, from *The Sclera in Systemic Disorders*, 2nd edition, Butterworth-Heinemann, 2004)

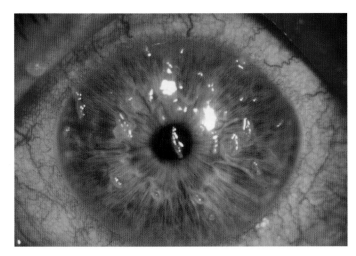

Fig. 2.4 Corneal filaments

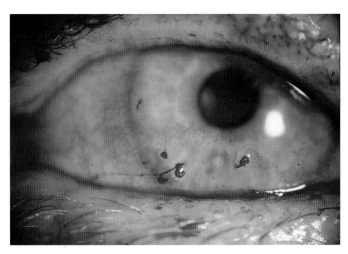

Fig. 2.6 Mucus plaques stained with rose bengal

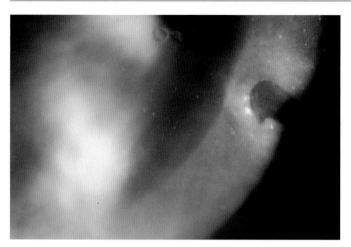

Fig. 2.7 Corneal melting

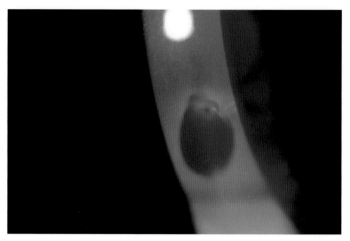

Fig. 2.9 Dry spot in a fluorescein-stained tear film

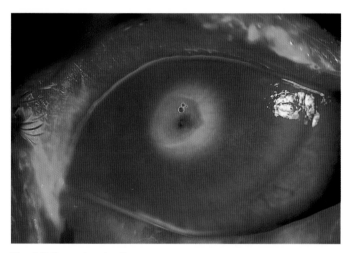

Fig. 2.8 Corneal perforation

> **NB:** There is no clinical test to confirm the diagnosis of evaporative dry eye. It is therefore a presumptive diagnosis based on the presence of meibomian gland disease. Tarsal transillumination to visualise the meibomian glands can give an indication of gland dropout.

It is suggested the tests are performed in the following order because the Schirmer strip paper can damage the ocular surface and cause staining.

Tear film break-up time

The tear film break-up time (BUT) is abnormal in aqueous tear deficiency and meibomian gland disorders. It is measured as follows:

- Fluorescein 2% or a sterile impregnated strip moistened with non-preserved saline is instilled into the lower fornix.

- The patient is asked to blink several times and then stop.

- The tear film is examined with a broad beam and a cobalt blue filter. After an interval of time, black spots or lines appear in the fluorescein-stained film, indicating the formation of dry areas (Fig. 2.9).

- The BUT is the interval between the last blink and the appearance of the first randomly distributed dry spot. The development of dry spots always in the same location may indicate a local corneal surface abnormality (e.g. epithelial basement membrane disease) rather than an intrinsic instability of the tear film. A BUT of less than 10 seconds is abnormal.

Ocular surface staining

1. **Fluorescein** stains corneal and conjunctival epithelium where there is sufficient damage to allow the dye to enter the tissues. In intensely dry eyes there may be no apparent staining due to dye quenching; staining can then be demonstrated by adding a drop of saline to the inferior fornix. A 2% solution or a moistened impregnated strip can be used.

2. **Rose bengal** is a dye that has an affinity for dead or devitalised epithelial cells that have a lost or altered mucus layer. Corneal filaments and plaques are also shown up more clearly by the dye and the use of a red-free filter may help visualisation. A 1% solution or a moistened impregnated strip can be used.

> **NB:** Rose bengal may cause intense stinging that can last for up to a day, particularly in patients with severe KCS. To minimise irritation, a very small drop should be used, immediately preceded by a drop of topical anaesthetic, and the excess washed out with saline.

3. **The pattern** of staining may aid diagnosis as follows:

- Interpalpebral staining of the cornea and conjunctiva is common in aqueous tear deficiency (Fig. 2.10).

- Superior conjunctival stain may indicate superior limbic keratoconjunctivitis.

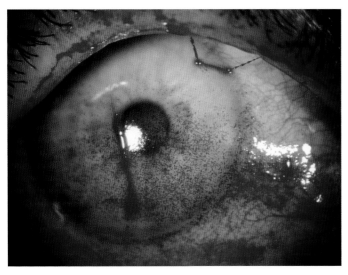

Fig. 2.10 Staining of the cornea and conjunctiva with rose bengal

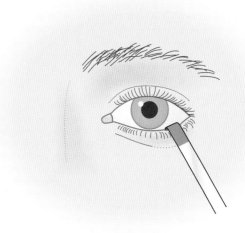

Fig. 2.11 Schirmer test

• Inferior corneal and conjunctival stain is often seen in patients with blepharitis or exposure.

Schirmer test

Schirmer test is a useful assessment of aqueous tear production. The test involves measuring the amount of wetting of a special (no. 41 Whatman) filter paper, 5 mm wide and 35 mm long. The test can be performed with or without topical anaesthesia. In theory, when performed with an anaesthetic (Schirmer 1), it measures basic secretion; without anaesthetic and with nasal stimulation (Schirmer 2), it measures maximum basic and reflex secretion. In practice, however, topical anaesthesia cannot abolish all sensory and psychological stimuli for reflex secretion. The test is performed as follows:

• The eye is gently dried of excess tears. If topical anaesthesia is applied, the excess should be removed from the inferior fornix with filter paper.

• The filter paper is folded 5 mm from one end and inserted at the junction of the middle and outer third of the lower lid, taking care not to touch the cornea or lashes (Fig. 2.11).

• The patient is asked to keep the eyes gently closed.

• After 5 minutes, the filter paper is removed and the amount of wetting from the fold measured.

• Less than 10 mm of wetting after 5 minutes without anaesthesia, and less than 6 mm with anaesthesia, is considered abnormal.

NB: Results can be variable and a single Schirmer test should not be used as the sole criterion for diagnosing dry eye, but repeatedly abnormal tests are highly supportive.

Other tests

The following tests are rarely performed in clinical practice.

1. **Fluorescein clearance test** and the tear function index may be assessed by placing 5 µl of fluorescein on the ocular surface and measuring the residual dye in a Schirmer strip placed on the lower lateral lid margin at intervals of 1, 10, 20 and 30 minutes. The presence of fluorescein on each strip is examined under blue light and compared with a standard scale or measured using fluorophotometry. In normal eyes, the value will have fallen to zero after 20 minutes. Delayed clearance is observed in all dry eye states.

2. **Lactoferrin** is the major protein secreted by the lacrimal gland. Tear lactoferrin is decreased in Sjögren syndrome and other lacrimal gland diseases. Commercially available immunoassay kits are available to measure lactoferrin in body fluids.

3. **Phenol red thread test** uses a thread impregnated with a pH-sensitive dye. The end of the thread is placed over the lower lid and the length that is wet (dye changes yellow to red in tears) is measured after 15 seconds. A value of 6 mm is abnormal. It is comparable to the Schirmer test but takes less time.

4. **Tear meniscometry** is a technique to quantify the height and thus the volume of the lower lid meniscus.

5. **Tear film osmolarity** measurement techniques are available as research tools.

6. **Impression cytology** to determine goblet cell numbers.

FURTHER READING

Afonso AA, Monroy D, Stern ME, et al. Correlation of tear fluorescein clearance and Schirmer test scores with ocular irritation symptoms. *Ophthalmology* 1999;106:803–810.

Bron AJ. Diagnosis of dry eye. *Surv Ophthalmol* 2001;45:S221–S226.

Feenstra RP, Tseng SC. Comparison of fluorescein and rose bengal staining. *Ophthalmology* 1992;99:605–617.

Feenstra RP, Tseng SC. What is actually stained by rose bengal? *Arch Ophthalmol* 1992;110:984–993.

Lee SH, Tseng SC. Rose bengal staining and cytologic characteristics associated with lipid tear deficiency. *Am J Ophthalmol* 1997;124:736–750.

Macri A, Pflugfelder S. Correlation of the Schirmer 1 and fluorescein clearance tests with the severity of corneal epithelial and eyelid disease. *Arch Ophthalmol* 2000;118:1632–1638.

Manning FJ, Wehrly SR, Foulks GN. Patient tolerance and ocular surface staining characteristics of lissamine green versus rose bengal. *Ophthalmology* 1995;102:1953–1957.

Nichols KK, Mitchell GL, Zadnik K. The repeatability of clinical measurements of dry eye. *Cornea* 2004;23:272–285.

Pflugfelder SC, Tseng SC, Yoshino K, et al. Correlation of goblet cell density and mucosal epithelial membrane mucin expression with rose bengal staining in patients with ocular irritation. *Ophthalmology* 1997;104:223–235.

TREATMENT

Dry eye is generally not curable and management is therefore structured around the control of symptoms and prevention of surface damage. The choice of treatment depends on the severity of the disease and involves one or more of the following measures alone or in combination.

Patient education

- Establishment of a realistic expectation of outcome and emphasis on the importance of compliance.
- Avoidance of toxic drugs or environmental factors; discontinue toxic topical medication if possible.
- Review of work environment.
- Emphasis on the importance of blinking whilst reading or using a VDU.
- Aids should be provided for patients with a loss of dexterity (e.g. rheumatoid arthritis). Plastic dropper bottles can be held in a nutcracker, as small unit dispensers may not be appropriate.
- Caution against laser refractive surgery.
- Discussion of management of contact lens intolerance.

Treatment of associated lid disease

- Treatment of blepharitis.
- Correction of lid margin abnormalities such as entropion, ectropion and trichiasis.
- Correction of abnormal globe position, lid retraction or exophthalmos in thyroid eye disease.
- Correction of corneal exposure from lagophthalmos.

Tear substitutes

Tear substitutes have a relatively simple formulation that cannot approximate the complex number of components and structure of the normal tear film. Their delivery is also periodic rather than continuous. Almost all are based on replacement of the aqueous phase of the tear film. There are no mucus substitutes, and paraffin is only an approximation to the action of tear lipids.

1. **Drops and gels** (see Table 2.2)

- Cellulose derivatives.
- Carbomers.
- Polyvinyl alcohol.
- Povidone.
- Sodium chloride.
- Sodium hyaluronate.
- Autologous serum.

2. **Ointments** containing petrolatum mineral oil can be used at bedtime.

NB: The preservatives are a potential source of toxicity, especially after punctal occlusion. Non-preserved drops should therefore be used whenever possible.

Mucolytic agents

Acetylcysteine 5% drops (Ilube) q.i.d. may be useful in patients with corneal filaments and mucous plaques. It may cause irritation following instillation. Acetylcysteine is also malodorous and has a limited bottle life, so it can be used only for up to 2 weeks. Debridement of filaments may also be useful.

Punctal occlusion

Punctal occlusion by reducing drainage, preserves natural tears and prolongs the effect of artificial tears. It is of greatest value in patients with moderate to severe KCS who have not responded to frequent use of topical treatment.

1. **Temporary** occlusion can be achieved by inserting commercially available collagen plugs into the canaliculi. The main aim is to ensure that epiphora does not occur following permanent occlusion.

- Initially the inferior puncta are occluded and the patient is reviewed after 1 or 2 weeks. If epiphora is induced, the plugs are removed.
- If the patient is now asymptomatic and without epiphora, the plugs are removed and the inferior canaliculi are permanently occluded (see below).

Table 2.2 Tear substitutes

Name	Primary agent	Product and Manufacturer	Preservative	Disadvantage
Acetylcysteine (mucolytic)	Acetylcysteine 5% + hypromellose 0.35%	Ilube (Alcon)	BAC	May sting
Cellulose derivatives	Carmellose (carboxymethylcellulose sodium 1%)	Celluvisc (Allergan)	Unpreserved	Deposits on lashes
	Hypromellose (hydroxypropylmethylcellulose HPMC)	Hypromellose 0.3% (Generic)	BAC or unpreserved	Short duration of action
		Hypromellose 0.32% (Artelac sdu Pharma Global)	Unpreserved	
		Hypromellose 0.5% (Isopto Plain Alcon)	BAC	Short duration of action Preservative limits frequency
		Hypromellose 1% (Isopto Alkaline)	BAC	Deposits on lashes Preservative limits frequency
	Hyetellose (Hydroxyethylcellulose (HECL) 0.44% drops + sodium chloride 0.35%	Minims Artificial Tears (Chauvin)	Unpreserved	Short duration of action
	Dextran 70 0.1% and hypromellose 0.3% drops	Tears Naturale (Alcon)	BAC	Preservative limits frequency
Carbomers (Polyacrylic acid)	Carbomer 980 0.2% gel	Gel Tears (Chauvin)	BAC	Preservative limits frequency
		Liposic (B & L)	Cetrimide	
		Viscotears (Novartis)	Cetrimide or unpreserved	
	Carbomer 974 0.25% gel	Liquivisc (Allergan)	BAC	Preservative limits frequency
Electrolyte solutions	Not declared	Thera Tears and others[f]	Unpreserved	No data available
HP guar	Hydroxypropyl and Guar	Systane[#]		
Lipids and oils	Yellow soft paraffin 80%, liquid paraffin 10%, wool fat 10%	Simple (Generic)	Unpreserved	
	White soft paraffin 57.3%, liquid paraffin 42.5%, wool alcohols 0.2%	LacriLube (Allergan)	Unpreserved	
	White soft paraffin 60%, liquid paraffin 30%, wool fat 10%	Lubritears (Alcon)	Unpreserved	
Polyvinyl alcohol	Polyvinyl alcohol (PVA) 1% drops	Hypotears (Novartis)	BAC	
	Polyvinyl alcohol (PVA) 1.4% drops	Liquifilm Tears (Allergan)	BAC or unpreserved*	
		Sno Tears (Chauvin)	BAC	
Povidone	Polyvinylpyrrolidone 5% drops	Oculotect (Novartis)	Unpreserved	
Saline	Sodium chloride 0.9% drops	Minims Sodium Chloride (Chauvin)	Unpreserved	
Serum	Autologous serum	Not commercially available	Unpreserved	Laboratory required
Sodium hyaluronate	Sodium hyaluronate 0.1% or 0.15% (usually contains Dextran)	Vismed, Vismed Gel, Vismed Light, Vislube (Cantor-Nissel) Hycosan (Bausch & Lomb) Aquify (Novartis) Oxyal (Santen) Fermavisc (NovartisPharma)[#]	Unpreserved	

Note: Product names apply to the United Kingdom. Some products may not be available in some countries.
BAC benzalkonium chloride. * Also contains Povidone 0.6%. # These products are CE marked and marketed as a device. f These products usually manufactured in the USA and imported (not evaluated by the FDA)
Preserved drops should not be used more than four times daily, which limits their use to mild dry eye states.

- In severe KCS, the inferior and superior canaliculi are plugged.

2. **Reversible** long-term occlusion lasting several months can be achieved with silicone plugs inserted into the vertical portion of the canaliculus (Fig. 2.12).

- Potential problems include extrusion, granuloma formation and distal migration; surgical removal is indicated rarely.

- Plugs that pass into the horizontal portion of the canaliculus cannot be visualised, and although they can usually be

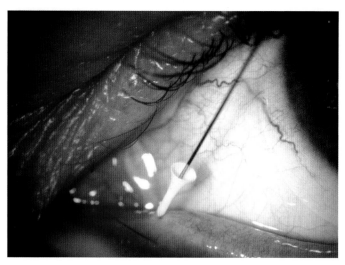

Fig. 2.12 Insertion of a silicone punctal plug

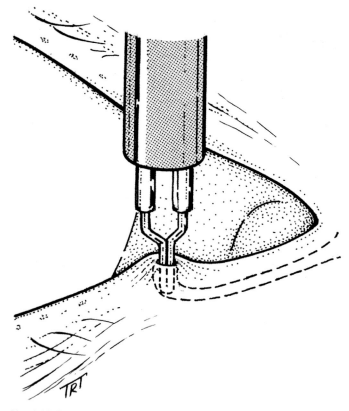

Fig. 2.13 Punctal occlusion using cautery

flushed out with saline if they cause epiphora, this is not always possible.

3. **Permanent** occlusion should be undertaken only in patients with severe dry eye with repeated Schirmer test values of 5 mm or less, and who have had a positive response to temporary plugs without epiphora. It should not be performed, if possible, in young patients who may have reversible pathology.

- Permanent occlusion is performed following punctal dilatation by coagulating the proximal canaliculus with cautery (Fig. 2.13); following successful occlusion, it is important to watch for signs of recanalisation.

- Laser cautery is less effective than thermal coagulation, with higher rates of recanalisation.

NB: All four puncta should not be occluded at the same session.

Anti-inflammatory agents

1. **Low-dose topical steroids** are effective supplementary treatment for acute exacerbations. The risks of long-term treatment must be balanced against the potential benefits of increased comfort.

2. **Topical ciclosporin** (0.05%, 0.1%) is a safe, well-tolerated agent that reduces T-cell-mediated inflammation of lacrimal tissue, resulting in an increase in the number of goblet cells and reversal of squamous metaplasia.

3. **Systemic tetracyclines** may control associated blepharitis and reduce inflammatory mediators in the tears (see Ch. 1).

Contact lenses

Although long-term contact lens wear may increase tear film evaporation, reduce tear flow, and increase the risk of infection, they have a role in the management of dry eye. These effects can be outweighed by the reservoir effect of fluid trapped behind the lens.

1. **Low water** content HEMA lenses may be successfully fitted to moderately dry eyes.

2. **Silicone** rubber lenses that contain no water and readily transmit oxygen are effective in protecting the cornea in extreme tear film deficiency. Deposition of debris on the surface of the lens can blur vision and be problematic. The continued availability of these lenses is in doubt.

3. **Occlusive** gas-permeable scleral contact lenses provide a reservoir of saline over the cornea. They can be worn on an extremely dry eye with exposure.

Conservation of existing tears

1. **Reduction of room temperature**, by avoiding central heating, to minimise evaporation of tears.

2. **Room humidifiers** may be tried but are frequently disappointing because the apparatus is incapable of significantly increasing the relative humidity of an average-sized room. A temporary local increase in humidity can be

achieved with moist chamber goggles or side shields to glasses, but they may be cosmetically unacceptable.

Other options

1. **Tarsorrhaphy** diminishes surface evaporation by reducing the palpebral aperture.

2. **Botulinum toxin injection** to the orbicularis muscle may help control the blepharospasm in severe dry eye. Injected at the median canthus, it reduces tear drainage, presumably by blocking lid movement.

3. **Oral cholinergic agonists** such as pilocarpine (5 mg q.i.d.) may reduce the symptoms of dry eye and dry mouth in patients with Sjögren syndrome. They may also cause blurred vision and intolerable sweating.

4. **Zidovudine**, an antiretroviral agent, may be beneficial in primary Sjögren syndrome.

5. **Submandibular gland transplantation** for extreme dry eye requires extensive surgery and tends to produce unacceptable levels of mucus in the tear film.

FURTHER READING

Calonge M. The treatment of dry eye. *Surv Ophthalmol* 2001;45:S227–239.

Geerling G, Sieg P, Bastian GO, et al. Transplantation of the autologous submandibular gland for most severe cases of keratoconjunctivitis sicca. *Ophthalmology* 1998;105:327–335.

Kunert KS, Tisdale AS, Gipson IK. Goblet cell numbers and epithelial proliferation in the conjunctiva of patients with dry eye syndrome treated with cyclosporine A. *Arch Ophthalmol* 2002;120:330–337.

Marsh P, Pflugfelder SC. Topical nonpreserved methylprednisolone therapy for keratoconjunctivitis sicca in Sjögren syndrome. *Ophthalmology* 1999;106:811–816.

Murube J, Murube E. Treatment of dry eye by blocking the lacrimal canaliculi. *Surv Ophthalmol* 1996;40:463–480.

Sahlin S, Chen E, Kaugesaar T, et al. Effect of eyelid botulinum toxin injection on lacrimal drainage. *Am J Ophthalmol* 2000;129:481–486.

Stevenson D, Tauber J, Reis BL. Efficacy and safety of cyclosporin A ophthalmic emulsion in the treatment of moderate-to-severe dry eye disease: a dose-ranging, randomized trial. The Cyclosporin A Phase 2 Study Group. *Ophthalmology* 2000;107:967–974.

Chapter 3

Conjunctivitis

INTRODUCTION

Anatomy

The conjunctiva is a transparent mucous membrane lining the inner surface of the eyelids and surface of the globe as far as the limbus. It has a dense lymphatic supply and an abundance of immunocompetent cells. Mucus from the goblet cells and secretions from the accessory lacrimal glands are essential components of the tear film. The conjunctiva is part of the defensive barrier against infection. The lymphatic drainage of the conjunctiva is to the preauricular and submandibular nodes, which corresponds to the drainage of the eyelids. The conjunctiva may be subdivided into the following (Fig. 3.1):

1. **The palpebral** conjunctiva starts at the mucocutaneous junction of the lid margins and is firmly attached to the posterior tarsal plates. The underlying tarsal blood vessels can be seen passing vertically from the lid margin and fornix.

2. **The forniceal** conjunctiva is loose and redundant and may be thrown into folds.

3. **The bulbar** conjunctiva covers the anterior sclera and is continuous with the corneal epithelium at the limbus. Radial ridges at the limbus form the palisades of Vogt. The stroma is loosely attached to the underlying Tenon capsule, except at the limbus, where the two layers fuse. A plica semilunaris (semilunar fold) is present nasally.

Histology

1. **The epithelium** is non-keratinising and about five cell layers thick. Basal cuboidal cells evolve into flattened polyhedral cells before they are shed from the surface. Goblet cells are located within the epithelium. They are most dense inferonasally and in the fornices, where they account for 5–10% of the basal cells.

2. **The stroma** (substantia propria) consists of richly vascularised loose connective tissue. The adenoid superficial layer does not develop until about 3 months after birth, hence the inability of the newborn to produce a follicular conjunctival reaction. The deep fibrous layer merges with the tarsal plates. The accessory lacrimal glands of Krause and Wolfring are located deep within the stroma.

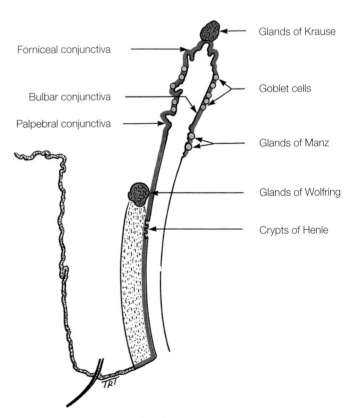

Forniceal conjunctiva

Bulbar conjunctiva

Palpebral conjunctiva

Glands of Krause

Goblet cells

Glands of Manz

Glands of Wolfring

Crypts of Henle

Fig. 3.1 Anatomy of the conjunctiva

Clinical evaluation

History

- Duration of symptoms, laterality, and potential precipitating or alleviating factors should be determined.

- All topical medications should be documented.

- A personal and family history of atopic disease (asthma, atopic dermatitis, hay fever) should be recorded.

- Recent contact lens wear.

Slit-lamp examination

- The lower tarsal conjunctiva, fornix and bulbar conjunctiva can be easily examined by gently retracting the lower lid on upgaze.

- The upper bulbar conjunctiva can be seen by retracting the upper lid on downgaze.

- The upper tarsal conjunctiva can be visualised after everting the upper lid.

- The upper fornix can be examined adequately only by double lid eversion with a Desmarres retractor; this may be necessary to exclude a retained foreign body.

- The caruncle and plica can be visualised in the primary position and on lateral gaze.

- The conjunctival blood vessels are roughly radial in orientation, as opposed to episcleral vessels that form a reticular pattern; they can be seen best with green light.

Signs of conjunctival inflammation

Clinical features of particular relevance to the differential diagnosis of conjunctival inflammation are: (a) symptoms, (b) discharge, (c) conjunctival reaction, (d) membranes, (e) associated keratopathy and (f) lymphadenopathy.

Symptoms

- Non-specific symptoms include lacrimation, gritty irritation, stinging and burning.

- Pain, photophobia and foreign body sensation suggest associated corneal involvement.

- Itching is the hallmark of allergic conjunctivitis, although it may also occur to a lesser extent in blepharitis and dry eye.

Discharge

- A watery discharge is composed of a serous exudate and tears, and occurs in acute viral or acute allergic conjunctivitis.

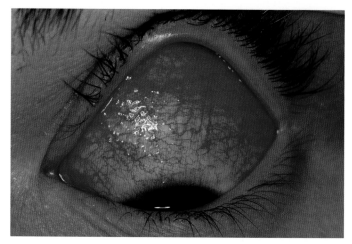

Fig. 3.2 Conjunctival injection in bacterial conjunctivitis (Courtesy of P J Saine)

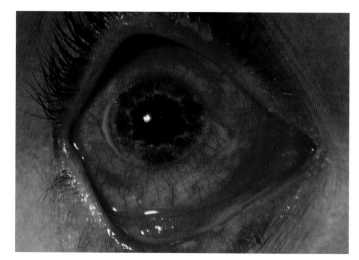

Fig. 3.3 Haemorrhagic conjunctivitis

- A mucoid discharge is typical of chronic allergic conjunctivitis and dry eye.

- A mucopurulent or purulent discharge occurs in acute bacterial or chlamydial infections.

NB: Patients often remove excessive discharge prior to examination.

Conjunctival reaction

1. **Conjunctival injection** that is diffuse, beefy-red and more intense away from the limbus is typical of bacterial infection (Fig. 3.2).

2. **Haemorrhagic conjunctivitis** (Fig. 3.3) often occurs with viral infections, although it may occasionally be present with bacterial infection with *Strep. pneumoniae*, *H. influenzae* and *N. meningitidis*.

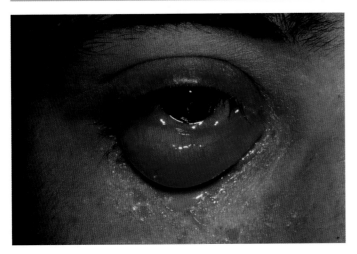

Fig. 3.4 Severe chemosis

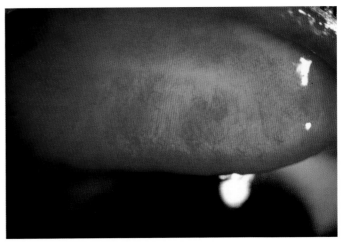

Fig. 3.5 Scarring of the tarsal conjunctiva

3. **Oedema** (chemosis) may occur when the conjunctiva is severely inflamed, producing a translucent swelling (Fig. 3.4). Severe oedema may protrude through the closed eyelids. Acute oedema usually indicates a hypersensitivity response whereas chronic change suggests orbital outflow constriction.

4. **Epithelial staining with rose bengal**

- Superior staining accompanies superior limbic keratoconjunctivitis.

- Interpalpebral or nasal conjunctival staining occurs in severe dry eye.

5. **Epithelial necrosis**

- Epithelial defects stain with fluorescein.

- Bulbar epithelial breakdown can develop in aminoglycoside toxicity.

- Necrosis may indicate acute disease in the presence of mucous membrane pemphigoid.

- Focal epithelial breakdown develops over conjunctival phlyctens.

6. **Subconjunctival scarring**

- Linear scarring over the upper tarsal plate may indicate previous trachoma or severe blepharitis (Fig. 3.5).

- Reticular pattern of scarring over the upper tarsal plate is seen in chronic allergic conjunctivitis.

- Loss of the plica, forniceal shortening and symblepharon are features of cicatrising conjunctivitis.

- Severe scarring may cause loss of goblet cells and cicatricial entropion.

7. **Follicular reaction**

a. **Histology** shows a subepithelial germinal centre of B lymphocytes with T lymphocytes (CD8+) in the periph-

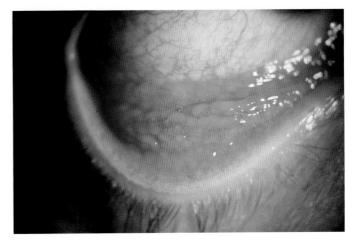

Fig. 3.6 Conjunctival follicles

ery. Inflammatory cells (plasma cells, macrophages and polymorphonuclear leucocytes) are found between follicles and indicate a delayed hypersensitivity response.

b. **Signs**

- Multiple, discrete, yellowish, slightly elevated lesions, most prominent in the fornices (Fig. 3.6).

- The size of each lesion is related to severity and duration of disease and can vary from 0.5 to 5 mm.

- Vessels normally pass over the surface of the follicle and as it increases in size, they are displaced peripherally.

c. **Causes**

- Viral conjunctivitis.

- Chlamydial conjunctivitis.

- Parinaud oculoglandular syndrome.

- Hypersensitivity to topical medications.

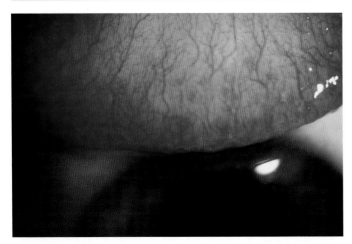

Fig. 3.7 Early papillary reaction

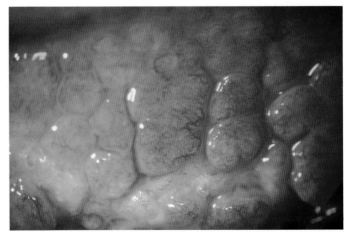

Fig. 3.9 Giant papillae

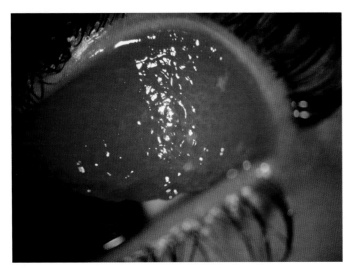

Fig. 3.8 Macropapillae

> **NB:** Small follicles are a normal finding in childhood (folliculosis), as are follicles in the fornices and at the margin of the upper tarsal plate in adults.

8. Papillary reaction

a. **Histology** shows hyperplastic conjunctival epithelium thrown into numerous folds or projections, with central vessels and a diffuse infiltrate of chronic inflammatory cells. Late changes include superficial stromal hyalinisation, scarring and the formation of crypts containing goblet cells.

b. **Signs.** Papillae can only develop in the palpebral and bulbar conjunctiva at the limbus where the conjunctiva is attached to the deeper fibrous layer.

• Micropapillae form a mosaic-like pattern of elevated red dots as a result of the central vascular channel (Fig. 3.7).

• Macropapillae (<1 mm) (Fig. 3.8) and giant papillae (>1 mm) (Fig. 3.9) develop with prolonged inflammation.

• Apical staining with fluorescein or the presence of mucus between giant papillae indicates active disease.

• Limbal papillae have a more gelatinous appearance; Trantas dots may develop at the apex in chronic allergic conjunctivitis.

c. **Causes**

• Chronic blepharitis.

• Allergic conjunctivitis.

• Bacterial conjunctivitis.

• Contact lens wear.

• Superior limbic keratoconjunctivitis.

• Floppy eyelid syndrome.

9. Infiltration represents cellular recruitment to the site of chronic inflammation and typically accompanies a papillary response. It is recognised by loss of detail of the normal tarsal vessels, especially on the upper lid (Fig. 3.10).

10. Membranes

a. **A pseudomembrane** consist of coagulated exudate adherent to the inflamed conjunctival epithelium (Fig. 3.11); it can be easily peeled off, leaving the epithelium intact.

b. **A true membrane** infiltrates the superficial layers of the conjunctival epithelium; attempted removal may be accompanied by tearing of the epithelium and bleeding.

c. **Causes**

• Severe adenoviral conjunctivitis.

• Gonococcal conjunctivitis.

• Ligneous conjunctivitis.

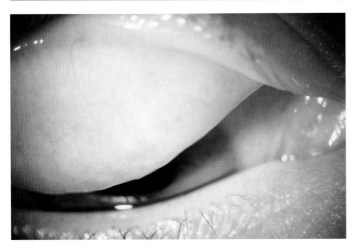

Fig. 3.10 Conjunctival infiltration

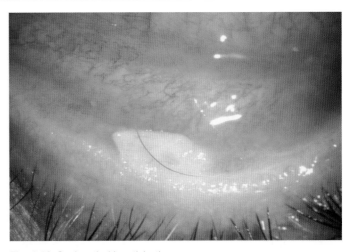

Fig. 3.12 Conjunctival keratinisation

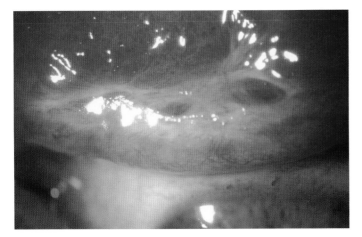

Fig. 3.11 Conjunctival pseudomembrane

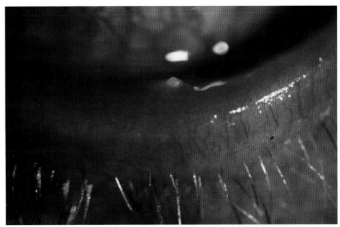

Fig. 3.13 Large concretion eroding the conjunctiva

- Acute Stevens–Johnson syndrome.
- Bacterial infection (*Streptococcus* sp., *Corynebacterium diphtheriae*).

NB: The distinction between a true membrane and a pseudomembrane is rarely clinically helpful; both can leave scarring following resolution.

11. **Keratinisation** is characterised by non-wetting patches of opaque epithelium (Fig. 3.12). Causes include chronic exposure, drying, or metaplasia following immune or chemical damage (conjunctival stem cell failure).

NB: Keratinisation of the caruncle is a common early sign of mucous membrane pemphigoid.

12. **Concretions** are yellowish discrete opacities beneath the tarsal conjunctiva. They often signify chronic posterior lid margin disease, but may be a normal ageing change. Occasionally, a large concretion may erode through the epithelium (Fig. 3.13) and abrade the cornea.

Lymphadenopathy

Causes of lymphadenopathy are viral, chlamydial and gonococcal infection, and Parinaud oculoglandular syndrome.

BACTERIAL CONJUNCTIVITIS

Acute bacterial conjunctivitis

Acute bacterial conjunctivitis is a common and usually self-limiting condition which is more frequent in children than in adults. In children, the most frequent isolates are *H. influenzae*, *Strep. pneumoniae* and *Moraxella catarrhalis* whereas in adults, *Staph. aureus*, *Strep. pneumoniae* and *H. influenzae* predominate. Spread of the infection is by direct eye contact with infected secretions.

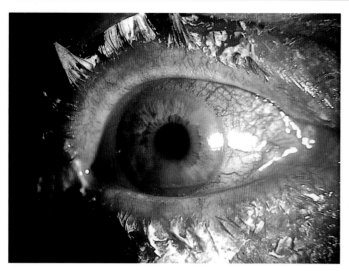

Fig. 3.14 Severe lid crusting in bacterial conjunctivitis

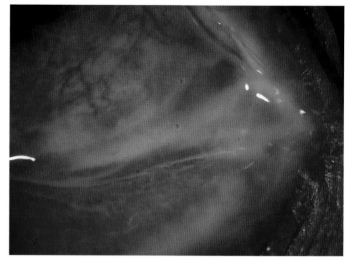

Fig. 3.16 Mucopurulent discharge in severe bacterial conjunctivitis

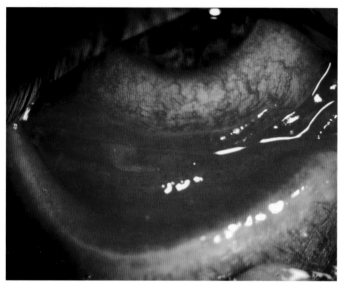

Fig. 3.15 Conjunctival injection in bacterial conjunctivitis

Diagnosis

1. Symptoms

- Acute onset of redness, grittiness, burning and discharge.

- Involvement is usually bilateral, although one eye may become affected 1–2 days before the other.

- On waking, the eyelids are frequently stuck together and difficult to open as a result of the accumulation of exudate during the night.

2. Signs

- Crusted and swollen eyelids, especially in children (Fig. 3.14).

- Diffuse conjunctival injection and an intense papillary reaction over the tarsal plates (Fig. 3.15).

- The discharge is initially watery, mimicking viral conjunctivitis, but later it becomes mucopurulent (Fig. 3.16).

- Superficial corneal punctate epithelial erosions are common.

3. Investigations are not routinely performed.

Treatment

About 60% of cases resolve within 5 days without treatment, but antibiotics are frequently administered to speed recovery and prevent reinfection. Before using topical antibiotics, it is important to clean the eyelids and lashes. In adults, broad-spectrum antibiotic drops are administered 2-hourly during the day for 5–7 days. Compliance in children is often better when using a gel or ointment. There is no evidence that any topical antibiotic is best at achieving clinical or microbiological cure.

1. **Fusidic acid** is a viscous gel which is useful for staphylococcal infections but not for most Gram-negative bacteria.

2. **Drops** include chloramphenicol, ciprofloxacin, ofloxacin, lomefloxacin, gentamicin, neomycin, framycetin and polymyxin B (in combination with bacitracin or trimethoprim).

3. **Ointments** provide higher concentrations for longer periods than drops but daytime use is limited because of blurred vision. Antibiotics available in ointment form include chloramphenicol, gentamicin, tetracycline, framycetin and polymyxin B (in combination with bacitracin or trimethoprim).

NB: Although the majority of cases of acute bacterial conjunctivitis are benign, children with *H. influenzae* conjunctivitis have a 25% risk of developing otitis. Patients infected with *N. gonorrhoeae* or *N. meningitidis* are at risk of corneal and systemic complications (see below).

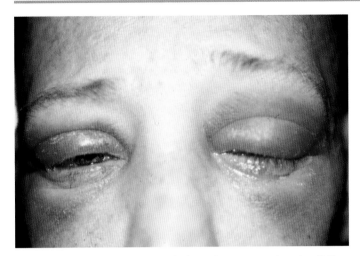

Fig. 3.17 Severe lid oedema and discharge in gonococcal conjunctivitis

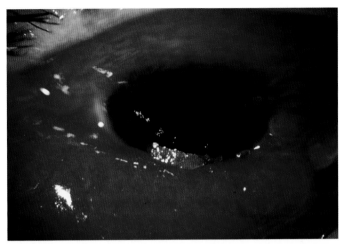

Fig. 3.19 Intense conjunctival hyperaemia and chemosis in gonococcal conjunctivitis

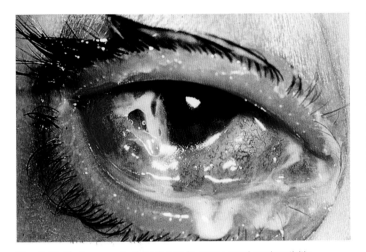

Fig. 3.18 Profuse purulent discharge in gonococcal conjunctivitis

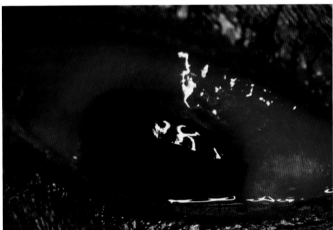

Fig. 3.20 Peripheral corneal ulceration in gonococcal keratoconjunctivitis

Gonococcal keratoconjunctivitis

Gonorrhoea is a venereal genitourinary tract infection caused by the Gram-negative diplococcus *N. gonorrhoeae*, which is capable of invading the intact corneal epithelium.

Diagnosis

1. **Presentation** is with acute, profuse conjunctival discharge.

2. **Signs**

- Severe lid oedema and tenderness (Fig. 3.17).

- Profuse purulent discharge (Fig. 3.18).

- Intense conjunctival hyperaemia, chemosis and frequently pseudomembrane formation (Fig. 3.19).

- Lymphadenopathy is prominent and, in severe cases, suppuration may occur.

- Peripheral corneal ulceration, often initially superior, ensues if conjunctivitis is not treated appropriately (Fig. 3.20).

- Central extension of ulceration (Fig. 3.21).

- Perforation and endophthalmitis (Fig. 3.22).

3. **Laboratory investigations**

- Gram stain shows Gram-negative kidney-shaped diplococci (Fig. 3.23).

- Culture on enriched media such as chocolate agar (Fig. 3.24) or Thayer–Martin medium.

- Polymerase chain reaction (PCR) for neisserial DNA.

Treatment

The patient should be hospitalised if there is corneal ulceration.

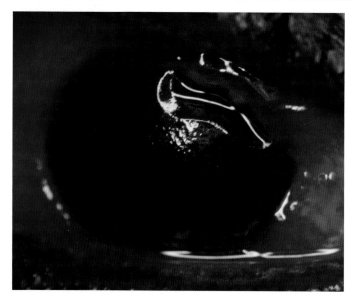

Fig. 3.21 Central extension of ulceration in gonococcal keratoconjunctivitis

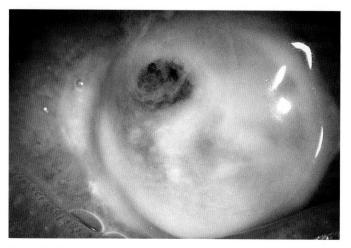

Fig. 3.22 Corneal perforation and endophthalmitis in gonococcal kerato-conjunctivitis

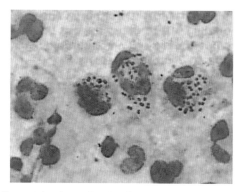

Fig. 3.23 Gram stain of pus showing Gram-negative kidney-shaped diplo-cocci which are mostly intracellular (Courtesy of Forbes and Jackson, from *Color Atlas and Text of Clinical Medicine*, 3rd edition, Mosby, 2003)

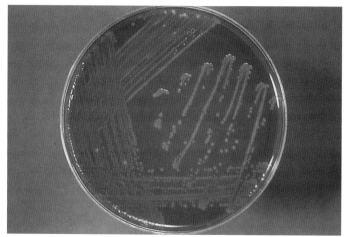

Fig. 3.24 Culture of *N. gonorrhoeae* on chocolate agar (Courtesy of Hart and Shears, from *Color Atlas of Medical Microbiology*, Mosby, 2004)

1. **Topical** gentamicin or bacitracin, initially every hour.

2. **Systemic**

- Intramuscular ceftriaxone 250 mg daily for 3 days or 1 g stat. Patients with keratitis require more aggressive treatment (up to 2 g intravenously for 3 days) than those with only conjunctival involvement.

- Intramuscular spectinomycin 1 g stat is an alternative on a named patient basis.

- Because of problems with multidrug resistance, it is important to determine local guidelines regarding antibiotic susceptibility and recommended treatment.

NB: Patients must be referred to a genitourinary department to be screened for associated chlamydial infection and contact tracing. Chlamydial co-infection is treated with doxycycline 200 mg daily for 1 week or azithromycin 1 g stat.

Meningococcal conjunctivitis

Pathogenesis

About 35% of the population are asymptomatic carriers of *N. meningitidis*. Meningococcal conjunctivitis is usually seen in children and is very rare in adults. It may be primary or secondary.

1. **Primary** conjunctivitis may appear as:

- Non-invasive disease.

- Invasive disease is characterised by fever, septicaemia and meningitis, which is fatal in 10–15% of cases. The risk of developing invasive disease increases 10–20 times if prophylactic systemic antibiotics are not given acutely.

2. **Secondary** conjunctivitis can be spread to the eye during end-stage septicaemia but is extremely rare.

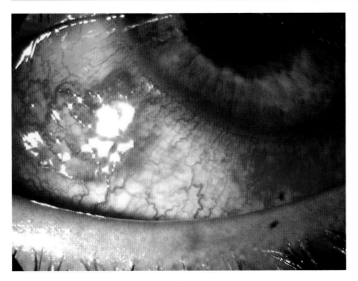

Fig. 3.25 Meningococcal conjunctivitis

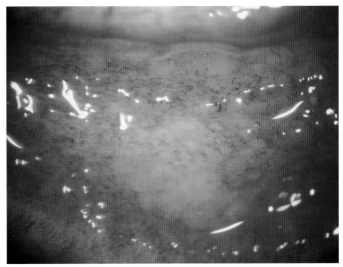

Fig. 3.26 Large follicles in the forniceal conjunctiva in chlamydial infection

Diagnosis

- Acute conjunctivitis which may be associated with subconjunctival haemorrhages and preauricular lymphadenopathy (Fig. 3.25).

- Keratitis develops in 30% of cases and may lead to ulceration and perforation.

Treatment

1. **Topical** treatment is with penicillin or cefotaxime drops.

2. **Systemic prophylaxis** should be given to reduce the risk of meningitis.

- Patients with conjunctivitis should receive oral ciprofloxacin 750 mg stat; alternatives include intramuscular ceftriaxone 250 mg or cefotaxime 500 mg.

- Close contacts of patients with invasive disease should receive oral ciprofloxacin 500 mg stat, but prophylactic treatment of contacts of those with primary conjunctivitis is not required.

Adult chlamydial conjunctivitis

Pathogenesis

Chlamydia are small, obligate intracellular bacteria, but, unlike other bacteria, they cannot replicate extracellularly and hence depend on host cells. They exist in two forms: a robust infective extracellular elementary body and a fragile intracellular replicating reticular body. Adult chlamydial (inclusion) conjunctivitis is an oculogenital infection caused by serotypes D–K of *Chlamydia trachomatis*. Transmission is by autoinoculation from genital secretions, although eye-to-eye spread may account for about 10% of cases. The incubation period is about 1 week.

Urogenital infection

1. **In males,** chlamydial infection is the most common cause of non-specific urethritis (NSU) and 'non-gonococcal urethritis' (NGU). It may also cause epididymitis and act as a trigger for Reiter disease.

2. **In females,** chlamydial infection may cause dysuria, pelvic inflammatory disease and perihepatitis (Fitz–Hugh–Curtis syndrome). Chronic salpingitis may result in infertility.

Diagnosis

1. **Presentation** is with a subacute onset of unilateral or bilateral redness, watering and discharge. Untreated, the conjunctivitis becomes chronic and may persist for several months.

2. **Signs**

- Watering or mucopurulent discharge.

- Large follicles are most prominent in the inferior fornix (Fig. 3.26) and may also involve the upper tarsal conjunctiva (Fig. 3.27).

- Peripheral corneal infiltrates may appear 2–3 weeks after the onset of conjunctivitis (Fig. 3.28).

- Tender preauricular lymphadenopathy.

- Neglected cases have less prominent follicles and develop mild conjunctival scarring and a superior pannus.

3. **Special investigations**

- PCR to detect chlamydial DNA is the investigation of choice.

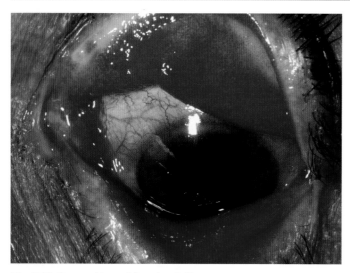

Fig. 3.27 Severe chlamydial conjunctivitis

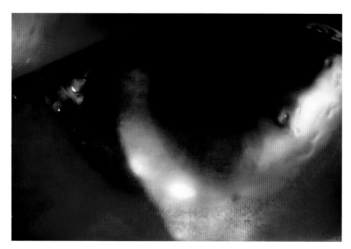

Fig. 3.28 Peripheral corneal infiltrates in chlamydial infection

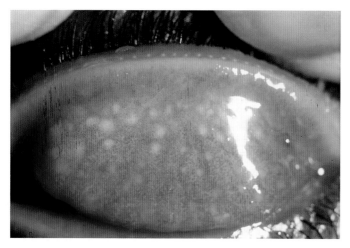

Fig. 3.29 Early active trachoma conjunctivitis

- Direct monoclonal fluorescent antibody microscopy of conjunctival smears is rapid and inexpensive but requires experience in interpretation.

- Standard single-passage McCoy cell culture requires at least 3 days.

NB: In view of the venereal nature of the disease, referral to a genitourinary clinic is mandatory for investigation and treatment of other possible sexually transmitted diseases.

Treatment

1. **Topical** erythromycin or tetracycline ointment initially for symptomatic relief.

2. **Systemic** therapy is with one of the following:

- Doxycycline 100 mg b.d. for 10 days.

- Azithromycin 1 g as a single dose is particularly effective because it acts intracellularly.

NB: Systemic therapy should not be started prior to genitourinary investigations.

Trachoma

Pathogenesis

Active trachoma is chronic conjunctival inflammation caused by infection with serotypes A, B, Ba and C of *C. trachomatis*. Initial infection is self-limiting and resolves without scarring. Repeated infection, particularly if associated with bacterial conjunctivitis, can lead to blindness. Trachoma is associated with poverty, overcrowding and poor hygiene. Sharing living space is also a risk factor, and there may be direct transmission from eye or nasal discharge. The fly is an important vector. Currently, trachoma is the leading cause of preventable blindness in the world. Blinding trachoma occurs in Africa, the Middle East, Asia, Australia and Central America. It affects approximately 150 million people worldwide, and about 5.5 million are at risk of blindness. Active trachoma is most common in children and up to 90% of pre-school children may be infected in hyper-endemic areas. The prevalence of active disease reduces to 5% in adults, with blinding sequelae more common in women.

Diagnosis

1. Active conjunctivitis

- Mixed follicular/papillary conjunctivitis associated with a mucopurulent discharge (Figs 3.29 and 3.30); in children under the age of 2 years, the papillary component may predominate.

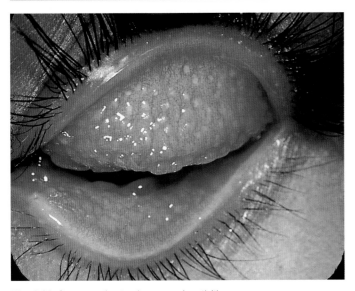

Fig. 3.30 Severe active trachoma conjunctivitis

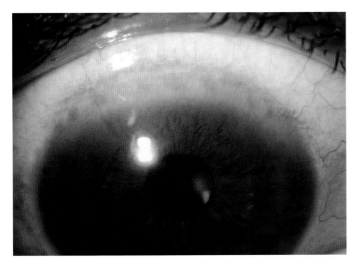

Fig. 3.31 Herbert pits

Fig. 3.32 Magnified view of Herbert pits; right eye shows stromal scarring; left eye shows pannus formation

- Superior conjunctival follicles at the upper limbus may resolve to leave a row of shallow depressions (Herbert pits) (Fig. 3.31).
- Keratitis ranges from superior epithelial keratitis to anterior stromal infiltrates and pannus formation (Fig. 3.32).

2. Chronic conjunctivitis

- Linear or stellate scars in milder cases (Fig. 3.33), or broad confluent scars (Arlt lines) (Fig. 3.34) in severe disease.

NB: The entire conjunctiva is involved, but the effects are most prominent on the upper tarsus.

3. Complications

- Trichiasis and secondary distichiasis (Fig. 3.35), and cicatricial entropion (Fig. 3.36).
- Dry eye caused by destruction of goblet cells and the ductules of the lacrimal gland.
- Corneal vascularisation, scarring (Fig. 3.37) and microbial infection.

Management

1. **Prevention** involves regular face washing and control of flies by spraying.

2. Antibiotics

- A single dose of azithromycin 20 mg/kg up to 1 g reduces rates of active trachoma, but may need to be repeated after 1 year.

R.E.

L.E.

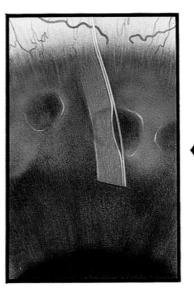

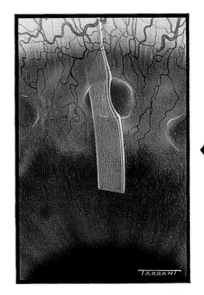

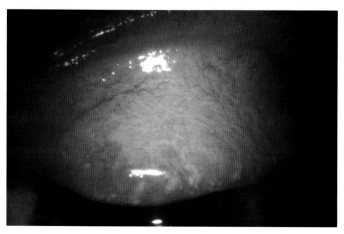

Fig. 3.33 Linear conjunctival trachomatous scarring

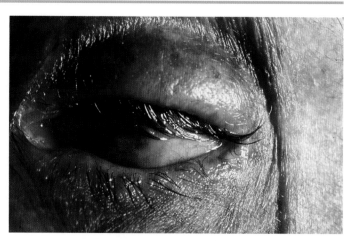

Fig. 3.36 Cicatricial upper lid entropion in trachoma (Courtesy of C Barry)

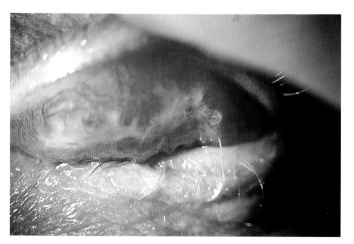

Fig. 3.34 More severe conjunctival trachomatous scarring (Arlt lines)

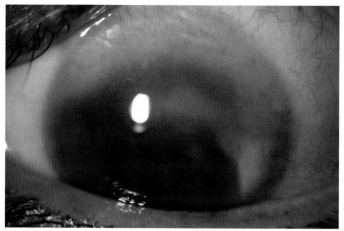

Fig. 3.37 Severe trachomatous corneal scarring

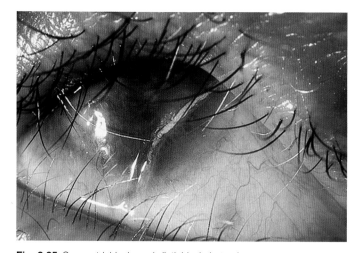

Fig. 3.35 Severe trichiasis and distichiasis in trachoma

Table 3.1 Modified WHO grading of trachoma

TF	= trachoma follicles with five or more (>0.5 mm) present on the superior tarsus
TI	= trachomatous inflammation diffusely involving the tarsal conjunctiva, which obscures 50% or more of the normal deep tarsal vessels
TS	= trachomatous conjunctival scarring
TT	= trachomatous trichiasis (at least one lash) touching the globe
CO	= corneal opacity over the pupil sufficient to blur iris details

3. **Surgery** is aimed at relieving trichiasis and maintaining complete lid closure.

The SAFE strategy for management	
S	Surgery for trichiasis
A	Antibiotics
F	Facial cleanliness
E	Environmental control

- Erythromycin 500 mg b.d. for 14 days is an alternative for women of childbearing age.

- Topical 1% tetracycline is less effective than oral treatment.

Ophthalmia neonatorum

Pathogenesis

Ophthalmia neonatorum (neonatal conjunctivitis) develops within 2 weeks of birth as the result of infection transmitted from mother to infant during delivery. It is serious because of the lack of immunity in the infant and immaturity of the ocular surface (no lymphoid tissue and relatively poor tear film).

1. **N. gonorrhoeae** is now an uncommon although serious cause in developed countries.

2. **C. trachomatis** accounts for the majority of cases in developed countries and may also cause pneumonitis, otitis and rhinitis.

3. **Other pathogens** include *Staph. aureus*, *Strep. pneumoniae*, *H. influenzae* and *Enterobacteriacae* (*Bacillus* sp., *E. coli* and *Klebsiella* sp.). Herpes simplex virus (typically HSV-2) is a rare cause and is usually associated with generalised viral infection including encephalitis.

Prophylaxis

Many developed countries (UK, Denmark, Sweden) have abandoned prophylaxis, while in others (USA, Canada) 0.5% erythromycin or 1% tetracycline ointment is used. Povidone-iodine (2.5%) is a cheap and effective agent against all of the common pathogens that cause ophthalmia neonatorum but is not commercially available.

Diagnosis

1. **Presentation** is usually between 3 and 19 days after birth.

2. **Signs**

- Usually bilateral eyelid oedema which may be severe in gonococcal infection.

- Discharge which is initially sero-sanguineous and later mucopurulent (Fig. 3.38).

- A papillary conjunctival reaction which may occasionally be associated with pseudomembranes.

- Corneal complications are more severe with *N. gonorrhoeae* infection and include corneal ulcer and perforation. *C. trachomatis*, if untreated, can cause conjunctival scarring and peripheral corneal pannus.

3. **Investigations**

- Gram stain of exudate for diplococci (gonorrhoea) and inclusion bodies (chlamydia).

- Cultures on chocolate agar or Thayer–Martin plates for *N. gonorrhoeae*.

- Immunofluorescence tests for chlamydia.

- PCR for chlamydial and neisserial DNA.

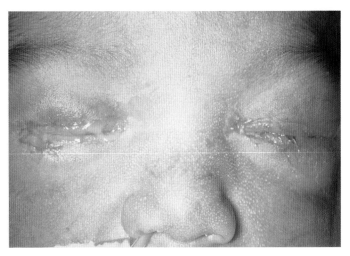

Fig. 3.38 Ophthalmia neonatorum

Treatment

Urgent treatment is indicated in association with a paediatric infectious diseases specialist.

1. **Chlamydial** infection is treated with oral erythromycin ethyl succinate (50 mg/kg/day) in four divided doses for 2 weeks. If chlamydial pneumonitis is suspected, treatment should be for 3 weeks. Erythromycin or tetracycline ointment is used in addition but not as sole therapy.

2. **Gonococcal** infection requires ceftriaxone 50 mg/kg/day intravenously or intramuscularly, or cefotaxime 100 mg/kg/day.

3. **Other bacterial** infections are treated with chloramphenicol or neomycin ointment q.i.d. Systemic antibiotics may be considered in severe cases.

4. **Herpes simplex** infection requires systemic aciclovir 30 mg/kg/day in divided doses for 14 days, and topical aciclovir five times daily.

NB: If chlamydia or gonorrhoea is confirmed, the parents and their partners must be investigated and treated by a genitourinary physician.

FURTHER READING

Andreoli CM, Wiley HE, Durand ML, et al. Primary meningococcal conjunctivitis in an adult. *Cornea* 2004;23:738–739.

Bodor FF. Conjunctivitis-otitis media syndrome: more than meets the eye. *Contemp Pediatr* 1989;6:55–60.

Garland SM, Malatt A, Tabrizi S, et al. Chlamydia trachomatis conjunctivitis, prevalence and association with genital tract infection. *Med J Aust* 1995;162:363–366.

Isenberg SJ, Apt L, Yoshimori R, et al. Povidone-iodine for ophthalmia neonatorum prophylaxis. *Am J Ophthalmol* 1994;118:701–706.

Katusic D, Petricek I, Mandic Z, et al. Azithromycin vs doxycycline in the treatment of inclusion conjunctivitis. *Am J Ophthalmol* 2003;135:447–451.

Mabey DCW, Solomon AW, Foster A. Trachoma. *Lancet* 2003;362:223–229.

Postema EJ, Remeijer L, van der Meijden WI. Epidemiology of genital chlamydial infections in patients with chlamydial conjunctivitis; a retrospective study. *Genitourin Med* 1996;72:203–205.

Seal DV, Barrett SP, McGill JI. Aetiology and treatment of acute bacterial infection of the external eye. *Br J Ophthalmol* 1982;66:357–360

Thylefors B, Negrel AD, Pararajasegaram R, et al. Global data on blindness. *Bull World Health Organ* 1995;73:115–121.

West S, Munoz B, Lynch M, et al. Impact of facewashing on trachoma in Kongwa, Tanzania. Lancet 1995;345:155–158.

Winceslaus J, Goh BT, Dunlop EMC, et al. Diagnosis of ophthalmia neonatorum. *Br Med J (Clin Res Ed)* 1987;295:1377–1379.

VIRAL CONJUNCTIVITIS

Adenoviral keratoconjunctivitis

Pathogenesis

Adenoviruses are icosahedral-shaped, unenveloped viruses with a linear, double-stranded DNA genome (Fig. 3.39). There are 51 subtypes that affect humans and many cause clinical infection. Viral subtyping permits epidemiological tracing of outbreaks.

1. **Adenoviral keratoconjunctivitis** is the most common external ocular viral infection that may be sporadic or occur in epidemics in hospitals, schools and factories. The spread of infection is facilitated by the ability of the virus to survive on dry surfaces and the fact that viral shedding may occur for 4–10 days before clinical disease is apparent.

2. **Transmission** of this highly contagious virus is by respiratory or ocular secretions, and dissemination is by contaminated towels or equipment such as tonometer heads. Following the onset of conjunctivitis, the virus is shed for about 12 days.

3. **Precautions** must be taken to avoid transmission following examination of patients with suspected adenoviral infection. Thorough washing of hands is important, as is meticulous disinfection of ophthalmic instruments. In addition, infected hospital personnel should not come into contact with patients, and busy eye departments should have a separate 'red eye room' for management of patients with conjunctivitis.

> **NB:** It is an occupational hazard of ophthalmologists.

Spectrum of infection

The spectrum of adenoviral eye infection varies from mild and almost subclinical disease, to full-blown infection with significant morbidity.

1. **Pharyngoconjunctival fever** is caused by serotypes Ad3, Ad7 and Ad11. It is spread by droplets within families with upper respiratory tract infection. Keratitis develops in about 30% of cases but is seldom severe.

2. **Epidemic keratoconjunctivitis** is caused by serotypes Ad8, Ad19 and Ad37, which cause severe disease; Ad4 causes mild disease. The virus is usually transmitted by hand-to-eye contact, instruments and solutions. Keratitis, which may be severe, develops in about 80% of cases.

Conjunctivitis

1. **Presentation** is usually with unilateral watering, redness, discomfort and photophobia; the contralateral eye is typically affected 1–2 days later, but less severely.

2. **Signs**

- Eyelid oedema.

- A mixed papillary/follicular conjunctivitis over the tarsal plates (Fig. 3.40).

- A marked follicular reaction in the fornices (Fig. 3.41).

- Severe infection may result in conjunctival haemorrhages, chemosis and pseudomembranes (Figs 3.42 and 3.43).

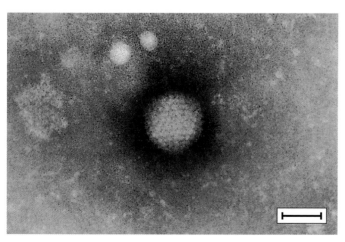

Fig. 3.39 Negative-stain electron micrograph of an adenovirus (Courtesy of Hart and Shears, from *Color Atlas of Medical Microbiology*, Mosby, 2004)

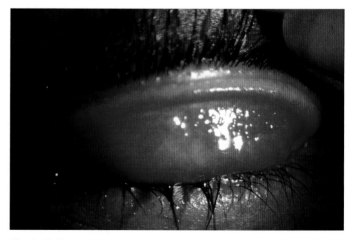

Fig. 3.40 Tarsal follicles and papillae in adenoviral conjunctivitis

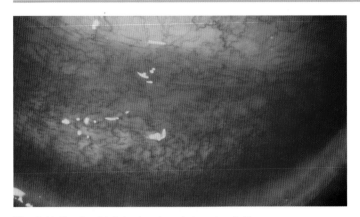

Fig. 3.41 Forniceal follicles in adenoviral conjunctivitis

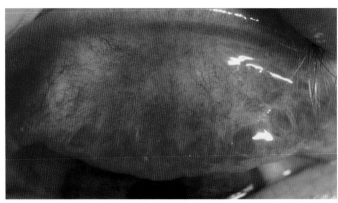

Fig. 3.44 Resolving conjunctival pseudomembrane

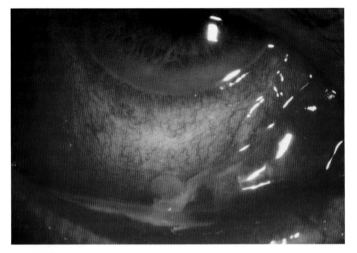

Fig. 3.42 Haemorrhagic conjunctivitis with chemosis and early pseudomembrane formation in severe adenoviral infection

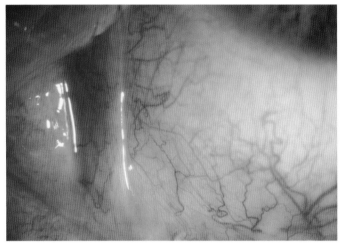

Fig. 3.45 Conjunctival scarring following adenoviral infection

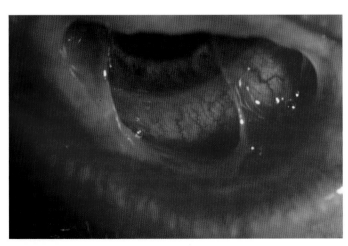

Fig. 3.43 Extensive pseudomembrane formation in severe adenoviral infection

- Tender preauricular lymphadenopathy.
- The pseudomembranes resolve (Fig. 3.44) but may leave mild conjunctival scarring (Fig. 3.45).

Keratitis

1. **Stage 1** occurs within 7–10 days of the onset of symptoms and is characterised by a punctate epithelial keratitis that resolves within 2 weeks (Fig. 3.46).

2. **Stage 2** is characterised by focal, white, subepithelial opacities that develop beneath the fading epithelial lesions (Fig. 3.47) that are thought to represent immune response to the virus.

3. **Stage 3** is characterised by anterior stromal infiltrates that gradually fade over months or years (Fig. 3.48).

Treatment

1. **Conjunctivitis** is treated symptomatically with artificial tears and cold compresses until spontaneous resolution occurs within 3 weeks. Topical steroids may be required for severe membranous conjunctivitis.

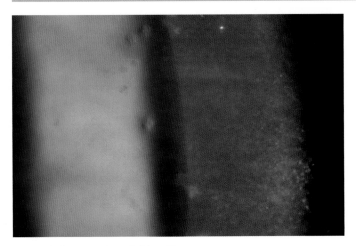

Fig. 3.46 Stage 1 adenoviral keratitis

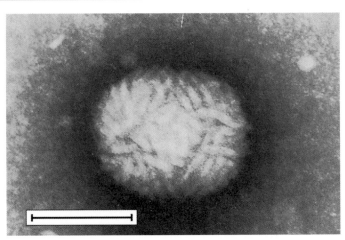

Fig. 3.49 Negative-stain electron micrograph of molluscum contagiosum virus, which is described as resembling a ball of string (Courtesy of Hart and Shears, from *Color Atlas of Medical Microbiology*, Mosby, 2004)

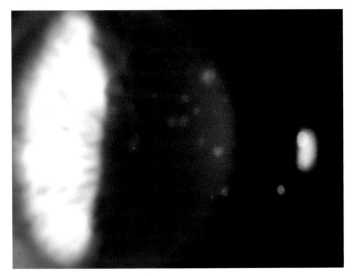

Fig. 3.47 Stage 2 adenoviral keratitis

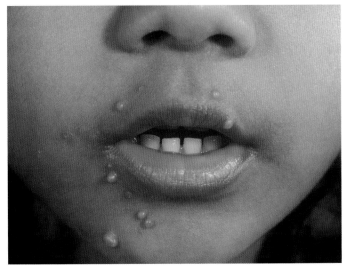

Fig. 3.50 Molluscum lesions in a child

2. **Keratitis** responds well to topical steroids. Unfortunately, they do not shorten the natural course of the disease but merely suppress the corneal inflammation, so that the lesions tend to recur if steroid therapy is discontinued prematurely.

Molluscum contagiosum conjunctivitis

Pathogenesis

Molluscum contagiosum is a skin infection caused by a human-specific double-stranded DNA poxvirus (Fig. 3.49) which typically affects otherwise healthy children, with a peak incidence between 2 and 4 years (Fig. 3.50). Transmission is by contact with infected people and then by auto-inoculation. Multiple, and occasionally confluent, lesions may develop in immunocompromised patients (Fig. 3.51). A distribution in the chinstrap region is common in HIV-positive patients.

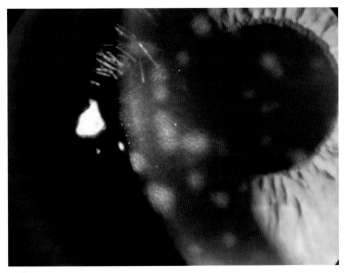

Fig. 3.48 Stage 3 adenoviral keratitis

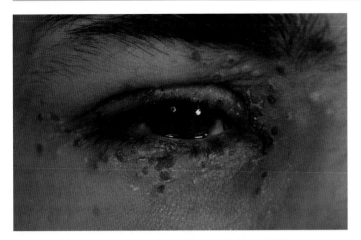

Fig. 3.51 Extensive molluscum lesions in a patient with AIDS

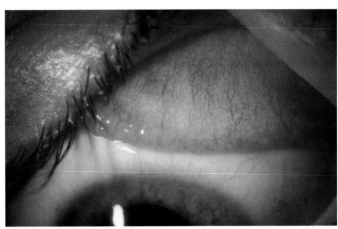

Fig. 3.53 Conjunctivitis in molluscum infection

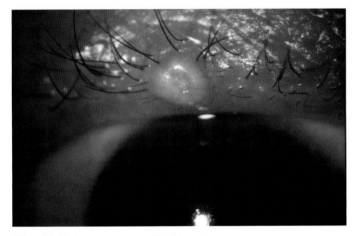

Fig. 3.52 Molluscum lesion on the lid margin

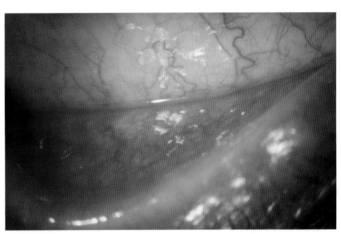

Fig. 3.54 Conjunctivitis associated with a molluscum lesion on the lower lid

Diagnosis

1. **Presentation** is with chronic, unilateral, ocular irritation and a mild discharge.

2. **Signs**

- A pale, waxy, umbilicated nodule on the lid margin (Fig. 3.52).

- Ipsilateral follicular conjunctivitis and mild mucoid discharge (Figs 3.53 and 3.54).

- Bulbar nodules may rarely occur in immunocompromised patients.

- Untreated longstanding cases may develop a fine epithelial keratitis or pannus.

Treatment

The lesions are self-limiting and removal may only be necessary for cosmetic reasons or secondary conjunctivitis.

1. **Preferred** treatment is by physical expression, which may be facilitated by making a small nick in the skin at the margin of the lesion with the tip of a needle.

2. **Other options** such as phenol ablation, cauterisation, cryotherapy or laser are more hazardous and liable to cause scarring, depigmentation or loss of lashes.

Acute haemorrhagic conjunctivitis

Pathogenesis

Acute haemorrhagic conjunctivitis is caused by enterovirus 70 or coxsackievirus A24. It has a rapid onset and resolution.

NB: The lash line should be examined carefully in patients with chronic conjunctivitis so as not to overlook a molluscum lesion (Fig. 3.55).

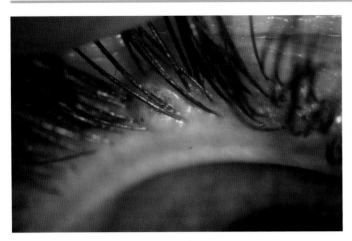

Fig. 3.55 Molluscum lesion in the lash line

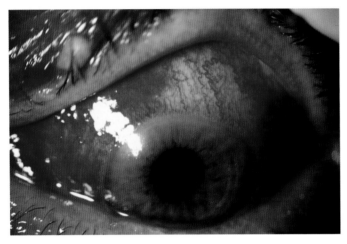

Fig. 3.56 Acute haemorrhagic conjunctivitis

The infection is spread by direct inoculation and the use of traditional eye medicines rather than by the usual faecal–oral route. Large outbreaks of acute haemorrhagic conjunctivitis occurred in Central Africa and Asia in the 1980s.

Diagnosis

1. **Presentation** is with acute onset of usually bilateral burning, watering, discharge and lid swelling. Some patients have a sore throat and malaise.

2. **Signs**

* Subconjunctival haemorrhages and follicular conjunctivitis (Fig. 3.56).

* Preauricular lymphadenopathy.

> **NB:** *N. meningitides* or herpes simplex infection may cause sporadic haemorrhagic conjunctivitis.

Management

There is no antiviral therapy for either agent. Management therefore involves limitation of infection by education and infection control.

FURTHER READING

Charteris DG, Bonshek RE, Tullo AB. Ophthalmic molluscum contagiosum: clinical and immunopathological features. *Br J Ophthalmol* 1995;79:476–481.

Elnifro EM, Cooper RJ, Klapper PE, et al. Diagnosis of viral and chlamydial keratoconjunctivitis: which laboratory test? *Br J Ophthalmol* 1999;83:622–627.

Gottsch JD. Surveillance and control of epidemic keratoconjunctivitis. *Trans Am Ophthalmol Soc* 1996;94:539–584.

Leahey AB, Shane JJ, Listhaus A, et al. Molluscum contagiosum eyelid lesions as the initial manifestation of acquired immunodeficiency syndrome. *Am J Ophthalmol* 1997;124:240–241.

Robinson MR, Udell IJ, Garber PF, et al. Molluscum contagiosum of the eyelids in patients with acquired immune deficiency syndrome. *Ophthalmology* 1992;99:1745–1747.

Sladden MJ, Johnston GA. Common skin infections in children. *BMJ* 2004;329:95–99.

Weller R, O'Callaghan CJ, MacSween RM, et al. Scarring in molluscum contagiosum: comparison of physical expression and phenol ablation. *BMJ* 1999;319:154.

ALLERGIC CONJUNCTIVITIS

Acute allergic rhinoconjunctivitis

Pathogenesis

Atopy is a genetically determined predisposition to mount an allergic response to environmental allergens. Acute rhino-conjunctivitis is the most common form of ocular and nasal allergy, affecting about 20% of the population. The following two clinical syndromes have been described, based on the pattern of exacerbations and the likely allergen:

1. **Seasonal allergic conjunctivitis** (hay fever), with onset during the spring and summer, is the commonest form. The most frequent allergens are tree and grass pollens, although the specific allergen varies with geographic location.

2. **Perennial allergic conjunctivitis** causes symptoms throughout the year, with exacerbation in the autumn, when exposure to house dust mites (*Dermatophagoides pteronyssinus*), animal dander and fungal allergens is greatest. It is less common and milder than seasonal allergic conjunctivitis.

Diagnosis

1. **Presentation** is with transient, acute attacks of redness, watering and itching, associated with sneezing and nasal discharge.

2. **Signs**, which resolve completely between attacks, are:

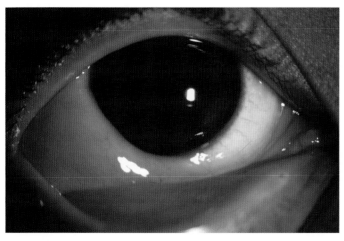

Fig. 3.57 Mild conjunctival hyperaemia and chemosis in acute allergic conjunctivitis

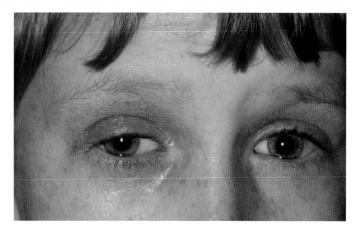

Fig. 3.59 Lid eczema of the lids in a patient with vernal disease

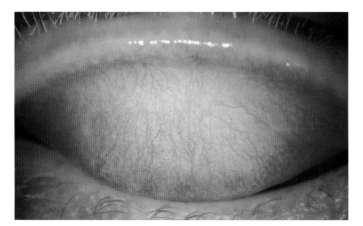

Fig. 3.58 Small superior tarsal papillae in acute allergic conjunctivitis

- Lid oedema.
- Conjunctival hyperaemia and chemosis (Fig. 3.57).
- Small papillae on the upper tarsal conjunctiva (Fig. 3.58).

Treatment

1. **Mast cell stabilisers** (sodium cromoglicate q.i.d., nedocromil sodium b.d. and lodoxamide b.d.) for long-term use. There is no difference in benefit of a particular preparation except frequency of instillation.

2. **Antihistamines** (levocabastine, azelastine, epinastine, emedastine, ketotifen, b.d or q.i.d) when the patients is symptomatic. They are as effective as mast cell stabilisers and there is no difference in benefit between different preparations.

3. **Combined antihistamines and mast cell stabilisers** (olopatadine and emedastine b.d.).

4. **Combined antihistamines and vasoconstrictors** (antazoline and xylometazoline) may provide temporary relief.

5. **Steroids** are effective but rarely indicated.

Vernal keratoconjunctivitis

Pathogenesis

Vernal keratoconjunctivitis (VKC) is a bilateral, recurrent disorder in which IgE and cell-mediated immune mechanisms play important roles. It primarily affects boys and usually presents in the first decade of life (mean age 7 years). Ninety-five per cent of cases remit by the late teens and the remainder develop atopic keratoconjunctivitis. VKC is rare in temperate regions but in sub-Saharan regions of Africa it is a significant public health problem. In temperate regions, about three-quarters of patients have associated atopy and two-thirds have a family history of atopy. Such patients often develop asthma and eczema in infancy. VKC may occur on a seasonal basis, with a peak incidence over late spring and summer, although there may be mild perennial symptoms.

Classification

1. **Palpebral** disease primarily involves the upper tarsal conjunctiva and may be associated with significant corneal disease as a result of the close apposition between the inflamed upper tarsal plates and corneal epithelium.

2. **Limbal** disease typically affects black and Asian patients.

3. **Mixed**, with signs of both palpebral and limbal disease.

Diagnosis

1. **Symptoms** consist of intense itching, which may be associated with lacrimation, photophobia, a foreign body sensation, burning and thick mucoid discharge. Constant blinking is also common and may be misdiagnosed as neurotic.

2. **Eyelids** may show eczema and fissuring at the canthi (Fig. 3.59).

3. **Palpebral disease**

- Diffuse papillary hypertrophy on the superior tarsus.

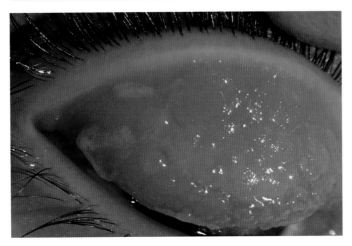

Fig. 3.60 Giant papillae in active vernal disease

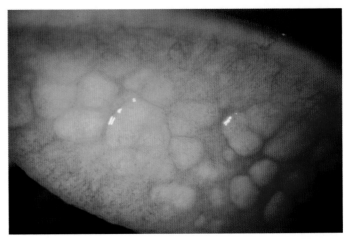

Fig. 3.63 Relatively inactive vernal disease

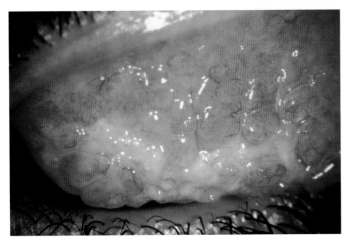

Fig. 3.61 Giant papillae and mucus in active vernal disease

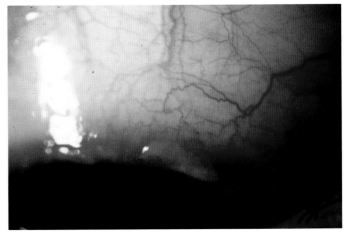

Fig. 3.64 Gelatinous limbal papillae in mild vernal limbitis

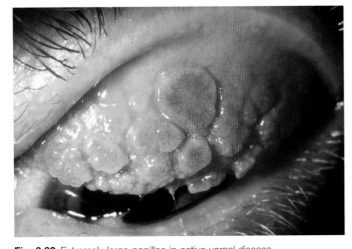

Fig. 3.62 Extremely large papillae in active vernal disease

- Giant papillae (>1 mm) have a flat-topped polygonal appearance reminiscent of cobblestones (Fig. 3.60).

- In active disease, the mucus lies between the papillae (Fig. 3.61).

- Extremely large papillae are uncommon (Fig. 3.62).

- Decreased disease activity is characterised by less conjunctival injection and mucus production (Fig. 3.63).

- In some cases, a fine reticulate pattern of subconjunctival scarring may develop, although this is rarely of clinical significance.

4. Limbal disease

- Gelatinous papillae on the limbal conjunctiva (Fig. 3.64).

- The papillae may be associated with discrete white spots at their apices (Trantas dots) (Figs 3.65–3.67).

- Conjunctival cysts may develop in chronic disease.

- In tropical regions, limbal disease may be severe and encroach onto the visual axis.

5. Keratopathy is more frequent in palpebral disease and may take the following forms:

- Punctate epithelial erosions involving the superior cornea are the earliest findings.

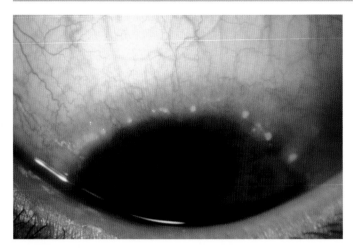

Fig. 3.65 Mild vernal limbitis with Trantas dots

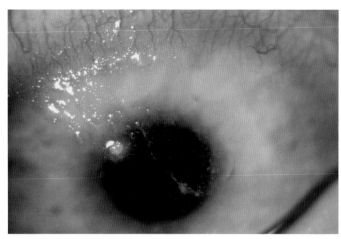

Fig. 3.68 Sheet of mucus in vernal disease

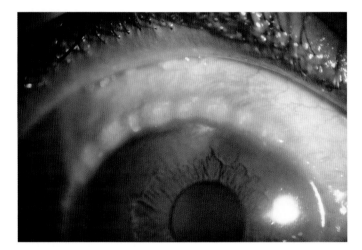

Fig. 3.66 More severe vernal limbitis

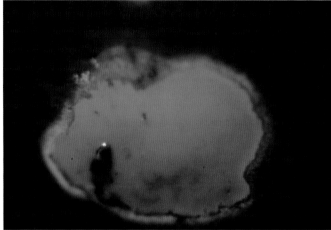

Fig. 3.69 Corneal macroerosion stained with fluorescein

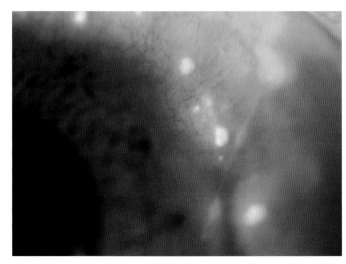

Fig. 3.67 Magnified view of Trantas dots

- A sheet of mucus on the superior cornea (Fig. 3.68).

- Epithelial macroerosions resulting from necrosis caused by toxins released from the inflamed conjunctiva (Fig. 3.69).

- Shield ulcers (Fig. 3.70) and plaques (Fig. 3.71) may develop in palpebral or mixed disease when the exposed Bowman layer becomes coated with mucus and calcium phosphate. This may results in poor wetting and delayed re-epithelialisation.

- Pseudogerontoxon can develop in recurrent limbal disease. It resembles a local area of arcus senilis adjacent to a previously inflamed segment of the limbus (Fig. 3.72).

- Peripheral superficial vascularisation, especially superior, may develop following chronic inflammation and mucus deposition in the absence of ulceration.

- Herpes simplex keratitis can be aggressive and occasionally bilateral.

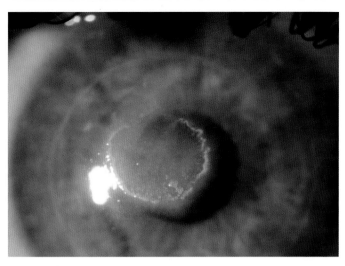

Fig. 3.70 Shield ulcer in vernal disease

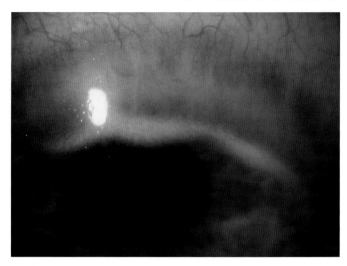

Fig. 3.72 Pseudogerontoxon in vernal disease

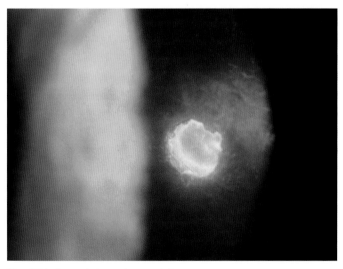

Fig. 3.71 Corneal plaque in vernal disease

NB: Patients with VKC have an increased incidence of keratoconus which is frequently complicated by hydrops. Other associations of atopic dermatitis are cataract and retinal detachment.

Management

1. Education and support

- Allergen avoidance, cool bedroom, synthetic bed-wear and removal of bedroom carpets.

- Awareness of time lost from school and impact on other family members.

- Reassurance of high probability of eventual resolution with a good visual outcome.

2. Topical

a. *Mast cell stabilisers* are rarely effective as sole treatment, but they reduce the need for steroids. Lodoxamide and nedocromil sodium are more effective than sodium cromoglicate.

b. *Antihistamines* when used in isolation are as effective as mast cell stabilisers.

c. *Steroids* are indicated mainly for keratopathy, although they may be required short-term for severe discomfort. Fluorometholone 0.1% is preferred as it has a low risk of causing ocular hypertension. Exacerbations should be treated intensively with prompt tapering. It is often possible to discontinue steroids between attacks. Monitoring intraocular pressure and the appearance of the optic disc is essential, particularly when a strong steroid (dexamethasone, prednisolone) is used. Blindness from cataract and glaucoma may occur where steroid treatment is unsupervised.

d. *Acetylcysteine* 5% to 20% is a mucolytic agent which is useful for mucous deposition and early plaque formation.

e. *Ciclosporin* 1% or 2% may be considered in steroid-resistant cases but is less effective than topical steroids and relapses occur rapidly after stopping.

3. Supratarsal steroid injection for non-compliant patients and those resistant to conventional therapy. The injection consists of 0.1 ml of either dexamethasone 4 mg/ml or triamcinolone 40 mg/ml after upper lid eversion. There is no clear difference in benefit between the two steroids.

4. Systemic

a. *Immunosuppressive agents* (steroids, ciclosporin and azathioprine) may be used in severe unremitting disease unresponsive to maximum tolerated topical therapy.

b. *Oral antihistamines* help sleep and reduce nocturnal eye rubbing.

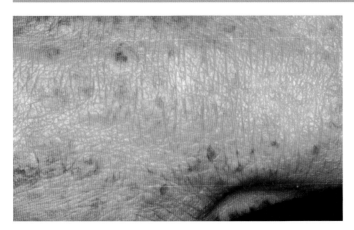

Fig. 3.73 Atopic dermatitis of the hand

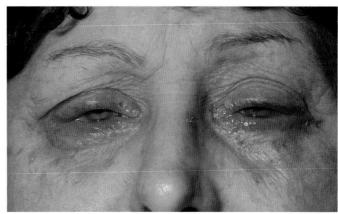

Fig. 3.74 Severe atopic dermatitis around the eyes

5. Surgery

a. **Superficial keratectomy** may be required to remove plaques. The epithelium is removed to the edge of the calcified region and a very superficial dissection performed. Medical treatment must be maintained until the cornea has re-epithelialised to prevent recurrences. Excimer laser phototherapeutic keratectomy is an alternative.

b. **An amniotic membrane overlay graft** with tarsorrhaphy or lamellar keratoplasty may be required for severe persistent epithelial defects with ulceration.

Atopic keratoconjunctivitis

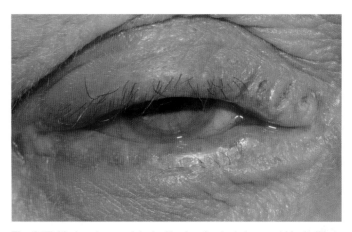

Fig. 3.75 Madarosis associated with chronic staphylococcal blepharitis in a patient with atopic dermatitis

Pathogenesis

Atopic keratoconjunctivitis (AKC) is a rare bilateral and symmetric disease that typically develops in young men following a long history of severe atopic dermatitis (Fig. 3.73). About 5% of patients have childhood vernal disease. AKC tends to be chronic and unremitting, with a low expectation of eventual resolution, and is therefore associated with significant visual morbidity. Patients are sensitive to a wide range of environmental airborne allergens.

Diagnosis

The diagnosis is clinical and there is no single laboratory test to distinguish AKC from VKC.

1. Symptoms are similar to those of VKC but often are more severe and unremitting.

2. Eyelids

- Red, thickened, macerated and fissured (Fig. 3.74).

- Chronic staphylococcal blepharitis and madarosis are common (Fig. 3.75).

- Tightening of the facial skin may cause lower lid ectropion and epiphora (Fig. 3.76).

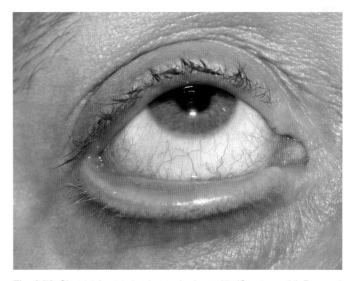

Fig. 3.76 Cicatricial ectropion in atopic dermatitis (Courtesy of A Pearson)

3. Conjunctiva

- Micropapillary conjunctivitis over the upper and lower tarsal plates and inferior fornix (Fig. 3.77).

- Giant papillae may develop with time (Fig. 3.78).

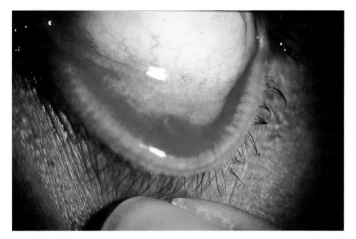

Fig. 3.77 Micropapillary conjunctivitis in atopic disease

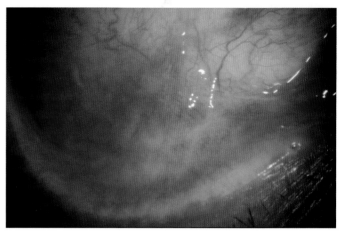

Fig. 3.80 Forniceal shortening in atopic disease

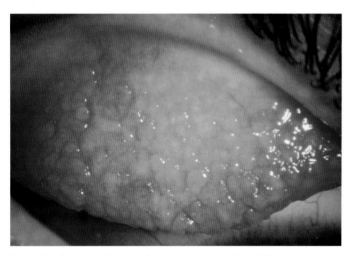

Fig. 3.78 Giant papillae in active atopic keratoconjunctivitis

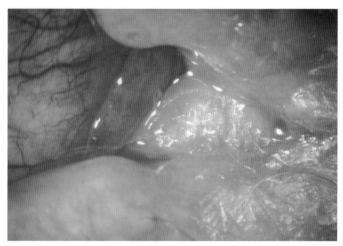

Fig. 3.81 Keratinisation of the conjunctiva in atopic disease

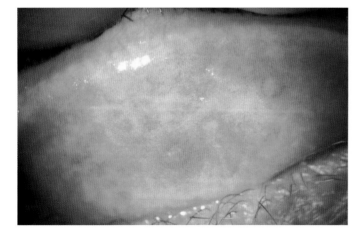

Fig. 3.79 Infiltration and scarring of the tarsal conjunctiva in atopic disease

- Scarring and infiltration of the tarsal conjunctiva results in a flattening of giant papillae and featureless appearance (Fig. 3.79).

- Cicatricial conjunctivitis may develop with inferior forniceal shortening (Fig. 3.80), symblepharon formation, and keratinisation of the caruncle (Fig. 3.81).

4. Keratopathy

- Punctate epithelial erosions over the inferior third of the cornea are common.

- Persistent epithelial defects (Fig 3.82).

- Plaque formation (Fig. 3.83).

- Peripheral superficial vascularisation in response to chronic surface inflammation.

- Predisposition to keratoconus (Fig. 3.84), secondary bacterial and fungal infection, and aggressive herpes simplex infection.

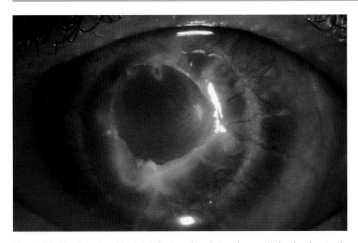

Fig. 3.82 Persistent epithelial defect and peripheral vascularisation in atopic disease

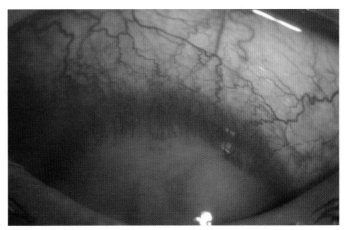

Fig. 3.84 Keratoconus with hydrops in atopic keratoconjunctivitis

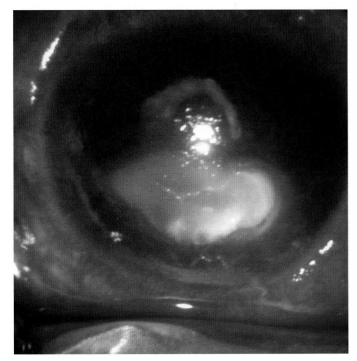

Fig. 3.83 Corneal plaque in atopic disease

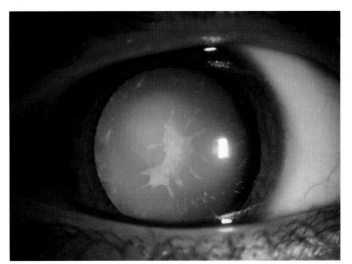

Fig. 3.85 Shield-like cataract in atopic disease

NB: Patients with atopic disease may also develop shield-like presenile cataracts (Fig. 3.85).

Management

Guidelines are similar to those of vernal disease, although AKC is less responsive and requires prolonged treatment.

1. Topical

a. Mast cell stabilisers are effective and should be used throughout the year as prophylaxis against exacerbation and as steroid-sparing agents.

b. Ketolorac combined with a mast cell stabiliser.

c. Antihistamines are less effective than in VKC.

d. Steroids are effective short term for severe exacerbations and keratopathy. A small number of patients require long-term low-dose therapy for reasonable control.

e. Acetylcysteine 5% or 10% for mucus deposition on the cornea.

f. Ciclosporin 1% or 2% is effective in some patients.

g. Antibiotics and lid hygiene should be used for associated staphylococcal blepharitis.

2. Supratarsal steroid injections should be considered when topical treatment is ineffective.

3. Systemic

a. Antihistamines for severe itching.

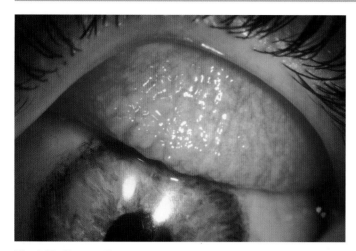

Fig. 3.86 Giant papillary conjunctivitis associated with an artificial eye

b. **Antibiotics** (doxycycline 50–100 mg daily for 6 weeks or azithromycin 500 mg once daily for 3 days) to reduce inflammation aggravated by blepharitis.

c. **Ciclosporin** (4 mg/kg) in severe cases.

NB: Because of the high carriage of *Staph. aureus* on the lid margins, cataract surgery is associated with an increased risk of endophthalmitis.

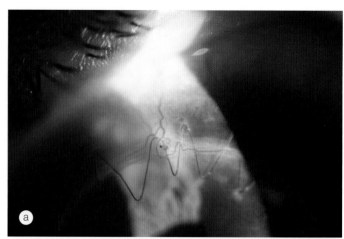

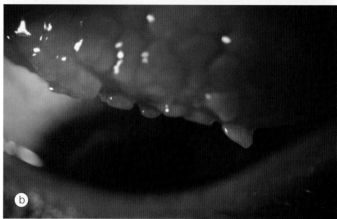

Fig. 3.87 (a) Loose corneal suture; (b) giant papillary conjunctivitis in the same patient

Giant papillary conjunctivitis

Pathogenesis

Giant papillary conjunctivitis (GPC) was originally described in association with soft contact lens wear, but has subsequently been recognised in association with a variety of mechanical stimuli of the tarsal conjunctiva, including ocular prosthesis (Fig. 3.86), exposed sutures (Fig. 3.87), scleral explants, corneal calcium deposits and filtering blebs. The risk of developing GPC is increased by deposition of mucus and cellular debris on the contact lens surface (lens spoliation). The tissue response is characteristic of allergy, although patients may not have any other features of atopy. Eosinophils and mucosal mast cells are found in the epithelium. GPC may develop in patients with mild allergic eye disease that is exacerbated by contact lens wear.

Diagnosis

1. **Symptoms** consist of a foreign body sensation, redness, itching and loss of contact lens tolerance. They are often worse when the contact lens has been removed.

2. **Signs**

- Excessive mobility of the contact lens with upper lid lens capture.

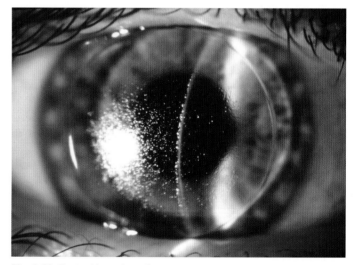

Fig. 3.88 Contact lens deposits

- Increased mucus production and coating of the contact lens (Fig. 3.88).

- Micropapillae on the superior tarsal conjunctiva.

- Macropapillae with focal scarring on the apices may develop in advanced cases (see Fig. 3.86).

Table 3.2 Summary of clinical findings in allergic conjunctivitis

	Acute		Chronic		Limited	
	SAC	**PAC**	**VKC**	**AKC**	**CLAGPC**	**Contact**
Pathogenesis	Type I		Type I and Type IV		Type 1 and Type IV Mechanical	Type IV
Allergen	Pollen, dander	House dust mite	Pollen, dander, house dust mite		Not known	Varies
Lids	Swelling		Ptosis Eczema	Thickened Loss of lashes Fissuring Ectropion Keratinisation	Ptosis	Swelling Scaling
Conjunctiva	Chemosis Papillae		Giant papillae Infiltration Mild scarring	Infiltration Sheet scarring Papillae	Macropapillae Giant papillae Focal scarring	Chemosis Injection
Cornea	Punctate epithelial keratitis		PEE superior Adherent mucus Macroerosion Plaque ulcer Vascularisation	PEE inferior Vascularisation Plaque ulcer	Usually nil	Usually nil

SAC, seasonal allergic conjunctivitis; PAC, perennial allergic conjunctivitis; VKC, vernal keratoconjunctivitis; AKC, atopic keratoconjunctivitis; CLAGPC, contact lens-associated giant papillary conjunctivitis; PEE, punctate epithelial erosions.

NB: In contrast to VKC, keratopathy is rare due to less secretion of toxic cytokines.

Treatment

1. **Removal of the stimulus**

- Stopping contact lens wear.

- Removal of exposed sutures, ocular prosthesis, etc.

2. **Cleaning contact lens or prosthesis**

- Use of daily disposable lenses.

- Rigid contact lenses may be easier to clean effectively.

- Protein-removing tablets.

- Polishing of prosthesis and cleaning with a detergent.

3. **Mast cell stabilisers**, which should be non-preserved in patients wearing soft contact lenses.

4. **Topical steroids** are rarely indicated but are safe to treat GPC associated with an ocular prosthesis.

Contact dermatitis

Pathogenesis

Contact dermatitis is an inflammatory response that usually follows exposure to a medication or preservative, cosmetics or metals. An irritant can also cause a non-allergic toxic dermatitis. Contact dermatitis is distinct from atopic dermatitis affecting the eyelid, and from a hypersensitivity reaction to a drug. The individual is sensitised on first exposure and develops an immune reaction on further exposure. Reaction is mediated by a delayed type IV hypersensitivity response.

Diagnosis

1. **History** of exposure and re-exposure to a potential allergen.

2. **Symptoms** include itching and tearing following exposure.

3. **Signs**

- Lid oedema, scaling, angular fissuring and tightness (Figs 3.89 and 3.90).

- Chemosis, redness and papillary conjunctivitis.

- Punctate corneal epithelial erosions.

Treatment

- Stopping exposure to the allergen, if it can be identified.

- Use of non-preserved drops, if sensitivity to preservatives suspected.

- Cold compress for symptomatic relief.

- Topical steroids may be helpful but are rarely required.

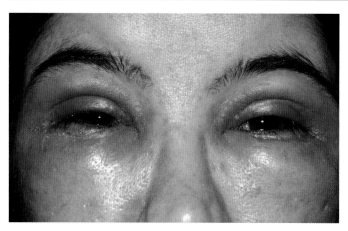

Fig. 3.89 Contact dermatitis

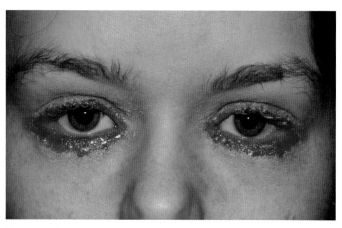

Fig. 3.90 Extremely severe contact dermatitis

- Oral antihistamine for severe cases.

- Care to avoid re-exposure (record in notes).

FURTHER READING

Akpek EK, Dart JK, Watson S, et al. A randomized trial of topical cyclosporin 0.05% in topical steroid-resistant atopic keratoconjunctivitis. *Ophthalmology* 2004;111:476–482.

Bonini S, Coassin M, Aronni S, et al. Vernal keratoconjunctivitis. *Eye* 2004;18:345–351.

Foster CS, Calonge M. Atopic keratoconjunctivitis. *Ophthalmology* 1990;97:992–1000.

Hingorani M, Moodaley L, Calder VL, et al. A randomized, placebo-controlled trial of topical cyclosporin A in steroid-dependent atopic keratoconjunctivitis. *Ophthalmology* 1998;105:1715–1720.

Rikkers SM, Holland GN, Drayton GE, et al. Topical tacrolimus treatment of atopic eyelid disease. *Am J Ophthalmol* 2003;135:297–302.

Tuft SJ, Dart JKG, Kemeny M. Limbal vernal keratoconjunctivitis: clinical characteristics and immunoglobulin E expression compared with palpebral vernal. *Eye* 1989;3:420–427.

Tuft SJ, Keenly DM, Dart JK, et al. Clinical features of atopic keratoconjunctivitis. *Ophthalmology* 1991;98:150–158.

Tuft SJ, Cree IA, Woods M, et al. Limbal vernal keratoconjunctivitis in the tropics. *Ophthalmology* 1998;105:1489–1493.

CICATRISING CONJUNCTIVITIS

Mucous membrane pemphigoid

Mucous membrane pemphigoid is a mucocutaneous blistering disease that affects women more commonly than men (2:1) with a mean age of onset in the sixth decade (see Ch. 8). Conjunctival disease (ocular cicatricial pemphigoid – OCP) is seen in 75% of cases with oral involvement but only in 25% of those with skin lesions; occasionally it occurs in isolation. OCP is always bilateral, but frequently asymmetric with regard to time of onset, severity and rate of progression.

Pathogenesis

An unknown trigger in genetically susceptible individuals causes autoantibody production against components of the basement membrane and hemidesmosomes. The result is a type II hypersensitivity response with IgG or IgA antibodies binding to the basement membrane zone and causing complement activation. Inflammatory cells are recruited by this reaction, causing separation of the epithelium from the underlying tissue. The release of cytokines in the tissue causes fibroblast activation and scarring resulting in conjunctival shrinkage and loss of components of the ocular surface (tears, mucin and meibomian gland function). The resultant damage causes keratinisation, corneal drying, epithelial defects, vascularisation and scarring. Dry eye is caused by a combination of destruction of goblet cells and accessory lacrimal glands as well as occlusion of the main lacrimal ductules.

Ocular features

1. **Presentation** is with an insidious onset of non-specific conjunctivitis with redness, irritation, burning and tearing.

NB: Because of the rarity of the condition, the diagnosis is often overlooked and treatment delayed.

2. **Conjunctiva**

- Papillary conjunctivitis associated with diffuse hyperaemia (Fig. 3.91).

- Limbitis (Fig. 3.92) and conjunctival necrosis (Fig. 3.93) require immediate treatment.

- Subconjunctival bullae are transient and rarely observed.

- Chronic conjunctivitis with fine lines of subconjunctival fibrosis (Fig. 3.94).

- Shallowing of the inferior fornices (Fig. 3.95).

- Flattening of the plica and keratinisation of the caruncle (Fig. 3.96).

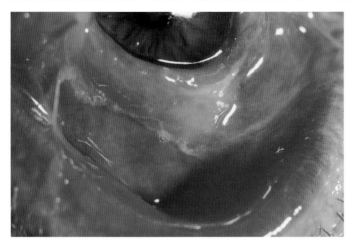

Fig. 3.91 Severe conjunctival hyperaemia in the acute stage of ocular cicatricial pemphigoid

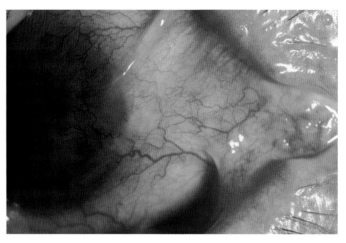

Fig. 3.94 Early subconjunctival fibrosis in ocular cicatricial pemphigoid

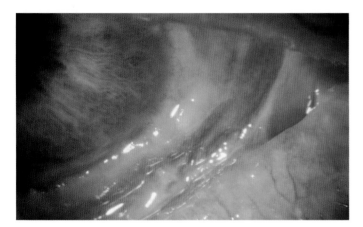

Fig. 3.92 Limbitis in ocular cicatricial pemphigoid

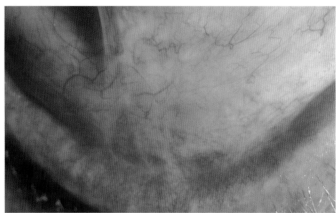

Fig. 3.95 Short inferior fornix in ocular cicatricial pemphigoid

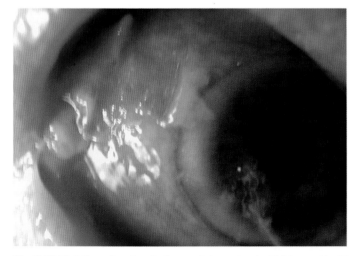

Fig. 3.93 Limbitis and conjunctival necrosis in ocular cicatricial pemphigoid

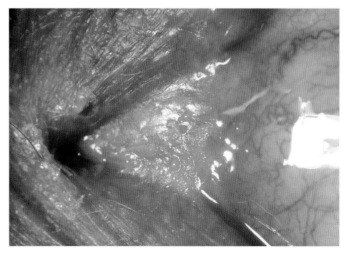

Fig. 3.96 Flat plica and keratinisation of the caruncle in ocular cicatricial pemphigoid

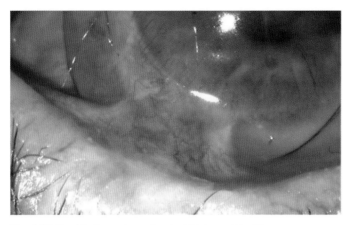

Fig. 3.97 Symblepharon in ocular cicatricial pemphigoid

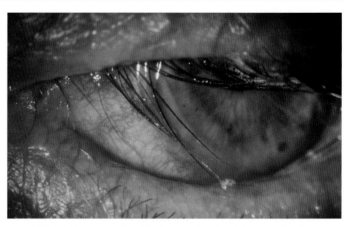

Fig. 3.99 Trichiasis and distichiasis in ocular cicatricial pemphigoid

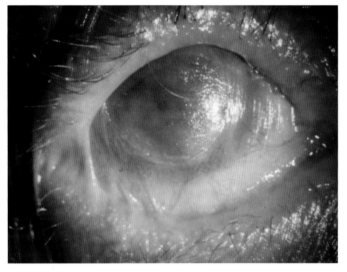

Fig. 3.98 Ankyloblepharon and keratinisation in advanced ocular cicatricial pemphigoid

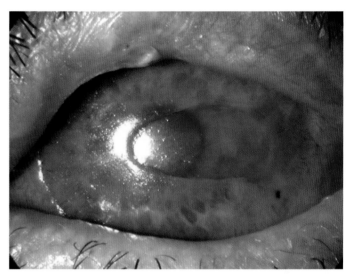

Fig. 3.100 Large corneal epithelial defect in ocular cicatricial pemphigoid

- Symblepharon (adhesion between the bulbar and palpebral conjunctiva) (Fig. 3.97).

- Ankyloblepharon (adhesions at the outer canthi between the upper and lower lids) (Fig. 3.98).

- The chronically progressive course of the disease may be interrupted by exacerbations characterised by diffuse conjunctival hyperaemia and oedema.

3. Lids

- Trichiasis and distichiasis (metaplastic lashes) (Fig. 3.99).

- Blepharitis and keratinisation of the lid margin.

4. Cornea

- Superficial punctate keratitis.

- Epithelial defects associated with drying and exposure (Fig. 3.100).

- Infiltration and peripheral vascularisation (Fig. 3.101).

- Keratinisation (Fig. 3.102 and see Fig. 3.98).

- 'Conjunctivalisation' of the cornea surface following damage to the limbus with epithelial stem cell failure (Fig. 3.103).

- End-stage disease is characterised by total symblepharon and corneal opacification (Fig. 3.104).

Investigations

1. **Conjunctival biopsy.** A 2 mm piece of bulbar conjunctiva adjacent to an inflamed site is removed but the tarsal conjunctiva should not be biopsied as it may stimulate aggressive scarring. Immunofluorescence shows linear deposition of immunoglobulin (IgG or IgA) or complement (C3) deposition at the conjunctival basement membrane.

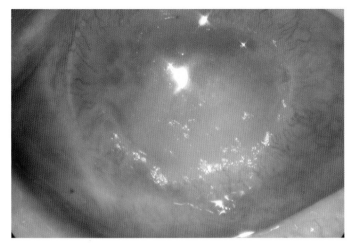

Fig. 3.101 Corneal infiltration and peripheral vascularisation in ocular cicatricial pemphigoid

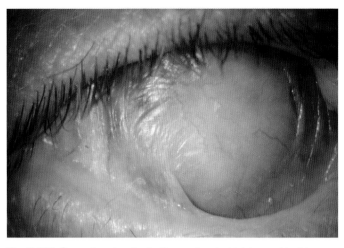

Fig. 3.103 Corneal conjunctivalisation ocular cicatricial pemphigoid

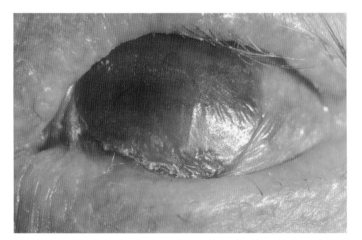

Fig. 3.102 Severe keratinisation in ocular cicatricial pemphigoid

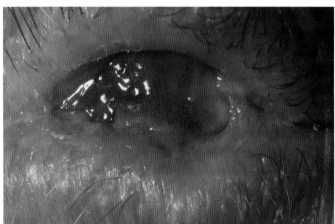

Fig. 3.104 End-stage ocular cicatricial pemphigoid

2. **Barium meal** examination and referral for possible endoscopy is indicated in patients with dysphagia.

3. **A dental opinion** is usually indicated as progressive gingivitis may develop (Fig. 3.105). It is also indicated in patients about to undergo keratoprosthesis implantation (see below).

Systemic treatment

Systemic treatment should be introduced incrementally until all signs of active disease have resolved. Initial treatment depends on activity at presentation. Unfortunately, although some patients are cured, about 30% progress inexorably to blindness despite maximum tolerated therapy.

1. Acute disease

- Systemic steroids (prednisolone 1–1.5 mg/kg) are essential to control limbitis and conjunctival necrosis, but must not be used as sole long-term therapy.

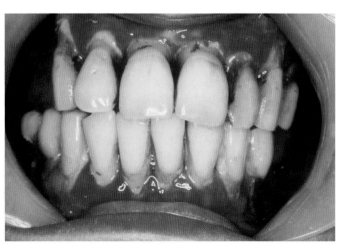

Fig. 3.105 Severe gingivitis in ocular cicatricial pemphigoid

- Cyclophosphamide (1–2 mg/kg) should be added to allow the steroid dose to be reduced.

2. Mild to moderate inflammation

- Dapsone 50 mg daily, increasing to 100 mg daily, if tolerated. It is important to check glucose-6-phosphate dehydrogenase and haemoglobin levels before starting therapy.

- Azathioprine or methotrexate if dapsone is contraindicated, although the onset of action is 2 or 3 weeks.

- Ciclosporin has been used, although data to support its effect are lacking.

3. Severe inflammation

- Cyclophosphamide should not be used for more than 12 months because of the risk of bladder carcinoma.

- Azathioprine or mycophenolate mofetil (CellCept) is suitable for long-term therapy.

- Monoclonal antibodies against the interleukin-2 receptor and intravenous immunoglobulin therapy have shown promising results in some patients.

Local treatment

- Topical steroids are used as adjunctive treatment.

- Artificial tears for surface drying; non-preserved if possible.

- Retinoic acid to reduce keratinisation.

- Subconjunctival mitomycin C injection if systemic immunosuppression is not possible, but the results in advanced disease are disappointing.

- Silicone rubber contact lenses may be used with caution to protect the cornea from aberrant lashes and drying.

- Rigid scleral contact lenses may be effective in holding a tear film in front of the cornea and protecting it from lid friction and exposure, but do not prevent forniceal scarring and symblepharon formation.

Surgery

Reconstructive surgery should be performed *only* after inflammation has been controlled. Even if the disease is quiescent, a course of systemic steroid should be considered.

- Trichiasis and distichiasis can be treated by cryotherapy, which may be combined with lid splitting to expose the lash follicles.

- Severe dry eyes may require punctal occlusion if the puncta are not already scarred.

- Large, recurrent, corneal defects may require tarsorrhaphy or botulinum toxin injection into the levator to induce ptosis.

- Entropion is best managed by a technique that does not incise conjunctiva, such as retractor plication.

- Keratinisation may be controlled by mucous membrane transplantation. Alternatively, amniotic membranes may be used, although the long-term success is worse.

- Keratoplasty is a high-risk procedure in a dry eye with corneal epithelial failure, because of frequent problems with re-epithelialisation. Lamellar grafts are preferred for perforations.

- Limbal stem cell transfer may be attempted for conjunctivalisation and keratinisation.

- Keratoprosthesis may be beneficial in end-stage disease (Fig. 3.106) although it may be associated with extrusion (Fig. 3.107).

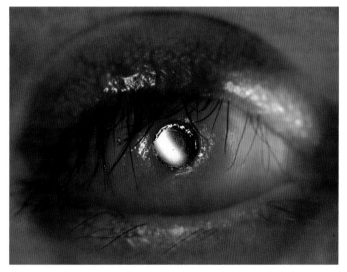

Fig. 3.106 Keratoprosthesis (Courtesy of C Liu and G Facinelli)

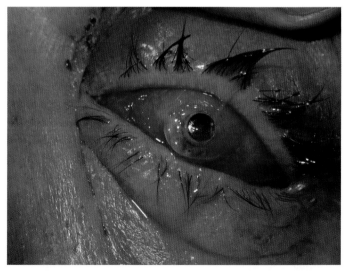

Fig. 3.107 Extrusion of a keratoprosthesis

• Cataract surgery may be technically difficult in the immobile eye with shallow fornices. A corneal section or 'open-sky' approach with a very large incision may be required.

Monitoring disease progress

The depth of the fornices should be measured regularly and the position of adhesions noted. The sum of the three readings for the distance from the inferior limbus to the centre of the lower posterior lid margin in three positions of gaze (up, right and left) is simple and reliable.

Drug-induced cicatrisation (pseudopemphigoid)

Pathogenesis

In some patients, exposure to medications triggers a response similar to ocular mucous membrane pemphigoid or trachoma. This is most frequently seen in patients using long-term topical medications for glaucoma or dry eye that contain benzalkonium chloride. The mechanism may involve toxicity and drug-induced autoimmunity to the epithelial basement membrane complex. Some cases may therefore be progressive even after the offending agent has been removed (drug-induced ocular pemphigoid).

Diagnosis

History of stinging or redness when using drops.

• A follicular conjunctivitis in early disease.

• Subepithelial fibrosis over the upper tarsal plate.

• Conjunctival keratinisation (Fig. 3.108).

• Shortening of the inferior fornices and symblepharon (Fig. 3.109).

• Other signs consistent with ocular cicatricial pemphigoid.

Management

• Withdrawal of suspect medications.

• Use of non-preserved drops and less toxic alternative medications, if possible.

• Immunosuppression may be necessary for severe and aggressive disease (drug-induced pemphigoid).

• Further treatment is as for ocular cicatricial pemphigoid.

Stevens–Johnson syndrome and toxic epidermal necrolysis

Stevens–Johnson syndrome and toxic epidermal necrolysis (Lyell disease) reflect different severity of the same mucocutaneous blistering disease process. Both are uncommon but potentially lethal conditions that may be associated with severe ocular complications. They have the same clinical signs, treatment and prognosis, although ocular involvement is much less common in toxic epidermal necrolysis. Males are affected more often than females, with a mean age of onset of 25 years.

Pathogenesis

The disease is thought to be either a delayed hypersensitivity response to drugs or a response to epithelial cell antigens modified by drug exposure. Specific drug metabolites may also play a role, suggesting a genetically determined enzyme deficiency. A wide range of drugs have been incriminated, including antibiotics, especially trimethoprim, analgesics, cold remedies, non-steroidal anti-inflammatory drugs, phenytoin and allopurinol. Infection with *Mycoplasma pneumoniae* also appears to be a risk factor. However, because symptoms often take 3 weeks to develop after exposure, in over 50% of cases the precipitating cause cannot be identified with certainty.

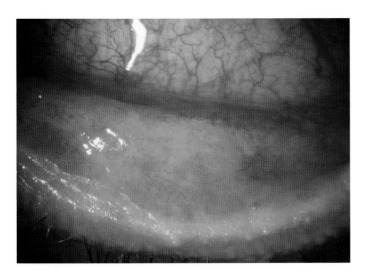

Fig. 3.108 Conjunctival keratinisation in pseudopemphigoid

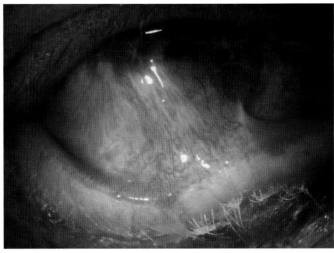

Fig. 3.109 Forniceal shortening and symblepharon in advanced pseudopemphigoid

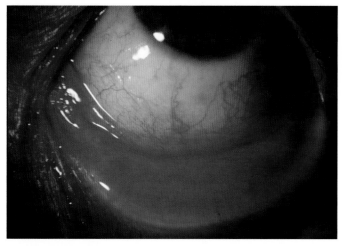

Fig. 3.110 Acute conjunctivitis in Stevens–Johnson syndrome

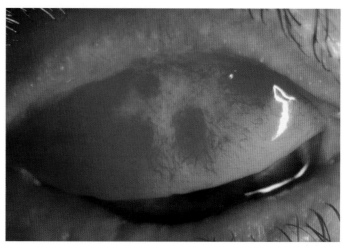

Fig. 3.112 Scarring of the upper tarsal plate in Stevens–Johnson syndrome

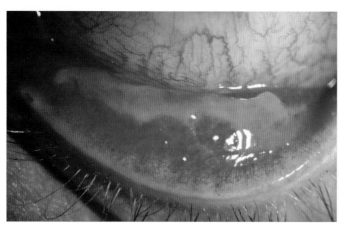

Fig. 3.111 Pseudomembranous conjunctivitis in Stevens–Johnson syndrome

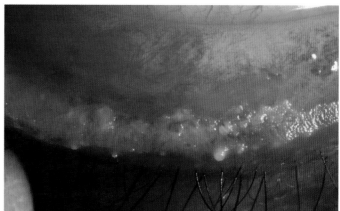

Fig. 3.113 Posterior lid margin disease and early conjunctival scarring in Stevens–Johnson syndrome

Ocular features

1. Acute disease

- Crusty eyelids associated with a transient, self-limiting papillary conjunctivitis (Fig. 3.110).

- Severe membranous or pseudomembranous conjunctivitis with patchy conjunctival infarction (Fig. 3.111).

2. Late disease

- Reticular scarring of the upper tarsal plate (Fig. 3.112).

- Posterior lid margin disease with opening of the meibomian orifices onto the ocular surface (Fig. 3.113).

- Conjunctival scarring, symblepharon formation and keratinisation (Fig. 3.114).

- Dry eye resulting from loss of goblet cells and destruction of lacrimal gland ductules (Fig. 3.115).

- Corneal keratinisation (Fig. 3.116).

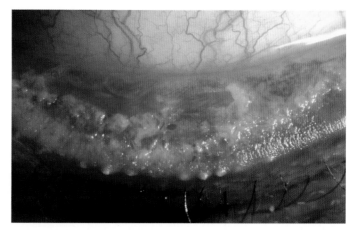

Fig. 3.114 Severe posterior lid margin disease with conjunctival scarring and keratinisation

- Keratopathy secondary to cicatricial entropion and aberrant lashes.

- Secondary bacterial or fungal keratitis.

- Corneal stem cell failure.

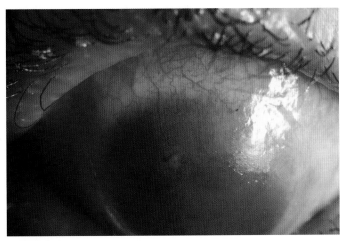

Fig. 3.115 Very dry vascularised cornea in Stevens–Johnson syndrome

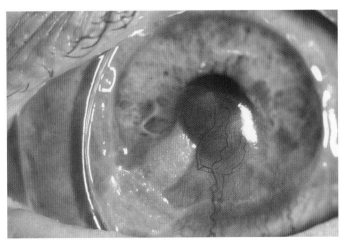

Fig. 3.117 Scleral ring in place in an eye with advanced disease

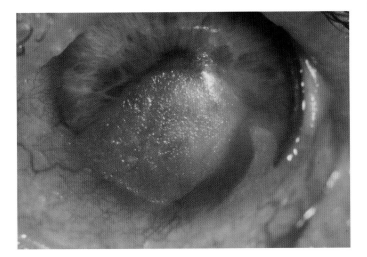

Fig. 3.116 Corneal keratinisation in Stevens–Johnson syndrome

3. Chronic ocular disease

- Lubrication and punctal occlusion for mild disease.

- Topical retinoic acid for keratinisation.

- Surgical removal of persistent keratin plaques abrading the cornea.

- Bandage contact lenses to maintain surface moisture and overcome irregular astigmatism. Gas-permeable scleral contact lenses for trichiasis and visual rehabilitation.

- Mucous membrane grafting and limbal cell transplantation.

- Lamellar corneal grafting is preferred to penetrating keratoplasty.

- Keratoprosthesis in end-stage disease.

NB: In contrast to ocular pemphigoid, immunosuppression is not required prior to conjunctival or lid surgery.

Treatment

1. Systemic disease. There is no specific treatment and management is similar to that of patients with severe burns, such as pain relief, maintenance of hydration, and treatment of infection. Debridement and replacement of sloughing skin may be required. Systemic steroids are contraindicated. Ciclosporin, thalidomide and immunoglobulins have been advocated, but without controlled trials to demonstrate a consistent effect.

2. Acute ocular disease

- Lubrication and prevention of exposure.

- Topical steroid and antibiotics.

- Lysis of conjunctival adhesions.

- A scleral ring, consisting of a large haptic lens with the central zone removed, may prevent symblepharon formation (Fig. 3.117).

Graft-versus-host disease
Pathogenesis

Graft-versus-host disease (GVHD) is a manifestation of stem cell transplantation for the treatment of leukaemias, severe anaemias and immune deficiencies. It is responsible for 50% of mortality after stem cell transplantation. Stem cells are derived from blood, bone marrow or umbilical cord. The host bone marrow is eradicated before transplant by irradiation or chemotherapy. Immunocompetent donor cells mount a response against host antigens. The host no longer has the ability to attack the grafted cells. Ocular symptoms are very common and they may be a presenting feature. Dry eye is primarily due to aqueous tear deficiency from lacrimal gland disease, but chemotherapy and total body irradiation may both contribute to ocular findings.

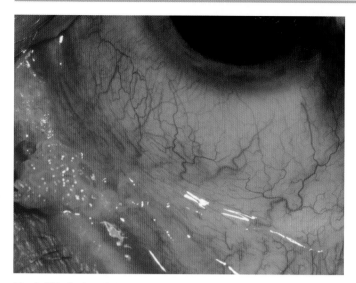

Fig. 3.118 Conjunctival papilloma in graft-versus-host disease

Diagnosis

1. Dry eye in up to 75%; it may persist after remission of GVHD.

2. Conjunctiva

- Pseudomembranous conjunctivitis.

- Cicatricial conjunctivitis.

- Viral infection with papillomavirus (Fig. 3.118) or herpes simplex.

3. Cornea

- Epithelial breakdown and persistent epithelial defect.

- Keratinisation.

- Microbial keratitis, which may be bilateral.

4. Other manifestations include cataract, related to irradiation and systemic corticosteroid, scleritis, central serous retinopathy and microvascular retinopathy.

Treatment

- Systemic steroids and ciclosporin or tacrolimus is usually indicated.

- Artificial tears or autologous serum drops for dry eye.

- Topical steroids or ciclosporin for dry eye and conjunctivitis.

- Topical retinoic acid 0.05% to reverse keratinisation.

- Punctal occlusion, bandage contact lens, tarsorrhaphy, amniotic membrane graft or keratoplasty may be required for persistent epithelial defect, infection and perforation. The visual outlook for these patients is poor.

FURTHER READING

Anderson NG, Regillo C. Ocular manifestations of graft versus host disease. *Curr Opin Ophthalmol* 2004;15:503–507.

Barabino S, Rolando M, Bentivoglio G, et al. Role of amniotic membrane transplantation for conjunctival reconstruction in ocular-cicatricial pemphigoid. *Ophthalmology* 2003;110:474–480.

Chiou AG-Y, Florakis GJ, Kazim M. Management of conjunctival cicatrizing diseases and severe ocular surface dysfunction. *Surv Ophthalmol* 1998;43:19–46.

Foster CS, Ahmed AR. Intravenous immunoglobulin therapy for ocular cicatricial pemphigoid: a preliminary study. *Ophthalmology* 1999;106:2136–2143.

Foster CS, Fong LP, Azar D, et al. Episodic conjunctival inflammation after Stevens-Johnson syndrome. *Ophthalmology* 1988;95:453–456.

Franklin RM, Kenyon KR, Tutschka PJ, et al. Ocular manifestations of graft-vs-host disease. *Ophthalmology* 1983;90:4–13.

Kerty E, Vigander K, Flage T, et al. Ocular findings in allogeneic stem cell transplantation without total body irradiation. *Ophthalmology* 1999;106:1334–1338.

Ng JS, Lam DS, Li CK, et al. Ocular complications of pediatric bone marrow transplantation. *Ophthalmology* 1999;106:160–164.

Power WJ, Ghoraishi M, Merayo-Lloves J, et al. Analysis of the acute ophthalmic manifestations of the erythema multiforme/Stevens-Johnson syndrome/toxic epidermal necrolysis disease spectrum. *Ophthalmology* 1995;102:1669–1676.

Power WJ, Neves RA, Rodriguez A. Increasing the diagnostic yield of conjunctival biopsy in patients with suspected ocular cicatricial pemphigoid. *Ophthalmology* 1995;102:1158–1163.

Power WJ, Saidman SL, Zhang DS, et al. HLA typing in patients with ocular manifestations of Stevens-Johnson syndrome. *Ophthalmology* 1996;103:1406–1409.

Rowsey JJ, Macias-Rodriguez Y, Cukrowski C. A new method for measuring progression in patients with ocular cicatricial pemphigoid. *Arch Ophthalmol* 2004;122:179–184.

Sami N, Letko E, Androudi S, et al. Intravenous immunoglobulin therapy in patients with ocular-cicatricial pemphigoid. *Ophthalmology* 2004;111:1380–1382.

Thorne JE, Anhalt GJ, Jabs DA. Mucous membrane pemphigoid and pseudopemphigoid. *Ophthalmology* 2004;111:45–52.

MISCELLANEOUS CONJUNCTIVITIS

Superior limbic keratoconjunctivitis (SLK)

SLK is an uncommon, usually bilateral, chronic disease of the superior limbus and bulbar conjunctiva. It typically affects middle-aged women who may have abnormal thyroid function, usually hyperthyroidism. SLK is probably under-diagnosed because symptoms are more severe than signs. The course can be prolonged, although remission eventually occurs without sequelae.

Pathogenesis

SLK appears to be the result of blink-related mechanical trauma from abnormal forces between the upper lid and superior bulbar conjunctiva, probably precipitated by tear film insufficiency. This results in loss of the ability of the lid to move freely over the conjunctiva and excess of conjunctival tissue. With increased movement of the conjunctiva, there is mechanical damage to both the tarsal and conjunctival surfaces.

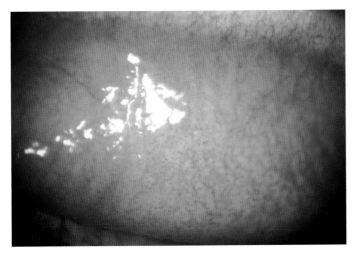

Fig. 3.119 Papillary hypertrophy in superior limbic keratoconjunctivitis

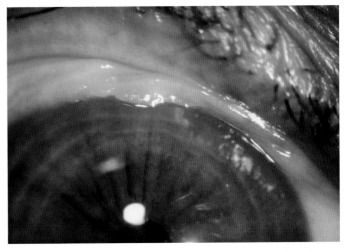

Fig. 3.121 Redundant conjunctiva in superior limbic keratoconjunctivitis

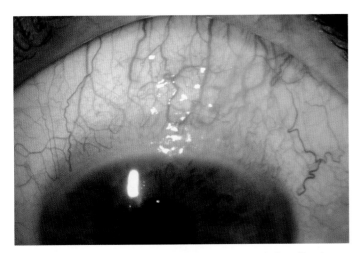

Fig. 3.120 Superior bulbar conjunctival injection and limbal papillary hypertrophy in superior limbic keratoconjunctivitis

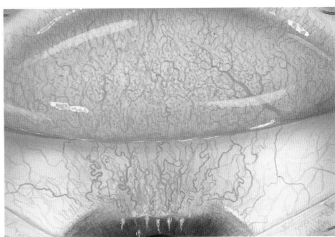

Fig. 3.122 Superior limbic keratoconjunctivitis with corneal filaments

Diagnosis

1. **Presentation** is with non-specific symptoms such as foreign body sensation, burning, photophobia and mucoid discharge.

2. **Conjunctiva**

- Papillary hypertrophy of the superior tarsus that may give rise to a diffuse velvety appearance (Fig. 3.119).

- Hyperaemia of the superior bulbar conjunctiva and limbal papillary hypertrophy which stains readily with rose bengal (Fig. 3.120).

- Light downward pressure on the upper lid results in a fold of redundant conjunctiva crossing the upper limbus (Fig. 3.121).

- Limbal palisades may be lost superiorly and petechial haemorrhages may be present.

- Keratinisation can be demonstrated on biopsy or impression cytology.

3. **Cornea**

- Superior punctate corneal epithelial erosions, often separated from the limbus by a zone of normal epithelium, are common.

- Superior filamentary keratitis develops in about one-third of cases (Fig. 3.122).

- A superior arcus may develop in longstanding disease.

4. **Keratoconjunctivitis sicca** is present in only about 50% of cases.

Treatment

The aim is to alter the abnormal mechanical interaction between the upper lid and the superior limbus. Conservative treatment should be tried initially, as the condition is usually self-limiting.

1. **Topical**

a. **Lubricants** to reduce friction between the lid and bulbar conjunctiva.

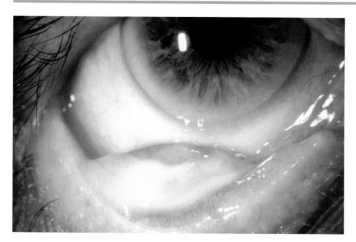

Fig. 3.123 Ligneous conjunctivitis

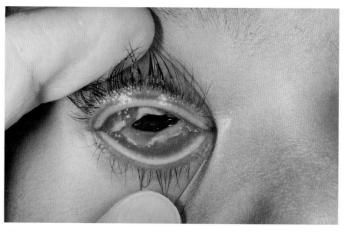

Fig. 3.124 Advanced ligneous conjunctivitis (Courtesy of U Raina)

b. **Mast cell stabilisers** (cromolyn, lodoxamide) and steroids to reduce any inflammatory component.

c. **Ciclosporin** 0.5% q.i.d. may be effective, possibly by controlling coexisting keratoconjunctivitis sicca.

d. **Acetylcysteine** 5% or 10% for filamentary keratitis.

e. **Retinoic acid** 0.05% to prevent keratinisation.

2. **Temporary superior punctal occlusion** is simple and usually effective.

3. **Soft contact lenses,** which intervene between the lid and the superior conjunctiva, may be useful. Interestingly, a unilateral lens may provide bilateral relief.

4. **Resection** of the superior limbal conjunctiva and Tenon capsule, either in a zone 2 mm from the superior limbus or at the upper margin of rose bengal staining, is usually effective in resistant disease. The mechanism is to remove excess conjunctiva and enable the remaining conjunctiva to grow on the sclera and not be mobile.

5. **Other modalities** include transconjunctival thermocautery or topical silver nitrate 0.5% to the affected area.

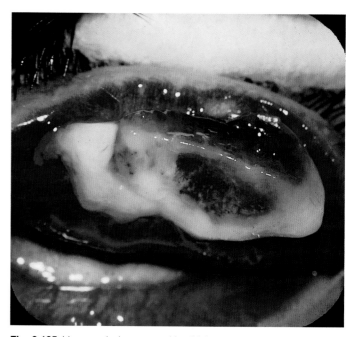

Fig. 3.125 Ligneous lesion covered by thick mucus

Ligneous conjunctivitis

Ligneous conjunctivitis is a very rare disorder characterised by recurrent, often bilateral, firm (woody) membranous lesions that predominantly affect the tarsal conjunctiva. Lesions may also develop in the periodontal tissue in the mouth, upper and lower respiratory tract, middle ear, and cervix. The condition may be associated with congenital occlusive hydrocephalus or juvenile colloid milium in sun-exposed areas. The disease may be triggered by relatively minor trauma or fever.

Pathogenesis

Ligneous conjunctivitis is an ocular manifestation of a systemic disorder, most frequently a homozygous or compound heterozygous mutation causing type I plasminogen deficiency transmitted as an autosomal recessive trait on chromosome 6. Markedly reduced extracellular fibrinolysis results in healing arrested at the stage of granulation tissue formation.

Clinical features

1. **Presentation** may be at any age, but more frequently in childhood.

2. **Signs**

- Gradual onset of a deep-red conjunctival mass (Figs 3.123 and 3.124).

- The lesions may be covered by a yellow–white thick mucoid discharge (Fig. 3.125).

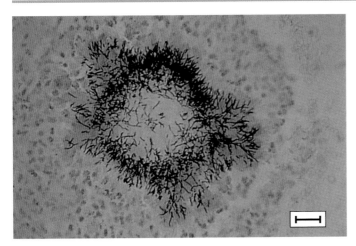

Fig. 3.126 A Gram stain of pus showing branching Gram-positive *Actinomyces israelii* (Courtesy of Hart and Shears, from *Color Atlas of Medical Microbiology*, Mosby, 2004)

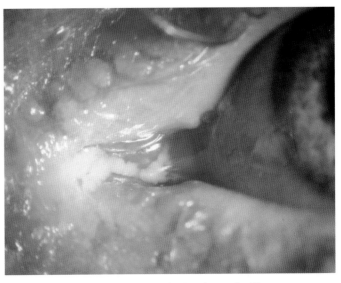

Fig. 3.127 Mucopurulent discharge in chronic canaliculitis

* Subepithelial deposits of hyaline-like material consisting predominantly of fibrin and granulation tissue.

* Corneal scarring, vascularisation, infection or melting may occur.

Treatment

1. **Surgical** removal with meticulous diathermy of the base of the lesion. Simple surgical removal without supplementary therapy results in rapid recurrences in the majority of cases.

2. **Topical**

* Following removal, immediate hourly heparin (5000 U/ml) and prednisolone 1% until the wound has re-epithelialised.

* Subsequently, heparin (1000 U/ml), which is tapered until all signs of inflammation have resolved.

* Regrowth requires long-term ciclosporin 2% and steroids.

3. **Other** modalities include:

* Intravenous or topical plasminogen (1 mg/ml) prepared from fresh frozen plasma.

* Oestrogenic contraceptive pill in women to increase residual plasminogen activity.

* Amniotic membrane transplantation to the conjunctiva after removal of the lesion.

* Prophylactic heparin treatment should be used prior to any subsequent ocular surgery.

Differential diagnosis

Other causes of conjunctival granulomas include foreign bodies, amyloid deposits, cat-scratch disease, ophthalmia nodosum, tuberculosis and Kimura disease.

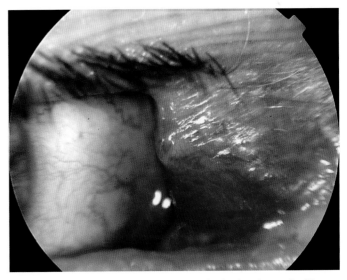

Fig. 3.128 Oedema of the superior canaliculus in chronic canaliculitis

Chronic canaliculitis

Chronic canaliculitis is an uncommon condition, frequently caused by *Actinomyces israelii*, which are anaerobic Gram-positive bacteria (Fig. 3.126). In most cases, there is no identifiable predisposition.

Diagnosis

1. **Presentation** is with unilateral epiphora associated with chronic mucopurulent discharge (Fig. 3.127), refractory to conventional treatment.

2. **Signs**

* Pericanalicular inflammation characterised by oedema of the canaliculus (Fig. 3.128).

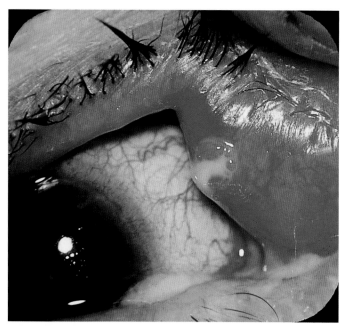

Fig. 3.129 Mucopurulent discharge on pressure over the canaliculus

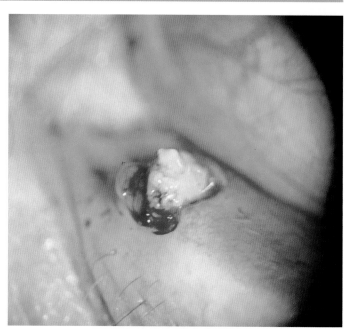

Fig. 3.131 Expressed sulphur granules in chronic canaliculitis

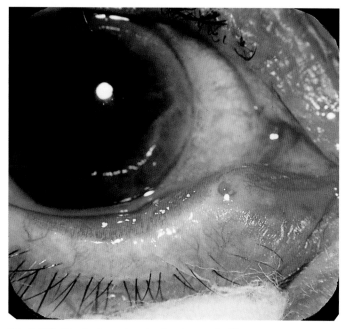

Fig. 3.130 'Pouting' punctum in chronic canaliculitis

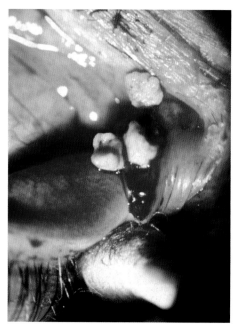

Fig. 3.132 Sulphur granules following canaliculotomy

- Mucopurulent discharge on pressure over the canaliculus (Fig. 3.129).

- A 'pouting' punctum is a diagnostic clue in mild cases (Fig. 3.130).

- Concretions consisting of sulphur granules may either be expressed on canalicular compression with a glass rod (Fig. 3.131) or become evident following canaliculotomy (Fig. 3.132).

NB: In contrast to dacryocystitis, there is no nasolacrimal duct obstruction, lacrimal sac distension or inflammation.

Treatment

1. **Topical antibiotics** such as ciprofloxacin q.i.d for 10 days may be tried initially, but are rarely curative.

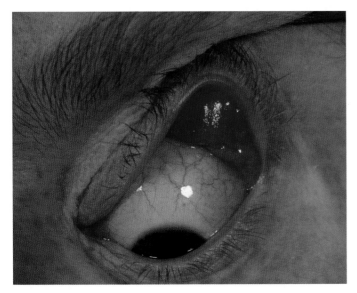

Fig. 3.133 Floppy eyelid syndrome with micropapillary conjunctivitis of the tarsal conjunctiva

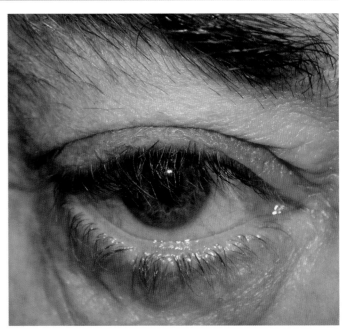

Fig. 3.134 Lash ptosis in floppy eyelid syndrome

2. Canaliculotomy (see Fig. 3.132) involving a linear incision into the conjunctival side of the canaliculus is the most effective treatment, although occasionally it may result in scarring and interference with canalicular function.

Differential diagnosis

1. **The 'giant fornix syndrome'** may also be a cause of chronic relapsing purulent conjunctivitis. This is due to retained debris in the upper fornix that is colonised by *Staph. aureus*, usually in elderly patients with levator disinsertion. Secondary corneal vascularisation is common. Treatment is with topical and systemic antibiotic.

2. **Other conditions** that may cause similar symptoms are a lacrimal diverticulum and a lacrimal stone.

Floppy eyelid syndrome

The floppy eyelid syndrome is an uncommon, unilateral or bilateral condition, which is frequently misdiagnosed. It typically affects very obese individuals who may also suffer from sleep apnoea. It is caused by eversion of the upper lid during sleep, allowing the tarsal conjunctiva to rub on the pillow. Mental retardation and keratoconus are reported associations.

Diagnosis

- Rubbery and loose upper eyelids which readily evert with gentle pressure on the skin below the brow (Fig. 3.133).

- Associated lash ptosis (Fig. 3.134) and lacrimal gland prolapse are common.

- Intense micropapillary conjunctivitis of the superior tarsal conjunctiva (see Fig. 3.133).

- Punctate keratopathy, filamentary keratitis or superior superficial neovascularisation may be present.

Treatment

- Mild cases may respond to nocturnal eye shields or taping of the lids.

- Severe cases require horizontal full-thickness upper lid shortening.

> **NB:** Treatment of sleep apnoea may relieve symptoms.

Parinaud oculoglandular syndrome

Parinaud oculoglandular syndrome is a rare condition characterised by chronic fever, unilateral granulomatous conjunctivitis with surrounding follicles (Fig. 3.135), and ipsilateral regional lymphadenopathy. It is virtually synonymous with cat-scratch disease (see Ch. 8) although several other agents have been associated, including tularemia, sporotrichosis, tuberculosis and acute *C. trachomatis* infection.

Kawasaki disease

Kawasaki disease (mucocutaneous lymph node syndrome) is an idiopathic paediatric vasculitis. It is the most common cause of acquired heart disease in children.

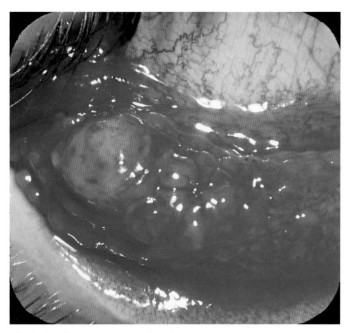

Fig. 3.135 Granulomatous conjunctivitis in Parinaud syndrome

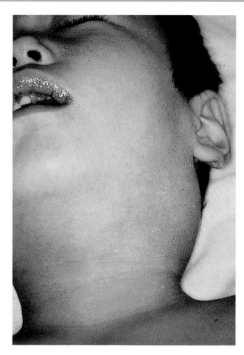

Fig. 3.137 Cervical lymphadenopathy in Kawasaki disease (Courtesy of Emond, Welsby and Rowland, from *Colour Atlas of Infectious Diseases*, Mosby, 2003)

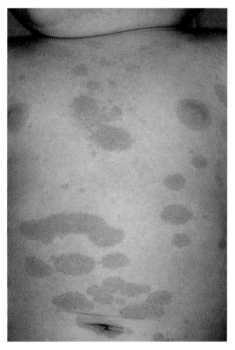

Fig. 3.136 Rash in Kawasaki disease (Courtesy of Emond, Welsby and Rowland, from *Colour Atlas of Infectious Diseases*, Mosby, 2003)

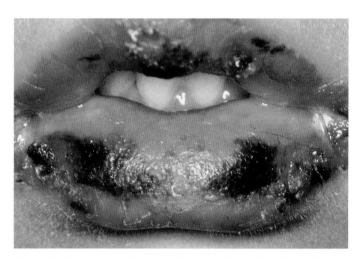

Fig. 3.138 Involvement of the lips in Kawasaki disease (Courtesy of Emond, Welsby and Rowland, from *Colour Atlas of Infectious Diseases*, Mosby, 2003)

Diagnosis

The diagnosis is made by the presence of fever over 5 days in association with at least four of the following:

* Bulbar conjunctival injection.

* Polymorphous rash (Fig. 3.136).

* Cervical lymphadenopathy (Fig. 3.137).

* Involvement of the lips (Fig. 3.138) and oral mucosa.

* Erythema and oedema of the extremities (Fig. 3.139) followed by periungual desquamation.

* Other features include extreme irritability and inflammation of a recent BCG scar.

Treatment

Treatment involves immunoglobulin and aspirin.

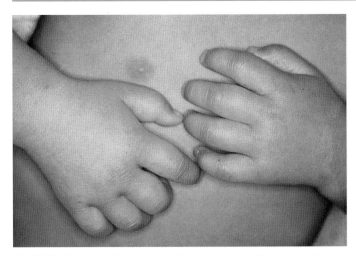

Fig. 3.139 Oedema of the hands in Kawasaki disease (Courtesy of Emond, Welsby and Rowland, from *Colour Atlas of Infectious Diseases*, Mosby, 2003)

FURTHER READING

Culbertson WW, Tseng SC. Corneal disorders in floppy eyelid syndrome. *Cornea* 1994;13:33–42.

De Cock R, Ficker LA, Dart JK, et al. Topical heparin in treatment of ligneous conjunctivitis. *Ophthalmology* 1995;102:1654–1659.

Harnden A, Alves B, Sheikh A. Rising incidence of Kawasaki disease in England: analysis of hospital admission data. *BMJ* 2002;324:1424–1425.

Moon DS, Goldbaum D, Fleischhauer J, et al. Eyelid, conjunctival, and corneal findings in sleep apnea syndrome. *Ophthalmology* 1999;106:1182–1185.

Nelson JD. Superior limbic keratoconjunctivitis (SLK). *Eye* 1989;3:1:80–89.

Perry HD, Doshi-Carnevale S, Donnenfeld ED, et al. Topical cyclosporine A 0.5% as a possible new treatment for superior limbic keratoconjunctivitis. *Ophthalmology* 2003;110:1578–1581.

Rose GE. The giant fornix syndrome. *Ophthalmology* 2004;111:1539–1545.

Rubin BI, Holland EJ, de Smet MD, et al. Response of reactivated ligneous conjunctivitis to topical cyclosporine. *Am J Ophthalmol* 1991;112:95–96.

Schuster V, Seregard S. Ligneous conjunctivitis. *Surv Ophthalmol* 2003;48:369–388.

Vecsei VP, Huber-Spitzy V, Arocker-Mettinger E, et al. Canaliculitis: difficulties in diagnosis, differential diagnosis and comparison between conservative and surgical treatment. *Ophthalmologica* 1994;208:314–317.

Watts P, Suresh P, Mezer E, et al. Effective treatment of ligneous conjunctivitis with topical plasminogen. *Am J Ophthalmol* 2002;133:451–455.

Yang H-Y, Fujishima H, Toda I, et al. Lacrimal punctal occlusion for the treatment of superior limbic keratoconjunctivitis. *Am J Ophthalmol* 1997;124:87.

Yokoi N, Komuro A, Maruyama K, et al. New surgical treatment for superior limbic keratoconjunctivitis and its association with conjunctivochalasis. *Am J Ophthalmol* 2003;135:303–308.

Chapter 4

Keratitis

INTRODUCTION

Anatomy

The average corneal diameter is 11.5 mm (vertical) and 12 mm (horizontal). The cornea consists of the following layers (Fig. 4.1):

1. **The epithelium** is stratified, squamous and non-keratinised, and comprises:

• A single layer of basal columnar cells attached by hemidesmosomes to the underlying basement membrane.

• Two to three rows of wing cells.

• Two layers of squamous surface cells.

• The surface area of the outermost cells is increased by microplicae and microvilli that facilitate the attachment of mucin and the tear film. After a lifespan of a few days, the superficial cells are shed into the tear film.

• The epithelial stem cells are principally located at the superior and inferior limbus, possibly in the palisades of Vogt, and are indispensable for the maintenance of healthy corneal epithelium. They also act as a junctional barrier,

preventing conjunctival tissue from growing onto the cornea.

> **NB:** Dysfunction or deficiency of limbal stem cells may result in chronic epithelial defects, overgrowth of conjunctival epithelium onto the corneal surface and vascularisation. Some of these problems may be treated by limbal cell transplantation.

2. **Bowman layer** is the acellular superficial layer of the stroma.

3. **The stroma** makes up 90% of corneal thickness. It is principally composed of regularly orientated layers of

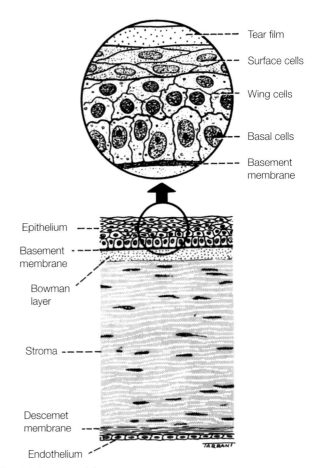

Tear film

Surface cells

Wing cells

Basal cells

Basement membrane

Epithelium

Basement membrane

Bowman layer

Stroma

Descemet membrane

Endothelium

TARRANT

Fig. 4.1 Anatomy of the cornea

collagen fibrils whose spacing is maintained by pro-teoglycan ground substance (chondroitin sulphate and keratan sulphate) with interspersed modified fibroblasts (keratocytes).

4. **Descemet membrane** is composed of a fine latticework of collagen fibrils. It consists of an anterior banded zone that is deposited in utero and a posterior non-banded zone laid down throughout life by the endothelium.

5. **The endothelium** consists of a single layer of hexagonal cells. It plays a vital role in maintaining corneal deturgescence. The cells cannot regenerate and they are arrested in the G1 phase of the cell cycle. The adult cell density is about 2500 cells/mm^2. The number of cells decreases at about 0.6% per year and neighbouring cells enlarge to fill the space as cells die. At a cell density of about 500 cells/mm^2, corneal oedema develops and corneal transparency is reduced.

Dendritic cells are bone marrow-derived antigen-presenting cells that are present in the peripheral corneal epithelium and anterior stroma. Small numbers of macrophages are also present in the posterior stroma. Dendritic cells are part of the immune defence mechanism and are thought to be essential for stimulation of corneal allograft rejection.

> **NB:** The cornea is the most densely innervated tissue in the body. The sensory supply is via the first division of the trigeminal nerve. There is a subepithelial and a stromal plexus of nerves. In eyes with corneal abrasions or bullous keratopathy, the direct stimulation of nerve endings causes pain, reflex lacrimation and photophobia.

Clinical evaluation

1. **A history** of corneal injury, childhood conjunctivitis or recent contact lens wear should be determined. The nature and timing of symptoms may provide important clues. It is important to systematically examine the patient for conditions that can predispose to corneal disease.

- The facial skin may have changes associated with corneal disease (e.g. eczema, rosacea, acne, seborrhoeic dermatitis).

- Joint, nose or ear deformities may be present in patients with autoimmune disease.

2. **Slit-lamp examination** should include the lids, conjunctiva and cornea.

- The lids should be examined for blepharitis, malposition, lagophthalmos and trichiasis.

- The conjunctiva should be examined for signs of papillary or follicular conjunctivitis, epithelial defect, scarring, shrinkage and discharge. The upper lid should be everted and double everted if necessary with a Desmarres retrac-

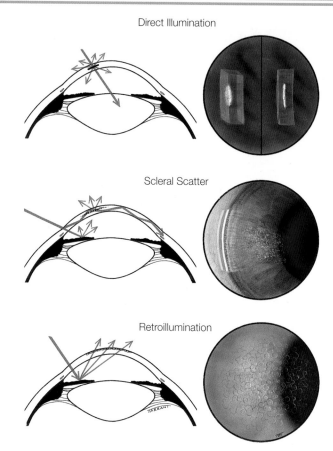

Direct Illumination

Scleral Scatter

Retroillumination

Fig. 4.2 Technique of slit-lamp biomicroscopy

tor. Limbitis is often associated with active corneal disease.

- The episcleritis and scleritis may be present with severe infection or autoimmune disease.

3. **The purpose** of slit-lamp examination of the cornea is to determine the position, depth and size of any abnormalities (Fig. 4.2).

- Direct illumination with diffuse light is used to detect gross abnormalities.

- A narrow, obliquely directed slit beam is used to visualise a cross-section of the cornea.

- Further narrowing of the beam to a very thin optical section that is moved across the cornea can determine the depth of a lesion.

- The height of the coaxial beam can be adjusted to measure the horizontal and vertical size of a lesion or associated epithelial defect.

- The use of a red-free filter makes red objects appear black, thereby increasing contrast when observing vascular structures or rose bengal staining. A cobalt blue filter is normally used in conjunction with fluorescein.

- Scleral scatter involves decentring the slit beam laterally so that the light is incident on the limbus with the micro-

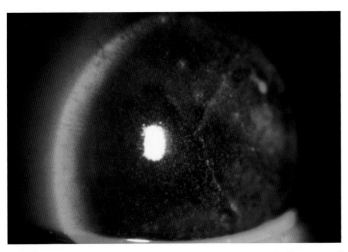

Fig. 4.3 Punctate epithelial erosions stained with fluorescein (Courtesy of A Bacon)

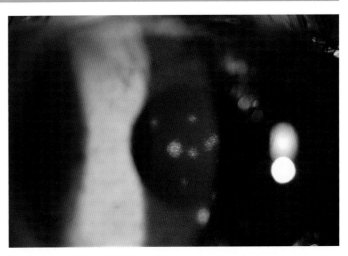

Fig. 4.4 Punctate epithelial keratitis

scope focused centrally. Light is then transmitted within the cornea by total internal reflection. A corneal stromal lesion will become illuminated because of forward light scatters. This technique is especially useful to detect subtle stromal haze, and cellular or lipid infiltration.

- Retroillumination uses reflected light from the iris or fundus after pupil dilation to illuminate the cornea. This allows the detection of fine epithelial and endothelial changes, cystic changes in the epithelium, keratic precipitates and small blood vessels.

- Specular reflection will show abnormalities of the endothelium such as reduced cell density and guttata. Pseudoguttata (dark events) probably represent endothelial cell oedema and inflammatory cells beneath the endothelial cell layer.

Signs of corneal inflammation

> **NB:** Because definitions vary between clinicians, it is recommended that signs are described or drawn wherever possible.

Superficial lesions

1. **Punctate epithelial erosions (PEE)** are tiny, epithelial defects that stain with fluorescein (Fig. 4.3) and with rose bengal. The lesions are non-specific and may develop in response to a wide variety of stimuli. Location may frequently indicate aetiology, for example:

- Superior in vernal disease, superior limbic keratoconjunctivitis, floppy eyelids and poorly fitting contact lenses.

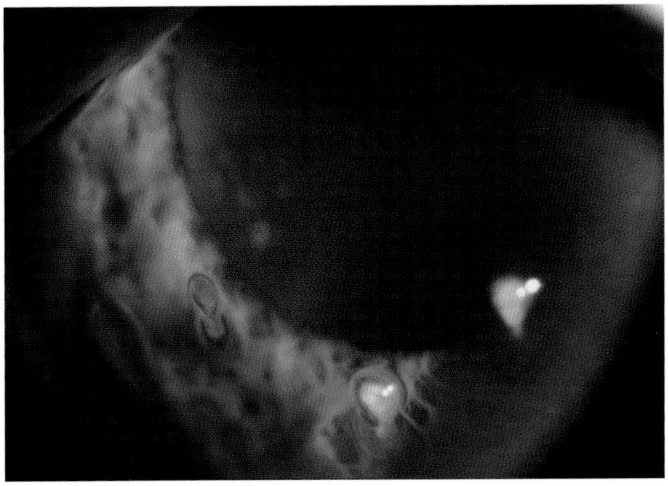

Fig. 4.5 Unstained corneal filaments

- Interpalpebral in dry eyes, reduced corneal sensation and exposure to ultraviolet light.

- Inferior in blepharitis, lagophthalmos, toxicity from drops and self-induced.

2. **Punctate epithelial keratitis (PEK)** is characterised by granular, opalescent, swollen epithelial cells, visible unstained (Fig. 4.4), which stain well with rose bengal but poorly with fluorescein. They are most commonly seen with adenoviral infection, but also develop with chlamydial infections, Thygeson superficial punctate keratitis and staphylococcal hypersensitivity.

3. **Mucus**

a. Filaments

- These consist of mucus strands lined with epithelium, attached at one end to the corneal surface; the unattached

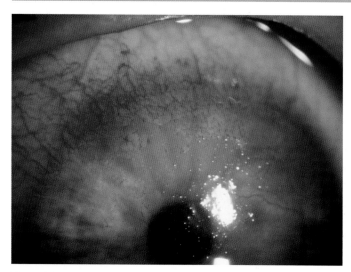

Fig. 4.6 Mucus sheet stained with rose bengal

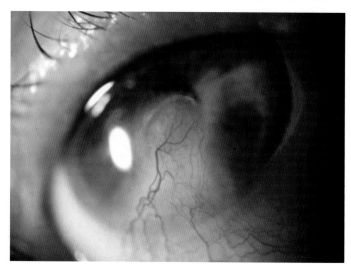

Fig. 4.8 Pannus

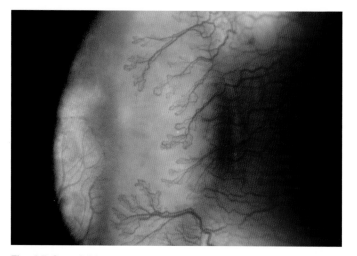

Fig. 4.7 Superficial vascularisation

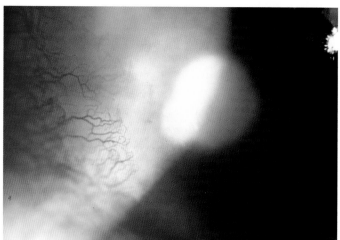

Fig. 4.9 Limbal infiltrate

end moves with each blink. Grey subepithelial opacities may be seen at the site of attachments (Fig. 4.5).

- They stain well with rose bengal but not fluorescein.

- Causes include dry eye, superior limbic keratoconjunctivitis, corneal epithelial instability, neurotrophic keratitis, eye patching and essential blepharospasm.

b. ***Diffuse*** mucus consists of adherent sheets, best detected by rose bengal (Fig. 4.6). It occurs in severe allergic disease and may precede epithelial breakdown (macroerosion).

4. Superficial neovascularisation is a feature of chronic ocular surface irritation (blepharitis, allergic conjunctivitis) or hypoxia (contact lens wear) (Fig. 4.7).

5. Pannus is a non-specific term that usually is applied to superficial neovascularisation accompanied by degenerative subepithelial change extending centrally from the limbus (Fig. 4.8); it follows chronic surface inflammation.

Stromal lesions

1. Infiltrates are focal areas of active stromal inflammation composed of accumulations of leucocytes and cellular debris.

a. ***Signs***

- Focal, granular, grey–white opacities, usually within the anterior stroma and associated with limbal or conjunctival hyperaemia (Fig. 4.9).

- Surrounding halo of less dense infiltration such that individual inflammatory cells may be discernible.

b. ***Causes***

- Non-infectious 'sterile keratitis' is the result of a hypersensitivity response to antigen. Risk factors include contact lens wear and blepharitis.

- Suppurative keratitis caused by bacteria, viruses, fungi and protozoa.

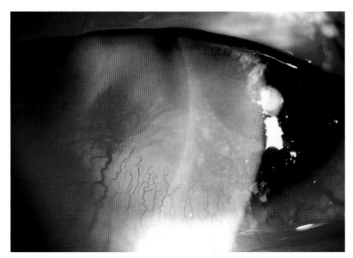

Fig. 4.10 Severe stromal neovascularisation seen on retroillumination

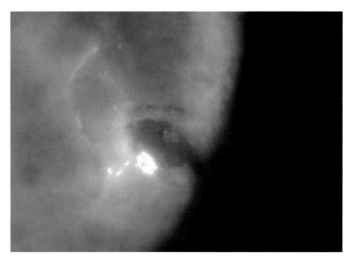

Fig. 4.12 Corneal ulceration

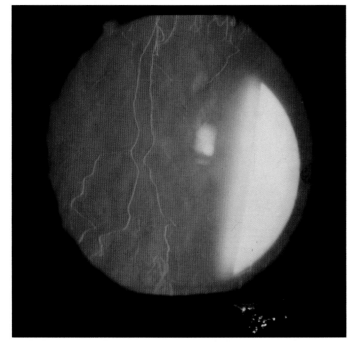

Fig. 4.11 Non-perfused 'ghost vessels' seen on retroillumination

> **NB:** The 'PEDAL' mnemonic is useful in distinguishing non-infectious from suppurative infiltrates. The latter are typically associated with more **P**ain, have larger **E**pithelial defects (>1 mm), have purulent **D**ischarge, are associated with **A**nterior chamber reaction (uveitis, hypopyon), and usually have a more central **L**ocation.

2. **Neovascularisation** (Fig. 4.10) occurs in response to a wide variety of stimuli. The venous blood vessels are easily seen, whereas the arterial feeding vessels are smaller and require high magnification. Non-perfused, deep vessels appear as 'ghost vessels', best detected by retroillumination (Fig. 4.11).

3. **Ulceration** (Fig. 4.12) is due to melting of the connective tissue in response to the release of proteases and matrix metalloproteinases (collagenases, gelatinases and stromolysins). These enzymes may be released from endogenous sources in response to inflammation or from exogenous organisms (bacteria, amoebae and fungi). The mechanisms may overlap, and the primary mechanism may change during the course of disease. The main stimuli are:

- Epithelial disease.

- Infection.

- Immune mechanisms.

> **NB:** Classification of melting disorders into *central* or *peripheral* can be a helpful aid in determining aetiology. In rheumatoid arthritis, a central melt is often the result of dry eye, whereas a peripheral melt is often immune-mediated.

4. **Lipid** deposition follows chronic inflammation with leakage from corneal new vessels (Fig. 4.13).

Documentation of clinical signs

A clinical diagram is useful to document the type and position of each change. The dimensions of epithelial opacities and stromal ulceration, and depth of new vessels and opacities should be recorded. Colour coding can be helpful (Fig. 4.14).

- Opacities such as scars and degenerations are drawn in black.

- Epithelial oedema is represented by fine blue circles, stromal oedema as blue shading, and folds in Descemet membrane as wavy blue lines.

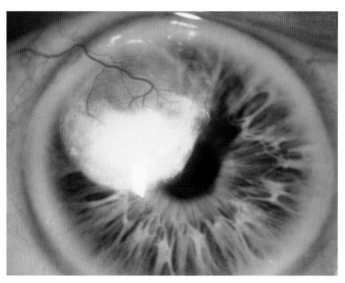

Fig. 4.13 Lipid degeneration

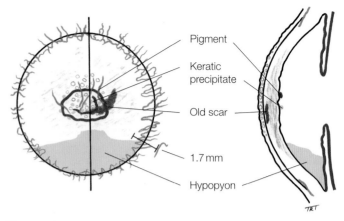

Fig. 4.14 Documentation of corneal lesions

- Hypopyon are shown in yellow.

- Blood vessels are then added in red. Superficial vessels are wavy lines that begin outside the limbus, and deep vessels are straight lines that begin at the limbus.

- Pigment such as iron rings and Krukenberg spindle are shown in brown.

Principles of treatment

The aim is to stop the disease process, eliminate any infectious agent, and limit associated corneal damage.

> **NB:** Have a working diagnosis on which to base treatment. Try to avoid unguided intervention and be prepared to modify the diagnosis.

Control of infection and inflammation

1. **Antimicrobial agents** should be started as soon as preliminary investigations have been completed. The initial choice of agent is determined by the likely aetiology, which is determined by the clinical examination (presumed bacterial, acanthamoebic, or fungal infection). Broad-spectrum treatment is used initially, with more selective agents introduced if necessary when the results of investigation are available.

2. **Topical steroids** should be used with caution because they may promote microbial growth and suppress corneal repair. They are contraindicated in active herpes simplex epithelial disease without effective antiviral cover.

3. **Systemic immunosuppressive agents** may be useful in certain forms of severe corneal ulceration and melting associated with systemic connective tissue disorders.

Promotion of re-epithelialisation

In eyes with a thin stroma, it is important to promote re-epithelialisation because thinning seldom progresses if the epithelium is intact. The following are the main methods of promoting re-epithelialisation:

1. **Reduction of exposure** to toxic medications and preservatives wherever possible.

2. **Lubrication** with unpreserved artificial tears and ointments.

3. **Eyelid closure** is particularly useful in exposure and neurotrophic keratopathies as well as in eyes with persistent epithelial defects. It can be achieved by one of the following methods:

- Taping the lids closed temporarily.

- Botulinum toxin injection into the levator muscle to induce a temporary ptosis.

- Lateral tarsorrhaphy (Fig. 4.15) or median canthoplasty.

4. **Bandage soft contact lenses** (Fig. 4.16) promote healing by mechanically protecting regenerating corneal epithelium from the constant rubbing of the eyelids.

5. **Amniotic membrane grafting** (Fig. 4.17) may be necessary for persistent unresponsive epithelial defects.

Other Measures

1. **Tissue adhesive** (cyanoacrylate) glue may be used to limit stromal ulceration and to seal small perforations. It is first applied onto a plastic patch, which is then applied to the area of thinning or perforation and a bandage contact lens inserted (Fig. 4.18).

2. **A conjunctival (Gundersen) flap** will cover the corneal ulceration is progressive and unresponsive (Fig. 4.19). This procedure is particularly suitable for chronic uni-

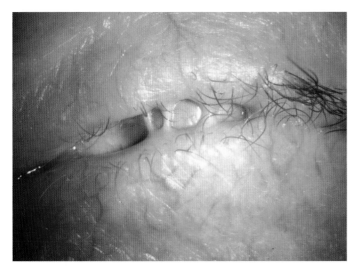

Fig. 4.15 Tarsorrhaphy

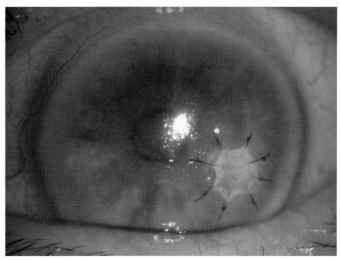

Fig. 4.17 Amniotic membrane graft over a persistent epithelial defect

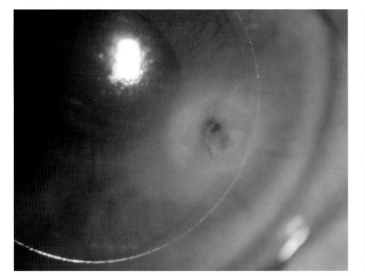

Fig. 4.16 Bandage contact lens in an eye with a small perforation

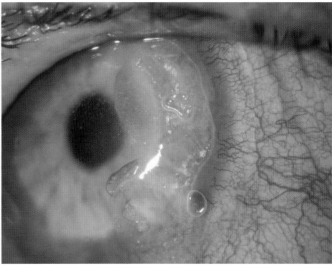

Fig. 4.18 Tissue glue under a bandage contact lens in an eye with severe peripheral thinning

lateral disease in which the prognosis for restoration of useful vision is poor.

3. **Limbal stem cell transplantation** may be required if there is stem cell deficiency following a variety of injuries such as chemical burns or cicatrising conjunctivitis. The source of the donor tissue may be the fellow eye (autograft) in unilateral disease or from a living or cadaver donor (allograft) when both eyes are affected.

4. **Keratoplasty** may be required to restore corneal transparency.

SUPPURATIVE BACTERIAL KERATITIS

Suppurative keratitis describes severe infection of the cornea characterised by an epithelial defect, infiltration, and other signs of inflammation. It is most frequently the result of bacterial or fungal infection, and less commonly viral or amoebic infection. However, there is wide geographic variation in the relative importance of different causes. In temperate areas, bacterial infection accounts for more than 95% of cases of suppurative keratitis, while in tropical regions, filamentary fungal infection can account for 50% of cases. Complications include corneal perforation, scleritis and endophthalmitis. Worldwide, suppurative keratitis accounts for 1.5 million new cases of unilateral blindness each year.

Pathogenesis

Pathogens

Bacterial keratitis is very uncommon in a normal eye and usually only develops when the ocular defences have been

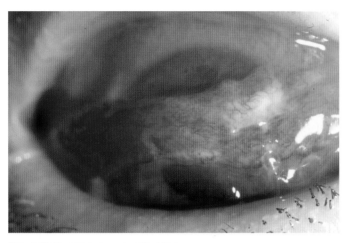

Fig. 4.19 Gundersen conjunctival flap

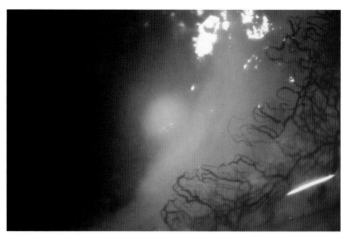

Fig. 4.20 Early bacterial keratitis

compromised. *N. gonorrhoeae, N. meningitides, C. diphtheriae* and *H. influenzae* can penetrate the apparently normal corneal epithelium. The virulence of the organism and the anatomic site of the infection determine the pattern of disease. The most common pathogens are:

1. ***P. aeruginosa***, which is a ubiquitous Gram-negative bacillus (rod) that flourishes in soil, vegetation and moist situations in the hospital environment. It is also a commensal of the gastrointestinal tract.

2. ***Staph. aureus***, which is a common Gram-positive and coagulase-positive commensal of the nares, skin and conjunctiva.

3. ***Strep. pyogenes***, which is a common Gram-positive commensal of the throat and vagina.

4. ***Strep. pneumoniae*** (pneumococcus), which is a Gram-positive commensal of the upper respiratory tract.

The relative contribution of various pathogens is dependent on region and local risk factors. Some bacteria that are considered normal flora of the ocular surface can become pathogens in the cornea (e.g. *Staph. epidermidis*, corynebacteria).

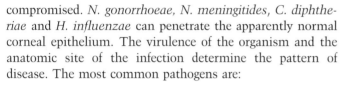

NB: Infection with *Pseudomonas* species and streptococci are often very aggressive.

Risk factors

1. **Contact lens wear**, particularly of soft lenses worn overnight, is the greatest risk factor for bacterial keratitis in developed countries. *Pseudomonas* species account for over 60% of cases. Infection is more likely if there is poor lens hygiene but it can also occur even if there is apparently meticulous lens care and with daily disposable lenses. The eye is exposed to high numbers of bacteria that can multiply in the contact lens case where they are protected from disinfection by bacterial biofilm. The corneal epithelium is also damaged by hypoxia and trauma and is then susceptible to infection. A diagnosis of bacterial keratitis must be considered in any contact lens user with an acutely painful red eye.

2. **Trauma** such as accidental injury, surgical (refractive surgery) and loose sutures. In developing countries, agricultural injury is the major risk factor for developing corneal infection.

3. **Ocular surface disease** such as herpes simplex keratitis, bullous keratopathy, dry eye, blepharitis, trichiasis, exposure, severe allergic eye disease and corneal anaesthesia. Ventilated patients are at risk of pseudomonal ulcers.

4. **Other factors** include topical or systemic immunosuppression, diabetes, vitamin A deficiency and measles.

Clinical features

1. **History**, with particular attention paid to the risk factors mentioned above.

2. **Presentation** is with pain, redness, photophobia, blurred vision, and discharge.

3. **Signs**, in chronological order:

- An epithelial defect associated with an infiltrate around the margin and base (Fig. 4.20) associated with circumcorneal injection.

- Enlargement of the infiltrate associated with stromal oedema and small hypopyon (Fig. 4.21).

- Severe infiltration with enlarging hypopyon (Fig. 4.22).

- Progressive ulceration may lead to corneal perforation, endophthalmitis (Fig. 4.23) and loss of the eye.

- Scleritis may develop with infections at the limbus.

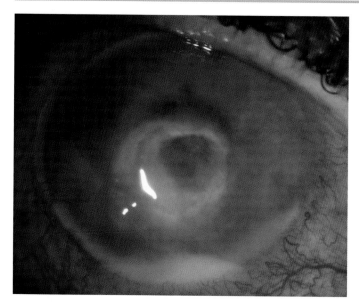

Fig. 4.21 More advanced bacterial keratitis with a small hypopyon

Table 4.1 Comparison between marginal and bacterial keratitis

	Marginal keratitis	Bacterial keratitis
Location	Peripheral	Central
Size	<1 mm	>1 mm
Epithelial defect	Small or absent	Present
Uveitis	Absent	Present

NB: If the cornea is opaque, an ultrasound scan should be performed to exclude endophthalmitis.

4. **Differential diagnosis** includes fungal keratitis, acanthamoeba keratitis, necrotic stromal herpes simplex keratitis, marginal keratitis (Table 4.1) and sterile inflammatory corneal infiltrates associated with contact lens wear.

Investigations

Microbiology

NB: Techniques and preferred culture media vary according to centres; liaison with the microbiologist is essential.

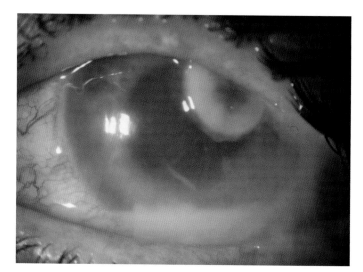

Fig. 4.22 Severe bacterial keratitis with a larger hypopyon

1. **Taking samples**

- A non-preserved topical anaesthetic is instilled.

- At the slit lamp, any loose mucus is wiped away from the surface of the ulcer.

- The margins and base of the lesion are scraped with either a heat-sterilised (Kimura) spatula, a blade, or the bent tip of a 21-gauge hypodermic needle.

- A thin smear is placed on a glass slide for Gram stain and microscopy.

NB: Do not use transport media, because the sample volume is typically tiny and isolation is unlikely.

2. **Gram staining**

- Differentiates bacterial species into 'Gram-positive' and 'Gram-negative' based on the ability of the dye (crystal violet) to penetrate the cell wall.

- Bacteria that take up crystal violet are Gram-positive (Fig. 4.24) and those that allow the dye to wash off are Gram-negative.

3. **Culture media.** The samples are plated onto selected media, taking care not to break the surface of the agar, and placed into an incubator until they are transferred to the laboratory.

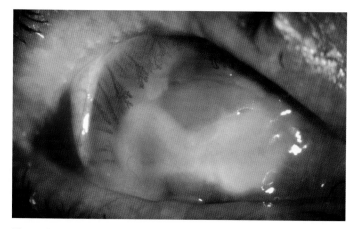

Fig. 4.23 Endophthalmitis secondary to bacterial keratitis (Courtesy of P Gilli)

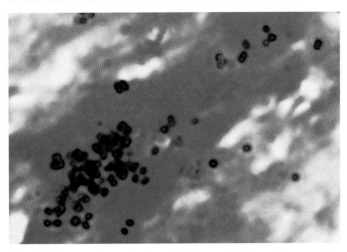

Fig. 4.24 Smear of pus showing staphylococci which are Gram-positive spherical cocci mostly arranged in clusters (Courtesy of Emond, Welsby and Rowland, from *Colour Atlas of Infectious Diseases*, Mosby, 2003)

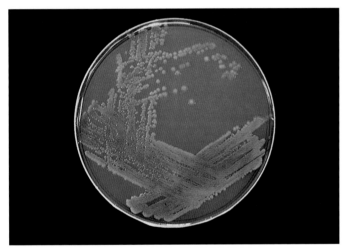

Fig. 4.25 *Staph. aureus* grown on blood agar, forming golden colonies with a shiny surface (Courtesy of Emond, Welsby and Rowland, from *Colour Atlas of Infectious Diseases*, Mosby, 2003)

- Blood agar (Fig. 4.25) is suitable for most bacteria and fungi except *Neisseria*, *Haemophilus* and *Moraxella* sp.

- Chocolate agar is used to isolate *Neisseria*, *Haemophilus* and *Moraxella* sp.

- Cooked meat broth for anaerobic and fastidious organisms.

- Brain heart infusion.

- For unresponsive ulcers, treatment should be stopped for 24 hours before rescraping the ulcer. Additional examinations should then include Ziehl–Nielson stain and Lowenstein–Jensen medium.

4. **Sensitivity report.** The plates should be transported to the laboratory as soon as possible, to increase the chances of isolating the offending organism. Generally, reports are

sent out at 1 or 2 days, 7 days and 2 weeks. When determining drug sensitivity for an isolated organism, the results are reported as:

- Susceptible: the organism is sensitive to the normal dose of the antimicrobial agent.

- Intermediate: the organism is likely to be sensitive to a high dose of the antimicrobial agent.

- Resistant: the organism is not sensitive to the antimicrobial agent at the tested dose.

NB: Most laboratories report sensitivity using a disc diffusion (Kirby–Bauer) method. The relevance of these results to topical antibiotics that can achieve a very high tissue level is uncertain.

Other investigations

1. **Polymerase chain reaction (PCR) techniques** are being developed but are not clinically available. They are so sensitive that it can be difficult to distinguish the signal of pathogen from contaminants or commensals.

2. **Corneal biopsy** should be considered for progressive keratitis suggestive of infection that is culture-negative. At the slit lamp or microscope, a 2 mm piece of tissue is removed from the margin of the ulcer by sharp dissection. The sample is bisected and half sent for histology (formaldehyde saline) and half sent in normal saline for homogenisation and culture.

Treatment

Bacterial keratitis has the potential to progress rapidly to corneal perforation. Even small axial lesions can cause surface irregularity and scar that can lead to significant loss of vision.

General principles

- The decision to treat is based on clinical grounds.

- Although the majority of ulcers will heal with empiric antibiotic treatment, cultures are recommended. The causative organism cannot be guessed reliably from the appearance of the ulcer.

- Treatment should be initiated even if Gram stain is negative and before the results of culture are available. The principle of treatment of bacterial keratitis is to achieve medical cure whilst minimising tissue destruction. Visual rehabilitation is performed after the inflammation and infection have been controlled.

- Topical application of antibiotics can achieve high tissue concentration and is the preferred route of administration. Initial treatment should be with broad-spectrum antibiotics to cover the most common causes of infection.

- Dual therapy involves a combination of two fortified antibiotics, typically an aminoglycoside and a cephalosporin, to cover common Gram-positive and Gram-negative pathogens. Fortified antibiotics are not commercially available and are not licensed for this form of administration. Dual therapy is associated with greater discomfort and toxicity.

- Monotherapy with a fluoroquinolone (i.e. ciprofloxacin 0.3% or ofloxacin 0.3%) is commercially available. Although they contain preservatives, toxicity is uncommon. Ciprofloxacin may be associated with white corneal precipitates, which may delay epithelial healing.

NB: Increasing resistance to fluoroquinolones has been reported (*Staphylococcus* sp. in the USA, and *Pseudomonas* sp. in India). A new generation of fluoroquinolones (e.g. moxifloxacin) has been introduced to address this. MRSA is an uncommon cause of bacterial keratitis and can usually be treated with vancomycin.

Preparation of fortified antibiotics

A standard parenteral or lyophilised antibiotic preparation is combined with a compatible vehicle such that the antibiotic does not precipitate.

1. **Gentamicin** 15 mg/ml (1.5%): 2 ml parenteral antibiotic (40 mg/ml) is added to 5 ml commercially available antibiotic ophthalmic solution (0.3%).

2. **Cefazolin, cefuroxime or ceftazidime** 50 mg/ml (5%): 500 mg parenteral antibiotic is diluted with 2.5 ml sterile water and added to 7.5 ml of preservative-free artificial tears. This is stable for 24 hours at room temperature or 96 hours if kept in a refrigerator.

NB: Potential problems with fortified antibiotics include cost, limited availability, possibly decreased sterility, short shelf-life and need for refrigeration.

Treatment regimen

1. **Topical antibiotics** are initially instilled at hourly intervals, day and night, for 24–48 hours. The frequency can be reduced to 2-hourly during waking hours for a further 48 hours, and then q.i.d. for 1 week. Treatment is continued until the epithelium has healed.

NB: It is important not to confuse failure of re-epithelialisation (persistent epithelial defect), resulting from toxicity, with continued infection.

Table 4.2 Antibiotics for treatment of keratitis

Isolate	Antibiotic	Concentration
Empiric treatment	Cefuroxime	5%
	+	
	Gentamicin	1.4%
	or	
	Fluoroquinolone	0.3%
Gram-positive cocci MRSA	Cefuroxime	0.3%
	Vancomycin	
	or	
	Teicoplanin	
Gram-negative rods	Gentamicin	1.4%
	or	
	Fluoroquinolone	0.3%
	or	
	Ceftazidime	5%
Gram-negative cocci	Fluoroquinolone	0.3%
	Ceftriaxone	5%
Mycobacteria	Amikacin	2%
	or	
	Clarithromycin	
Nocardia	Amikacin	2%
	or	
	Trimethorim +	1.6%
	Sulfamethoxazole	8%

2. **Oral antibiotics** (ciprofloxacin 750 mg twice daily for 7–10 days) is not usually necessary. Exceptions are threatened or actual corneal perforation, or a peripheral ulcer in which there is scleral extension. Oral therapy is also indicated for isolates for which there are potential systemic complications (e.g. *N. meningitides*).

3. **Subconjunctival antibiotics** are only indicated if there is poor compliance with topical treatment. Intensive topical treatment and subconjunctival injection achieve similar corneal levels.

4. **When to change antibiotics?**

- The initial regimen should be changed only if a resistant pathogen is isolated and ulceration is progressing.

- There is no need to change initial therapy if this has induced a favourable response, even if cultures show a resistant organism.

3. **Mydriatics** (atropine 1% or cyclopentolate 1%) are used to prevent the formation of posterior synechiae and to reduce pain from ciliary spasm.

4. **Topical steroids** increase the risk of bacterial keratitis when used in eyes with ocular surface disease. If they have been used prior to the onset of keratitis, there is an

increased risk of treatment failure. If infection is uncontrolled, they should be stopped until it has been controlled. The benefit in using topical steroid in established bacterial keratitis is unproven. The following guidelines apply:

- Steroids should not be introduced until the sensitivity of the isolate to antibiotics has been demonstrated and fungal infection excluded.

- Steroids can potentiate coexisting fungal or herpes infection, and may make elimination of acanthamoeba infection more difficult.

- Steroids reduce inflammation and can rapidly make the eye more comfortable. However, their use probably does not affect the amount of scar formation or the final visual outcome.

- Topical steroids may help to prevent rejection following infection of a corneal graft.

Causes of failure

1. **Incorrect diagnosis** caused by inappropriate cultures.

- The most common causes are unrecognised infection with herpes simplex virus (HSV), fungi, acanthamoeba and atypical mycobacteria.

- The cultures should be repeated using special media such as Lowenstein–Jensen (mycobacteria) and non-nutrient agar seeded with *E. coli* (acanthamoeba).

- If cultures are still negative, it may be necessary to perform corneal biopsy for histology and culture, or excisional keratoplasty.

2. **Inappropriate choice of antibiotics.**

3. **Drug toxicity**, particularly following frequent instillation of fortified aminoglycosides, may cause conjunctival necrosis and white corneal precipitates which delay corneal epithelial healing. There may be increasing discomfort, redness and discharge, despite eradication of infection.

4. **Gram-negative ulcers** may show increased inflammation during the first 48 hours, despite appropriate treatment.

Visual rehabilitation

1. **Lamellar keratoplasty** may be required for residual dense corneal scarring.

2. **Rigid contact lenses** may be required for irregular astigmatism, but only 3 months after re-epithelialisation of the ulcer.

3. **Cataract surgery** may be required, because secondary lens opacities are common following severe inflammation.

FURTHER READING

Alexandrakis G, Alfonso EC, Miller D. Shifting trends in bacterial keratitis in South Florida and emerging resistance to fluoroquinolones. *Ophthalmology* 2000;107:1497–1502.

Alexandrakis G, Haimovici R, Miller D, et al. Corneal biopsy in the management of progressive microbial keratitis. *Am J Ophthalmol* 2000;129:571–576.

Buehler PO, Schein OD, Stamler JF, et al. The increased risk of ulcerative keratitis among disposable soft contact lens users. *Arch Ophthalmol* 1992;110:1555–1558.

Carmichael TR, Gelfand Y, Welsh NH. Topical steroids in the treatment of central and paracentral ulcers. *Br J Ophthalmol* 1990;74:528–531.

Cheng KH, Leung SL, Hoekman HW, et al. Incidence of contact-lens-associated microbial keratitis and its related morbidity. *Lancet* 1999;354:181–185.

Dart JKG. Predisposing factors in microbial keratitis: the significance of contact lens wear. *Br J Ophthalmol* 1988;72:926–930.

Garg P, Sharma S, Rao GN. Ciprofloxacin-resistant Pseudomonas keratitis. *Ophthalmology* 1999;106:1319–1323.

Hyndiuk RA, Eiferman RA, Caldwell DR, et al. Comparison of ciprofloxacin ophthalmic solution 0.3% to fortified tobramycin-cefazolin in treating bacterial corneal ulcers. Ciprofloxacin Bacterial Keratitis Study Group. *Ophthalmology* 1996;103:1854–1862.

Matthews TD, Frazer DG, Minassian DC, et al. Risks of keratitis and patterns of use with disposable contact lenses. *Arch Ophthalmol* 1992;110:1559–1562.

Prajna NV, George C, Selvaraj S, et al. Bacteriologic and clinical efficacy of ofloxacin 0.3% versus ciprofloxacin 0.3% ophthalmic solutions in the treatment of patients with culture-positive bacterial keratitis. *Cornea* 2001;20:175–178.

O'Brien TP. Management of bacterial keratitis: beyond exorcism towards consideration of organism and host factors. *Eye* 2003;17:957–974.

O'Brien TP, Maguire MG, Fink NE, et al. Efficacy of ofloxacin vs cefazolin and tobramycin in the therapy for bacterial keratitis. Report from the Bacterial Keratitis Study Research Group. *Arch Ophthalmol* 1995;113:1257–1265.

Ofloxacin Study Group. Ofloxacin monotherapy for the primary treatment of microbial keratitis. A double-masked, randomised, controlled trial with conventional dual therapy. *Ophthalmology* 1997;104:1902–1909.

Rodman RC, Spisak S, Sugar A, et al. The utility of culturing corneal ulcers in a tertiary referral center versus a general ophthalmology clinic. *Ophthalmology* 1997;104:1897–1901.

Schein OD, Buehler PO, Stamler JF, et al. The impact of overnight wear on the risk of contact lens-associated ulcerative keratitis. *Arch Ophthalmol* 1994;112:186–190.

Tuft SJ, Matheson M. In vitro antibiotic resistance in bacterial keratitis in London. *Br J Ophthalmol* 2000;84:687–691.

Van Gelder RN. Applications of the polymerase chain reaction to diagnosis of ophthalmic disease. *Surv Ophthalmol* 2001;46:248–258.

Wilhelmus KR. Indecision about corticosteroids for bacterial keratitis: an evidence-based update. *Ophthalmology* 2002;109:835–842.

FUNGAL KERATITIS

Fungi are micro-organisms that have rigid walls and multiple chromosomes containing DNA and RNA. The main types are: (a) *filamentous* fungi, which are multicellular organisms that produce tubular projections known as hyphae, and (b) *yeasts*, which are ovoid unicellular organisms that reproduce by budding and may occasionally form hyphae or pseudohyphae (Fig. 4.26).

Fungal keratitis is rare in temperate countries but is a major cause of visual loss in tropical and developing countries. In some hot and humid regions, it accounts for 50% of cases, the vast majority due to filamentous infection.

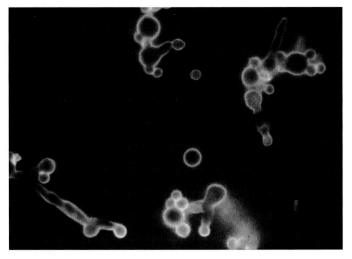

Fig. 4.26 *Candida albicans* showing germ tubes and pseudohyphae

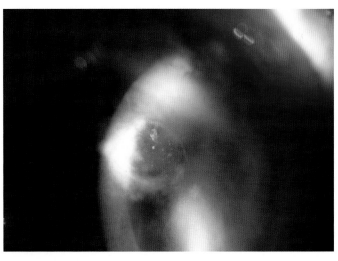

Fig. 4.27 Early filamentous keratitis

Pathogenesis

- The primary risk factors are trauma (65% of cases in tropical areas), particularly with vegetable matter, chronic ocular surface disease and epithelial defects, diabetes, systemic immunosuppression, and hydrophilic contact lenses. Topical steroid use may also be a risk factor for developing disease as well as enhancing fungal growth in established cases. Male agricultural workers in developing countries are at particular risk.

- Fungal infection can elicit a severe inflammatory response that can cause stromal necrosis and melting. Filamentous fungi can penetrate Descemet membrane, and corneal perforation is common. Once in the anterior chamber, the infection is very difficult to eradicate and aggressive surgery is usually required.

- The most common pathogens in tropical climates are filamentous fungi (*Aspergillus* sp., *Fusarium solani* and *Scedosporium* sp.). Yeasts (*Candida* sp.) are responsible for most cases in temperate climates.

Clinical features

The diagnosis is often delayed unless there is a high index of suspicion.

1. **Presentation** is with gradual onset of foreign body sensation, photophobia, blurred vision and discharge. Patients often have a history of trauma or chronic ocular surface disease.

2. **Signs** vary with the infectious agent. In early disease there tends to be less redness and lid swelling than with bacterial infection.

a. Filamentous keratitis

- A grey–yellow stromal infiltrate with indistinct margins (Fig. 4.27).

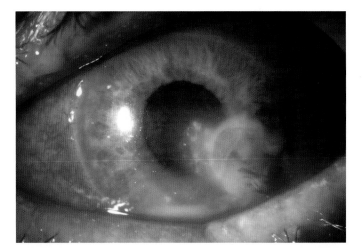

Fig. 4.28 Filamentous keratitis with several small satellite lesions and a small hypopyon

- Progressive infiltration, often surrounded by satellite lesions, and hypopyon (Figs 4.28–4.30).

b. Candida keratitis is characterised by a yellow–white infiltrate associated with dense suppuration (Figs 4.31 and 4.32).

Investigations

Laboratory examination should be performed before starting antifungal therapy. Filamentous fungi tend to proliferate anterior to Descemet membrane and a deep stromal biopsy may be required (similar in technique to performing a trabeculectomy – the excised deep tissue is sent for culture). Sometimes, the diagnosis can only be confirmed following anterior chamber tap or excisional keratoplasty.

1. **Gram and Giemsa** staining are equally sensitive (Fig. 4.33).

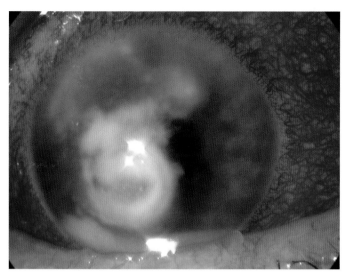

Fig. 4.29 Severe filamentous keratitis with large satellite lesions

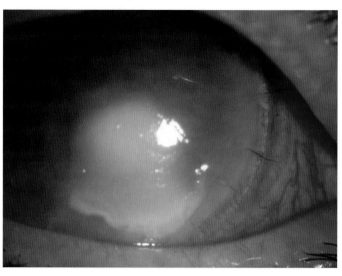

Fig. 4.32 Advanced candida keratitis

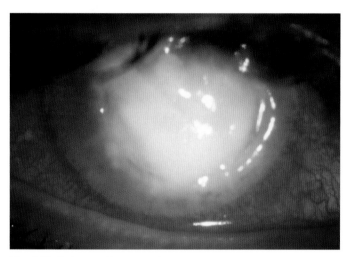

Fig. 4.30 End-stage filamentous keratitis

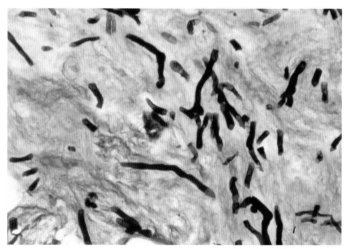

Fig. 4.33 Gram-stained *Candida albicans* showing pseudohyphae (Courtesy of Hart and Shears, from *Colour Atlas of Medical Microbiology*, Mosby, 2004)

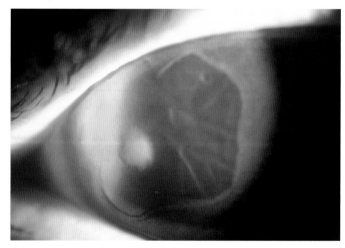

Fig. 4.31 Early candida keratitis

2. **Lactophenol cotton-blue** staining is effective when laboratory resources are limited (Fig. 4.34).

3. **Cultures** should be taken and plated on Sabouraud dextrose agar (Fig. 4.35), although most fungi will also grow on blood agar or in enrichment media at 27°C. Sensitivity testing can be performed in reference laboratories but the relevance of results to clinical effectiveness is uncertain.

4. **Confocal microscopy** can be used to visualise filamentous fungi.

5. **Histology** involving periodic acid–Schiff (PAS) stain and Gemorri/Grocott silver stain of corneal tissue are the most sensitive. Other techniques can be used (e.g. calcofluor white, which requires access to a fluorescent microscope).

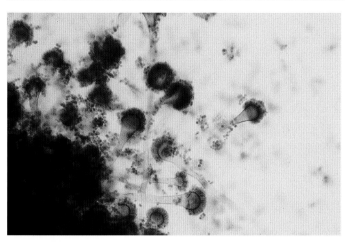

Fig. 4.34 Lactophenol cotton blue-stained preparation of *Aspergillus fumigatus* showing conidiophore and microconidia hyphae (Courtesy of Hart and Shears, from *Colour Atlas of Medical Microbiology*, Mosby, 2004)

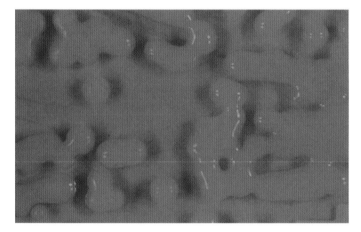

Fig. 4.35 *Candida albicans* growing on Sabouraud dextrose agar (Courtesy of Hart and Shears, from *Colour Atlas of Medical Microbiology*, Mosby, 2004)

Treatment

1. **Removal of the epithelium** over the lesion enhances penetration of antifungal agents. Similarly, a superficial keratectomy may help debulk the lesion.

2. **Topical treatment** should be given initially (hourly for 48 hours, reducing as signs permit). As most antifungals are only fungistatic, treatment should be continued for several weeks.

   a. *Filamentous* infection is treated with natamycin 5% or econazole 1%. Amphotericin B 0.15% and miconazole 1% are alternatives.

   b. *Candida* infection is usually treated with econazole 1%. Natamycin 5%, fluconazole 2%, amphotericin B 0.15% and clotrimazole 1% are alternatives.

NB: A broad-spectrum antibiotic should also be used, as bacterial co-infection is common.

3. **Systemic** antifungals may be required for severe keratitis or endophthalmitis. Preferred treatment options are itraconazole or voriconazole, 100 mg daily with a loading dose of 200 mg. Liver function should be monitored. Systemic amphotericin B, if indicated, has to be given intravenously (0.1 mg/kg). Miconazole and ketaconazole can also be given systemically. Oral fluconazole is effective against yeasts.

4. **Grafting**

   a. *Excisional penetrating keratoplasty* may be required in unresponsive cases. Because fungal filaments can extend beyond the clinical margins of the ulcer, a clear margin of 1 to 2 mm of normal cornea must be excised around the

Table 4.3 Antifungal agents for treatment of keratitis

Group		Topical	Systemic	Activity
Polyenes		Natamycin 5%	Amphotericin B	Filamentous (not Fusarium) and yeasts
		Amphotericin B 0.15%		
Azoles	Imidazole	Miconazole 1%	Miconazole	Filamentous and yeasts
		Clotrimazole 1%		
		Ketaconazole 1%	Ketaconazole	
	Pyrimidine	Flucytosine 1%		
	Triazole	Fluconazole 1%	Fluconazole	Yeasts
		Econazole 1% or 2%	Itraconazole	Filamentous and yeasts
			Voriconazole	
Antiseptics		Chlorhexidine 0.02%		May be effective if antifungals unavailable
		Povidone iodine 5%		
		Silver sulfadiazine 1%		

edges of the ulcer. Even so, recurrence at the margin of the graft develops in about one-third of cases. In the presence of corneal perforation or invasion of the anterior chamber, amphotericin B 0.05 μg in 0.1 ml should be injected intracamerally at the end of the procedure.

b. **Corneoscleral grafts** may be required in extensive corneal involvement, to achieve clearance. Peripheral iridectomy should be performed at the time of surgery, to prevent iris bombe. The iris and lens should be removed if these are involved.

FURTHER READING

Alexandrakis G, Haimovici R, Miller D, et al. Corneal biopsy in the management of progressive microbial keratitis. *Am J Ophthalmol* 2000;129:571–576.

Bharathi MJ, Ramakrishnan R, Vasu S, et al. Epidemiological characteristics and laboratory diagnosis of fungal keratitis: a three-year study. *Indian J Ophthalmol* 2003;51:315–321.

Gopinathan U, Garg P, Fernandes M, et al. The epidemiological features and laboratory results of fungal keratitis: a 10-year review at a referral eye care center in South India. *Cornea* 2002;21:555–559.

Hwang DG. Lamellar flap corneal biopsy. *Ophthalmic Surg* 1993;24:512–515.

Johns KJ, O'Day DM. Pharmacologic management of keratomycosis. *Surv Ophthalmol* 1988;33:178–188.

Leck AK, Thomas PA, Hagan M, et al. Aetiology of suppurative corneal ulcers in Ghana and south India, and epidemiology of fungal keratitis. *Br J Ophthalmol* 2002;86:1211–1215.

Prajna NV, John RK, Nirmalan PK, et al. A randomised clinical trial comparing 2% econazole and 5% natamycin for the treatment of fungal keratitis. *Br J Ophthalmol* 2003;87:1235–1237.

Rehman MR, Johnson GJ, Husain R, et al. Randomised trial of 0.2% chlorhexidine gluconate and 2.5% natamycin for fungal keratitis in Bangladesh. *Br J Ophthalmol* 1998;82:919–925.

Rosa RH Jr, Miller D, Alfonso EC. The changing spectrum of fungal keratitis in South Florida. *Ophthalmology* 1994;101:1005–1013.

Srinivasan M. Fungal keratitis. *Curr Opin Ophthalmol* 2004;15:321–327.

Thomas PA. Tropical ophthalmomycoses. In: Seal DV, Bron AJ, Hay J, eds. *Ocular Infection: Investigation and Treatment in Practice*. London: Martin Dunitz; 1998:121–142.

Thomas PA. Fungal infections of the cornea. *Eye* 2003;17:852–862.

HERPES SIMPLEX KERATITIS

Herpetic eye disease is the major cause of unilateral corneal scarring worldwide, and is the most common infectious cause of corneal blindness in developed countries. As many as 60% of corneal ulcers in developing countries may be the result of HSV and 10 million people worldwide may have herpetic eye disease.

Pathogenesis

Herpes simplex virus

HSV is enveloped with a cuboidal capsule and a linear double-stranded DNA genome (Fig. 4.36). The two subtypes are HSV-1 and HSV-2, which reside equally in almost all ganglia, and local factors favour HSV-1 reactivation from the trigeminal ganglion. Detection by PCR of HSV in the trigeminal ganglion increases from 18% at 20 years to almost 100% in

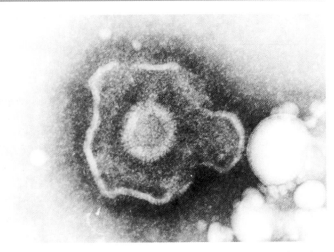

Fig. 4.36 Negative-stain electron micrograph of herpes simplex virus (Courtesy of Hart and Shears, from *Colour Atlas of Medical Microbiology*, Mosby, 2004)

people over 60 years of age. However, in lower socio-economic groups, 70–80% have HSV-1 antibodies by adolescence. Only about 20–25% of individuals with HSV antibodies have a clinical history of disease. HSV-1 primarily causes infection above the waist that may affect the face, lips and eyes, whereas HSV-2 causes venereally acquired infection (genital herpes). Rarely, HSV-2 may be transmitted to the eye through infected secretions, either venereally or at birth (ophthalmia neonatorum). HSV transmission is facilitated in conditions of crowding and poor hygiene.

Primary infection

Primary infection (no previous viral exposure) usually occurs by droplet transmission, or, less frequently, by direct inoculation. Due to protection bestowed by maternal antibodies, it is uncommon during the first 6 months of life. Most cases are probably subclinical or only cause mild fever, malaise and upper respiratory symptoms. Children may develop blepharoconjunctivitis (Fig. 4.37), which is usually benign and self-limited although corneal microdendrites develop in a minority of cases.

Recurrent infection

Recurrent disease (reactivation in the presence of cellular and humoral immunity) occurs as follows:

- After primary infection, the virus is carried to the sensory ganglion for that dermatome (e.g. trigeminal ganglion), where a latent infection is established.

- Subclinical reactivation can periodically occur when HSV is shed and patients are contagious. Stimuli such as fever, hormonal change, ultraviolet radiation, trauma and trigeminal injury may cause a clinical reactivation, when the virus replicates and is transported in the sensory axons to the periphery, where there is recurrent disease.

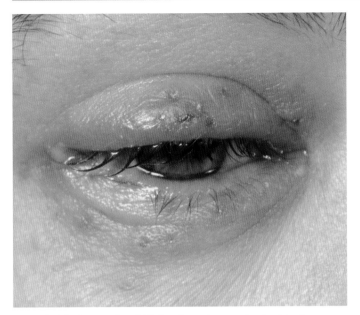

Fig. 4.37 Blepharoconjunctivitis in primary herpes simplex infection

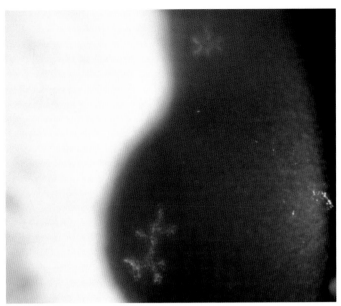

Fig. 4.38 Two early dendritic ulcers

- The pattern of disease (herpes labialis, herpes keratitis) depends on the site of reactivation, which may be remote from the site of primary infection. Hundreds of reactivations can occur during a lifetime. The rate for ocular recurrence of HSV after one episode is estimated to increase from 10% at 1 year to 23% at 2 years and to about 50% at 10 years. The more the number of previous attacks, the greater the risk of recurrence.

- The pattern of disease changes, and stromal disease accounts for only 2–6% of initial infection but 20–48% of recurrent disease. Visual complications are therefore associated with recurrent HSV.

- After the first episode, about 35% of the patients have a recurrent herpetic ulcer; 25% experience disciform or irregular stromal keratouveitis; 5% develop ocular hypertension; 6% develop scarring sufficient to decrease visual acuity. The risk of recurrence after stromal disease is about 10 times greater than that after epithelial disease.

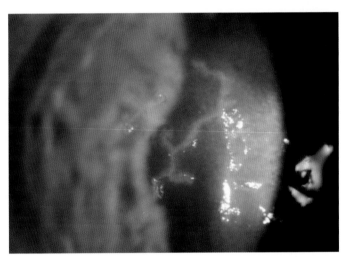

Fig. 4.39 Large unstained dendritic ulcer

NB: Risk factors for severe disease, which may be bilateral and frequently recurrent, include atopic eye disease, childhood, AIDS, malnutrition, measles and malaria. Inappropriate use of topical steroids may enhance the development of geographic ulceration (see below).

Epithelial keratitis

Epithelial (dendritic, geographic) keratitis is the result of virus replication and it is the most common presentation.

Diagnosis

1. **Presentation** may be at any age, with mild discomfort, watering and blurred vision.

2. **Signs**, in chronological order:

- Opaque epithelial cells arranged in a coarse punctate or stellate pattern (Fig. 4.38).

- Central desquamation results in a linear-branching (dendritic) ulcer, most frequently located centrally (Fig. 4.39).

- The ends of the ulcer have characteristic terminal buds and the bed of the ulcer stains well with fluorescein (Fig. 4.40).

- The virus-laden cells at the margin of the ulcer stain with rose bengal (Figs 4.41 and 4.42).

- Corneal sensation is reduced.

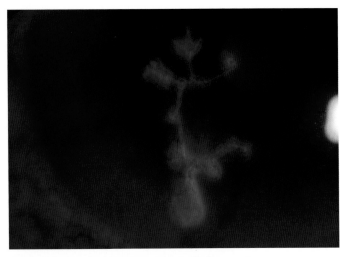

Fig. 4.40 Large dendritic ulcer stained with fluorescein

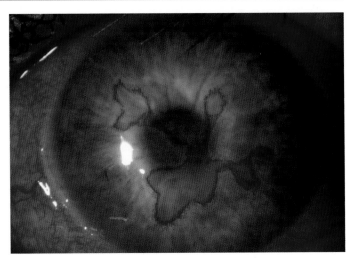

Fig. 4.42 Geographic dendritic ulcer stained with rose bengal

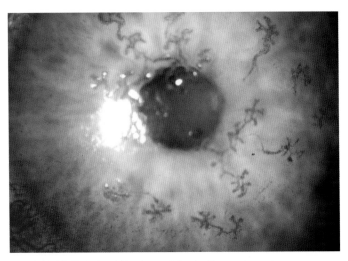

Fig. 4.41 Multiple dendritic ulcers stained with rose bengal

Treatment

Treatment of HSV disease is with purine or pyrimidine analogues that are incorporated to form abnormal viral DNA. Idoxuridine and vidarabine (Ara-A) are poorly soluble and relatively toxic, but are still used in regions where low cost is essential. Trifluridine (TFT) and aciclovir (Zovirax) have low toxicity and the latter can be used systemically. Both are active against HSV-1 and HSV-2.

1. **Topical** antiviral agents most frequently used are trifluorothymidine, aciclovir and vidarabine, which are similar in relative effectiveness. Aciclovir 3% ointment is used five times daily. The drug is relatively non-toxic, even when given for up to 60 days, because it acts preferentially on virus-laden epithelial cells. It is therefore suitable as antiviral cover for steroids in the management of disciform keratitis, which requires more prolonged treatment than simple dendritic ulceration (see below). Aciclovir penetrates intact corneal epithelium and stroma, achieving therapeutic levels in the aqueous humour, and can therefore be used to treat stromal herpetic keratitis. On this treatment, 99% will be resolved by 2 weeks. Other topical antiviral agents are available (e.g. ganciclovir 0.15% gel) but are no more effective.

> **NB:** Oral aciclovir does not hasten healing when used in combination with topical treatment. After epithelial HSV, a 3-week course of oral aciclovir 400 mg five times daily does not prevent stromal disease.

- Topical steroid treatment may allow progressive enlargement of the ulcer to a geographic or 'amoeboid' configuration (see Fig. 4.42).

- Following healing, there may be persistent punctate epithelial erosions which resolve spontaneously and should not be mistaken for persistent active infection.

- Mild subepithelial scarring may develop after healing.

3. **Culture** can be taken by debridement of the ulcer. This relies on a characteristic cytopathic effect in tissue culture, which can be used to distinguish HSV-1 from HSV-2; PCR is also available.

4. **Differential diagnosis** of dendritic ulceration includes herpes zoster keratitis, healing corneal abrasion (pseudodendrite), acanthamoeba keratitis, and toxic keratopathies secondary to topical medication.

2. **Debridement** may be used for dendritic but not geographic ulcers. The corneal surface is wiped with a sterile cellulose sponge 2 mm beyond the edge of the ulcer since pathology extends well beyond the visible dendrite. The removal of the virus-containing cells protects adjacent

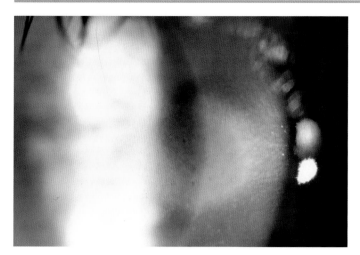

Fig. 4.43 Epithelial oedema in disciform keratitis

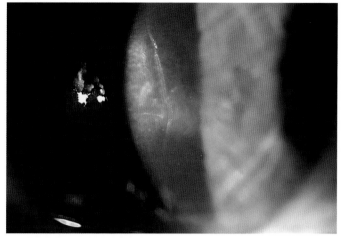

Fig. 4.45 Folds in Descemet membrane in disciform keratitis

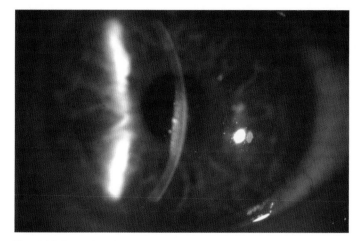

Fig. 4.44 Stromal oedema and keratic precipitates in disciform keratitis

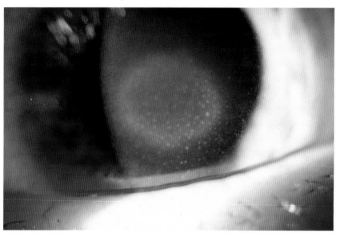

Fig. 4.46 Wesseley ring and keratic precipitates in disciform keratitis

healthy epithelium from infection and also eliminates the antigenic stimulus for stromal inflammation. An antiviral agent must be used in conjunction to prevent recurrence.

3. **Signs of treatment toxicity** include superficial punctate erosions, follicular conjunctivitis and punctal occlusion.

4. **Outcome**. The majority of lesions heal by 14 days irrespective of treatment. Eccentric lesions may be associated with superficial vascularisation extending centrally from the limbus, prolonged healing and early recurrences.

> **NB:** The majority of dendritic ulcers will eventually heal spontaneously without treatment.

Disciform keratitis

The exact aetiology of disciform keratitis (endotheliitis) is controversial. It may be an HSV infection of keratocytes or endothelium, or hypersensitivity reaction to viral antigen in the cornea. There is not always a past history of dendritic ulceration.

Clinical features

1. **Presentation** is with a gradual onset of blurred vision.

2. **Signs**

- A central zone of stromal oedema, often with overlying epithelial oedema (Fig. 4.43); occasionally, the lesion is eccentric.

- Keratic precipitates underlying the oedema (Fig. 4.44).

- Folds in Descemet membrane in severe cases (Fig. 4.45).

- A surrounding (Wessely) immune ring of stromal haze signifies deposition of viral antigen and host antibody complexes (Fig. 4.46).

- The intraocular pressure may be elevated despite only mild anterior uveitis.

- Healed lesions often have a faint ring of stromal opacification and thinning.

- Corneal sensation is reduced.

Treatment

1. **Initial** treatment of lesions involving the visual axis is with topical steroids and antiviral cover, both q.i.d. As improvement occurs, the frequency of administration of both is reduced in parallel over not less than 4 weeks.

2. **Subsequent.** Prednisolone 0.5% once daily is generally considered a safe dose at which to stop topical antiviral cover. A small number of patients require a very-low-dose steroid to prevent reactivation. In these cases, logarithmic reductions in steroid concentrations (0.3%, 0.1%, etc.) are available in some centres but have no proven benefit over a weak steroid such as fluorometholone 0.1% used on alternate days. Periodic attempts should be made to stop medication altogether.

> **NB:** There is no benefit in adding oral aciclovir to the topical steroid and antiviral therapy. Steroid-sparing treatment involves topical flurbiprofen 0.03% or topical ciclosporin combined with a topical antiviral agent.

Stromal necrotic keratitis

Viral antigen is detectable in stromal disease but viral replication is not thought to be an important component. Lymphocytes (Th1), antigen-presenting cells and polymorphonuclear neutrophils are critical for viral clearance, but they also mediate tissue destruction.

Clinical features

1. **Symptoms** are progressive discomfort and visual loss.

2. **Signs**

- Stromal necrosis and melting, often with profound interstitial opacification (Fig. 4.47).

- Associated anterior uveitis with keratic precipitates underlying the area of active stromal infiltration.

- If inappropriately treated, scarring, vascularisation and lipid deposition may result (Fig. 4.48).

> **NB:** Acute deterioration and melting might indicate secondary microbial infection.

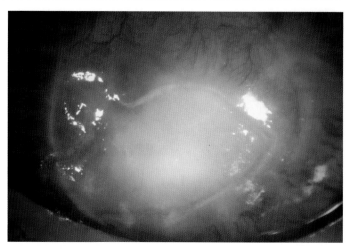

Fig. 4.47 Stromal necrotic herpetic keratitis

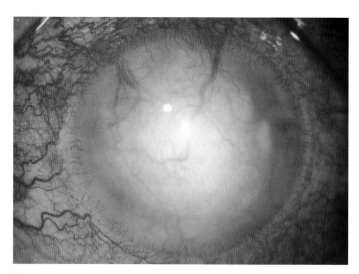

Fig. 4.48 Vascularisation and extensive lipid deposition in end-stage stromal necrotic herpetic keratitis

Treatment

- The primary goal is to achieve epithelial recovery. If possible, drops that may be toxic should be reduced, and oral aciclovir considered instead.

- Protection of the ocular surface from drying by the frequent use of non-preserved artificial tears.

- Inflammation should be reduced with topical steroids. Although this may make the eye comfortable more quickly, there is no evidence that the final visual outcome is improved.

- Further strategies to control corneal melting are described below.

Metaherpetic ulceration

Metaherpetic ulceration is caused by failure of re-epithelialisation resulting from devitalisation of the stroma and epithelial toxicity rather than viral replication.

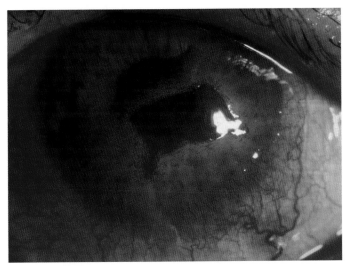

Fig. 4.49 Metaherpetic ulceration stained with rose bengal

1. Signs

- A non-healing epithelial defect after prolonged topical treatment (Fig. 4.49).

- There may be stromal ulceration, although necrosis is not a major feature.

- The stroma beneath the defect is grey and opaque.

- Other signs of inflammation (redness, uveitis) may be mild.

2. Treatment is that of persistent epithelial defects, as follows:

- Reduce exposure to toxic drops and preservatives.

- Frequent topical lubrication with non-preserved drops.

- Minimal use of topical steroid to control any inflammatory component.

- Bandage contact lens or temporary tarsorrhaphy as necessary.

Prophylaxis

The aim of prophylaxis is to reduce the frequency or severity of recurrences. Oral aciclovir (400 mg b.d.) reduces the rate of recurrent epithelial and stromal keratitis (see below) by about 45%, but this effect reduces or even disappears when the drug is stopped. The benefit of prophylaxis is greatest in patients with multiple recurrences and should be offered in the following cases:

- Frequent debilitating recurrences.

- Bilateral disease.

- Disease in an only eye.

- Corneal surgery with prior history of herpetic eye disease.

- Corneal surgery in the presence of severe atopy, even in patients without previous herpetic keratitis.

Complications

1. **Secondary infection.** Herpetic eye disease is a major predisposing factor for microbial keratitis.

2. **Secondary glaucoma** which may progress undetected if there is a poor view of the optic disc. Corneal thinning may give rise to a falsely low reading on applanation.

3. **Cataract** secondary to inflammation or prolonged steroid use.

4. **Iris atrophy** secondary to keratouveitis.

Keratoplasty for herpetic disease

Recurrence of herpetic eye disease on the graft and rejection threaten the survival of corneal grafts. Survival can be improved by preventing reactivation by prophylactic treatment after surgery.

1. **Topical** antivirals given during a rejection episode may reduce epithelial viral reactivation but may be toxic and delay re-epithelialisation.

2. **Oral** aciclovir (400 mg b.d.) should be used for patients undergoing penetrating keratoplasty. The duration of treatment and the optimum dose are not known. Immunohistochemistry should be performed on the excised tissue to confirm the presence of herpes antigen.

FURTHER READING

Barron BA, Gee L, Hauck WW, et al. Herpetic Eye Disease Study. A controlled trial of oral acyclovir for herpes stromal keratitis. *Ophthalmology* 1994;101:1871–1872.

Ficker LA, Kirkness CM, Rice NS, et al. The changing management and improved prognosis for corneal grafting in herpes simplex keratitis. *Ophthalmology* 1989;96:1587–1596.

Herpetic Eye Disease Study Group. A controlled trial of oral acyclovir for the prevention of stromal keratitis or iritis in patients with herpes simplex virus epithelial keratitis. The Epithelial Keratitis Trial. *Arch Ophthalmol* 1997;115:703–712.

Herpetic Eye Disease Study Group. Predictors of recurrent herpes simplex virus keratitis. *Cornea* 2001;20:123–128

Holland EJ, Schwartz GS. Classification of herpes simplex virus keratitis. *Cornea* 1999;18:144–154.

Liesegang TJ. Herpes simplex virus epidemiology and ocular importance. *Cornea* 2001;20:1–13.

Liesegang TJ, Melton LJ, Daly PJ, et al. Epidemiology of ocular herpes simplex. Incidence in Rochester, Minn, 1950 through 1982. *Arch Ophthalmol* 1989;107:1160–1165.

Moyes AL, Sugar A, Musch DC, et al. Antiviral therapy after penetrating keratoplasty for herpes simplex keratitis. *Arch Ophthalmol* 1994;112:601–607.

Remeijer L, Doornenbal P, Geerards AJ, et al. Newly acquired herpes simplex virus keratitis after penetrating keratoplasty. *Ophthalmology* 1997;104:648–652.

Uchoa UB, Rezende RA, Carrasco MA, et al. Long-term acyclovir use to prevent recurrent ocular herpes simplex virus infection. *Arch Ophthalmol* 2003;121:1702–1704.

Van Rooij J, Rijneveld WJ, Remeijer L, et al. Effect of oral acyclovir after penetrating keratoplasty. A placebo-controlled multicentre trial. *Ophthalmology* 2003;110:1916–1919.

Wilhelmus KR. Interventions for herpes simplex virus epithelial keratitis. *Cochrane Database Syst Rev* 2001;(1):CD002898

Wilhelmus KR, Coster DJ, Donovan HC, et al. Prognosis indicators of herpetic keratitis. Analysis of a five-year observation period after corneal ulceration. *Arch Ophthalmol* 1981;99:1578–1582.

Wilhelmus KR, Gee L, Hauck WW, et al. Herpetic Eye Disease Study. A controlled trial of topical corticosteroids for herpes simplex stromal keratitis. *Ophthalmology* 1994;101:1883–1896.

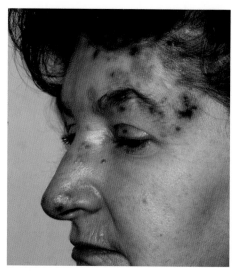

Fig. 4.50 Involvement of the side and tip of the nose (Hutchinson sign) in herpes zoster ophthalmicus

HERPES ZOSTER OPHTHALMICUS

Introduction

Pathogenesis

The varicella-zoster virus (VZV) causes chickenpox (varicella) and shingles (herpes zoster). VZV and HSV belong to the same subfamily of the herpes virus group and are morphologically identical but antigenically different. After the initial attack of chickenpox, the virus travels in a retrograde manner to the dorsal root and cranial nerve sensory ganglia, where it can remain dormant for decades. From there, it can reactivate after VZV-specific cellular immunity has faded, to cause shingles.

Mechanisms of ocular involvement

Ocular damage may be caused by the following mechanisms.

- Direct viral invasion may result in epithelial keratitis and conjunctivitis.

- Secondary inflammation and occlusive vasculitis may cause stromal keratitis, uveitis, scleritis and episcleritis.

- Reactivation causes necrosis and inflammation in the affected sensory ganglia, causing corneal anaesthesia that may result in neurotrophic keratitis.

- The mechanism of post-herpetic neuralgia is uncertain. Inflammation and destruction of the peripheral nerves or central ganglia, or altered signal processing in the CNS have been proposed.

Risk of occular involvement

- Involvement of the external nasal nerve (Hutchinson sign) (Fig. 4.50), which supplies the side of the tip and the side and the root of the nose, correlates significantly with subsequent development of ocular inflammation and corneal denervation because it is the terminal branch of the nasociliary nerve. Eye involvement may rarely occur when the disease affects the maxillary nerve.

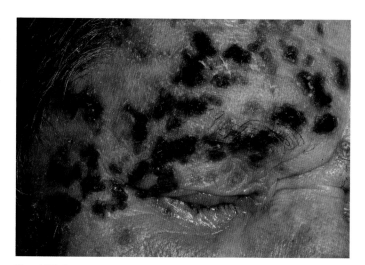

Fig. 4.51 Scattered lesions in herpes zoster ophthalmicus

- Herpes zoster ophthalmicus (HZO) occurs most frequently in the sixth and seventh decades. In the elderly, the signs and symptoms are more severe and last longer. Patients with AIDS also tend to have more severe disease. There is, however, no correlation between severity of ocular complications and age, sex, and severity of the skin rash.

Acute systemic disease

Clinical features

1. **A prodromal phase** lasting 3 to 5 days with tiredness, fever, malaise and headache precedes the appearance of the rash. Symptoms involving the dermatome of the ophthalmic nerve vary from superficial itching, tingling or burning sensation to a severe deep, boring or lancing pain that is either constant or intermittent. Older patients with

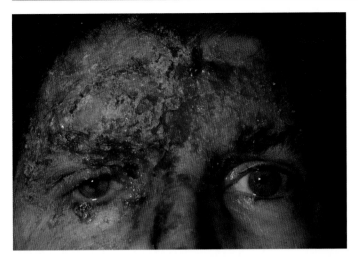

Fig. 4.52 Confluent haemorrhagic lesions in herpes zoster ophthalmicus

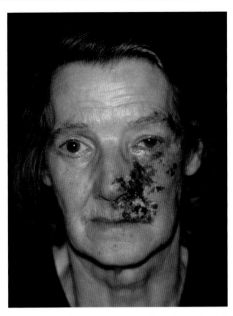

Fig. 4.54 Herpes zoster involving the maxillary branch of the trigeminal nerve

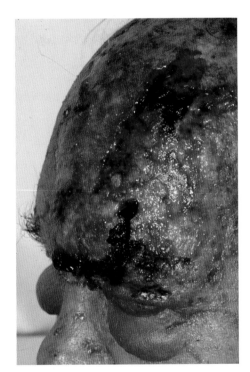

Fig. 4.53 Haemorrhagic bullae with necrosis in herpes zoster ophthalmicus

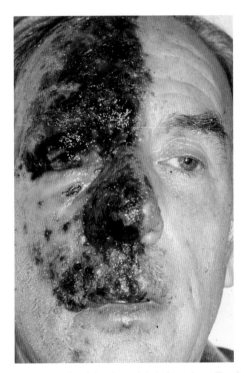

Fig. 4.55 Herpes zoster involving the ophthalmic and maxillary branches of the trigeminal nerve

severe pain and larger area of involvement are at particular risk of post-herpetic neuralgia.

2. **Skin lesions** appear initially as a painful erythema with a maculopapular rash. Within 24 hours, groups of vesicles appear, and these become confluent over 2 to 4 days. The vesicles often pass through a pustular phase (not necessarily indicative of secondary infection) before they crust and dry after 2 to 3 weeks. New crops of vesicles may appear in immunodeficient patients. The acute erythematous phase may be confused for cellulitis or contact dermatitis.

- The lesions vary in distribution, density and severity. They may be discrete and scattered (Fig. 4.51). Large, confluent and deep lesions with haemorrhagic bullae and tissue necrosis are more common in immunodeficiency (Figs 4.52 and 4.53). The lesions may involve one or more of the cutaneous branches of the trigeminal nerve (Figs 4.54 and 4.55).

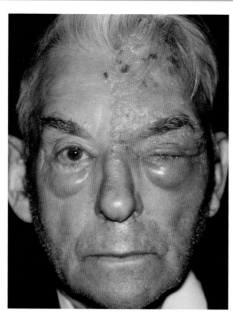

Fig. 4.56 Bilateral lid oedema in a patient with left herpes zoster ophthalmicus

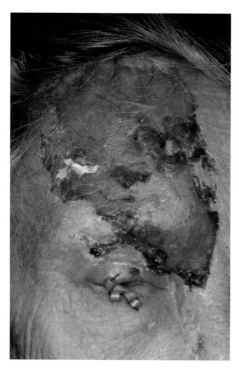

Fig. 4.57 Extensive skin necrosis following herpes zoster ophthalmicus

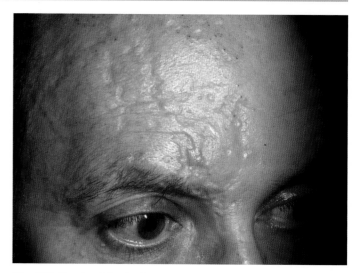

Fig. 4.58 Scarring following herpes zoster ophthalmicus

1–2 weeks. Such patients often have lymphoma, other malignancies or may be immunosuppressed.

• The development of shingles in children or young adults (<50 years) should prompt a search for immunodeficiency or malignancy. HIV infection should be excluded.

NB: People with shingles can transmit chickenpox to non-immune individuals. Contact with non-immune or immunosuppressed individuals should be avoided until crusting is complete.

Treatment

1. **Oral aciclovir** (800 mg five times daily for 3 to 7 days given within 72 hours of onset) is the treatment of choice. Patients presenting with new vesicles after 72 hours should also be treated to reduce the severity of acute HZO and the risk of post-herpetic neuralgia at 6 months. The incidence of late ophthalmic complications is also reduced by about 50%.

2. **Intravenous aciclovir** (5–10 mg/kg t.i.d.) is only indicated for encephalitis. The duration of treatment should be extended for the elderly or immunosuppressed. Aciclovir resistance has been reported in immunosuppressed patients receiving low-dose therapy to prevent recurrences. Foscarnet is then the treatment of choice.

3. **Other oral antiviral agents.** Valaciclovir 1 g t.i.d., famciclovir 750 mg daily and brivudine 125 mg daily are more expensive but have a more convenient dosing and are as effective as aciclovir 800 mg five times daily.

4. **Systemic steroids** (prednisolone 40 to 60 mg per day) should be used only in conjunction with systemic antivirals. They have a moderate effect at reducing acute pain

• The rash has a dermatomal distribution and respects the midline, although inflammatory oedema may cross the midline and give rise to the impression of bilateral involvement (Fig. 4.56).

• Skin lesions may leave extensive tissue destruction (Fig. 4.57) and depigmented scars (Fig. 4.58).

• Occasionally the rash may develop generalised mucocutaneous features and the patient become severely ill within

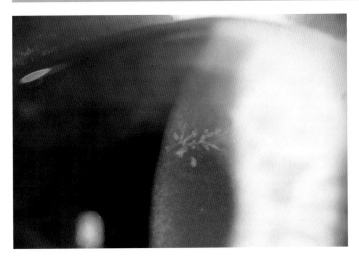

Fig. 4.59 Small unstained dendritic lesion in acute herpes zoster ophthalmicus

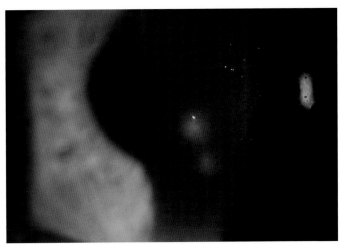

Fig. 4.61 Nummular keratitis in herpes zoster ophthalmicus

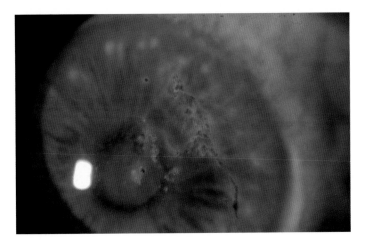

Fig. 4.60 Larger dendritic lesions stained with fluorescein in herpes zoster ophthalmicus

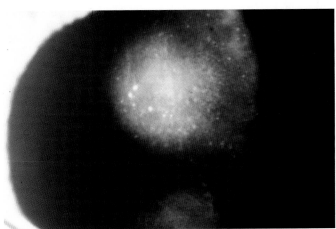

Fig. 4.62 Magnified view of a nummular lesion showing surrounding stromal haze

and accelerating skin healing, but have no effect on the incidence or severity of post-herpetic neuralgia.

5. **Symptomatic** treatment of skin lesions is by drying, antisepsis and cold compresses. The benefit of topical antibiotic/steroid combinations is uncertain.

Acute ocular disease

1. **Acute epithelial keratitis** develops in about 50% of patients within 2 days of the onset of the rash and resolves spontaneously a few days later. It is characterised by small, fine, dendritic lesions (Fig. 4.59) which, in contrast to herpes simplex dendrites, have tapered ends without terminal bulbs. The lesions stain with fluorescein (Fig. 4.60) and rose bengal. Treatment is with a topical antiviral, if appropriate.

2. **Conjunctivitis** is common and always associated with lid margin vesicles. Treatment is not required in the absence of corneal disease.

3. **Episcleritis** occurs at the onset of the rash and usually resolves spontaneously.

4. **Scleritis** and sclerokeratitis are uncommon and may develop at the end of the first week. If indolent, oral flurbiprofen (Froben) 100 mg t.i.d. may be required.

5. **Nummular keratitis** usually develops about 10 days after the onset of the rash. It is characterised by fine granular subepithelial deposits surrounded by a halo of stromal haze (Figs 4.61 and 4.62). The lesions fade in response to topical steroids but recur if treatment is discontinued prematurely.

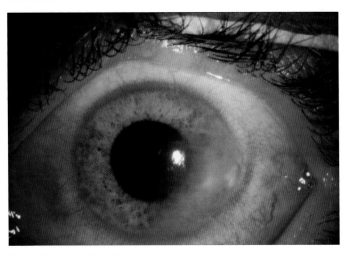

Fig. 4.63 Stromal keratitis in herpes zoster ophthalmicus

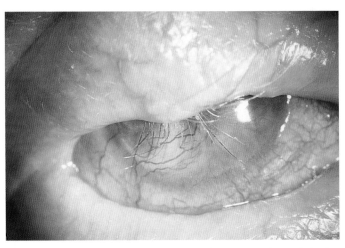

Fig. 4.65 Cicatricial ptosis, entropion, trichiasis and corneal vascularisation following herpes zoster ophthalmicus

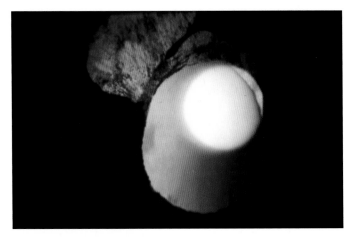

Fig. 4.64 Sectoral iris atrophy following herpes zoster anterior uveitis

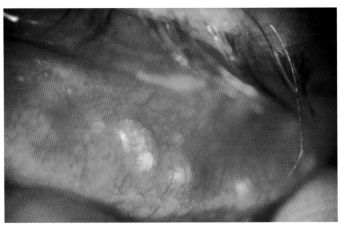

Fig. 4.66 Lipid-filled granulomata and subconjunctival scarring in herpes zoster ophthalmicus

6. **Stromal keratitis** develops 3 weeks after the onset of the rash in about 5% of cases (Fig. 4.63). It responds to topical steroids, but often becomes chronic.

7. **Disciform keratitis** is less common than with HSV infection but may lead to corneal decompensation. Treatment is with topical steroids.

8. **Anterior uveitis** is frequently associated with sectoral iris ischaemia and atrophy (Fig. 4.64).

9. **Neurological complications**

- Cranial nerve palsies affecting the third (most common), fourth and sixth nerves usually recover within 6 months.

- Optic neuritis is very rare.

- Guillain–Barré syndrome and encephalitis are rare and occur only with severe infection.

- Contralateral hemiplegia is also rare, usually mild and typically develops 2 months after the rash.

Chronic ocular disease

Clinical features

1. **Lid scarring** may result in ptosis, cicatricial entropion, trichiasis, madarosis and notching of the lid margin (Fig. 4.65).

2. **Lipid-filled granulomata** under the tarsal conjunctiva and subconjunctival scarring (Fig. 4.66).

3. **Scleritis** may become chronic and lead to patchy scleral atrophy (Fig. 4.67).

4. **Mucous plaque keratitis** develops in about 5% of cases, most commonly between the third and sixth months. It is characterised by the sudden appearance of elevated mucous plaques that stain with rose bengal (Fig. 4.68). When they assume a dendrite-like configuration (Fig. 4.69), they may be confused with herpes simplex dendritic ulcers. Treatment involves a combination of topical

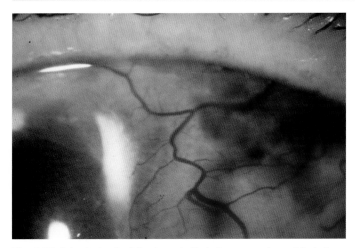

Fig. 4.67 Scleral atrophy following scleritis in herpes zoster ophthalmicus

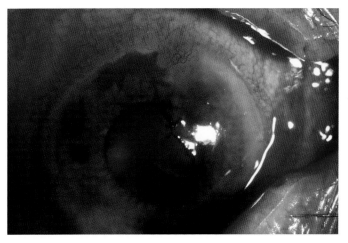

Fig. 4.69 Severe dendritic-like mucus plaque keratitis stained with rose bengal

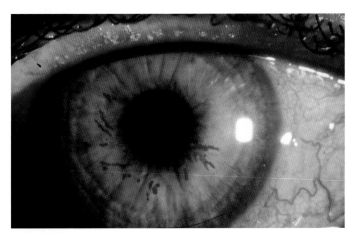

Fig. 4.68 Mucus plaque keratitis stained with rose bengal

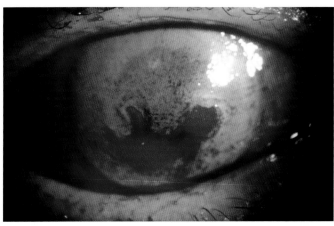

Fig. 4.70 Epithelial defect stained with rose bengal in neurotrophic keratitis

steroids and acetylcysteine. HZV antigen may be present and antiviral treatment may also be effective. Untreated, plaques resolve after a few months, leaving a faint diffuse corneal haze.

5. **Neurotrophic keratitis** with reduced sensation develops in about 50% of cases. It may rarely lead to severe ulceration, secondary bacterial infection and even perforation (Fig. 4.70).

6. **Lipid degeneration** (see Fig. 4.13) may develop in eyes with persistent severe nummular or disciform keratitis.

Post-herpetic neuralgia

Clinical features

Post-herpetic neuralgia is pain that persists after the rash has healed, usually defined as an interval of 3 months. It is rare in children but may develop in up to 75% of patients over 70 years of age. Pain may be constant or intermittent, worse at night and aggravated by minor stimuli (allodynia), touch and heat. It generally improves slowly with time, with only 2% of patients being affected after 5 years. Neuralgia may lead to depression, sometimes of sufficient severity to present the danger of suicide and can significantly impair the quality of life. Patients severely affected should be referred to a special pain clinic.

Treatment

Cold compress, topical capsaicin (depletes substance P) or local anaesthetic (lidocaine 5%) creams may be effective. Systemic treatment should be increased in steps as follows:

• Simple analgesics such as paracetamol up to 4 g daily

• Stronger analgesics such as codeine up to 240 mg daily.

• Amitriptyline 10–25 mg at night, increasing gradually to 75 mg daily if appropriate.

• Carbamazepine 400 mg daily for lancinating pain.

NB: Non-steroidal anti-inflammatory drugs are ineffective.

Relapsing phase

In the relapsing phase, lesions may reappear years after acute disease. On occasion, the acute episode may have been forgotten and lid scarring may be the only diagnostic clue. Reactivation of keratitis, episcleritis, scleritis or iritis can occur. Low-dose topical steroid (fluorometholone 0.1% daily) is effective after the acute event has been controlled.

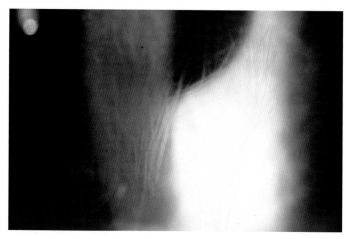

Fig. 4.71 Deep perfused stromal new vessels

FURTHER READING

Colin J, Prisant O, Cochener B, et al. Comparison of the efficacy and safety of valaciclovir and acyclovir for the treatment of herpes zoster ophthalmicus. *Ophthalmology* 2000;107:1507–1511.

Cunningham AL, Dworkin RH. The management of post-herpetic neuralgia. *BMJ* 2000;321:778–779.

Gnann JW Jr, Whitley RJ. Clinical practice. Herpes zoster. *N Engl J Med* 2002;347:340–346.

Gross G, Schofer H, Wassilew S, et al. Herpes zoster guideline of the German Dermatology Society (DDG). *J Clin Virol* 2003;26:277–289.

Helgason S, Petursson G, Gudmundsson S, et al. Prevalence of postherpetic neuralgia after a first episode of herpes zoster: prospective study with long term follow up. *BMJ* 2000;321:794–796.

Hoang-Xuan T, Buchi ER, Herbort CP, et al. Oral acyclovir for herpes zoster ophthalmicus. *Ophthalmology* 1992;99:1062–1067.

Liesegang TJ. Diagnosis and therapy of herpes zoster ophthalmicus. *Ophthalmology* 1991;98:1216–1229.

Liesegang TJ. Herpes zoster virus infection. *Curr Opin Ophthalmol* 2004;15:531–536.

Pavan-Langston D, Yamamoto S, Dunkel EC. Delayed herpes zoster pseudodendrites. Polymerase chain reaction detection of viral DNA and a role for antiviral therapy. *Arch Ophthalmol* 1995;113:1381–1385.

Severson EA, Baratz KH, Hodge DO, et al. Herpes zoster ophthalmicus in Olmsted County, Minnesota: have systemic antivirals made a difference? *Arch Ophthalmol* 2003;121:386–390.

Vafai A, Berger M. Zoster in patients infected with HIV: a review. *Am J Med Sci* 2001;321:372–380.

Vazquez M. Varicella zoster virus infections in children after the introduction of live attenuated varicella vaccine. *Curr Opin Pediatr* 2004;16:80–84.

Wareham D. Postherpetic neuralgia. *Clin Evid Concise* 2004;11:208–210.

Womack L, Liesegang T. Complications of herpes zoster ophthalmicus. *Arch Ophthalmol* 1983;101:42–45.

Zaal MJ, Volker-Dieben HJ, D'Amaro J. Prognostic value of Hutchinson's sign in acute herpes zoster ophthalmicus. *Graefes Arch Clin Exp Ophthalmol* 2003;241:187–191.

INTERSTITIAL KERATITIS

Interstitial keratitis (IK) is an inflammation of the corneal stroma without primary involvement of the epithelium or endothelium. In developed countries, it is most often associated with congenital syphilis (*Treponema pallidum*) but it may also be associated with a wide variety of infective causes such as tuberculosis, Lyme disease, leprosy and virus infection. All patients with IK should have treponemal serology, irrespective of the absence or presence of other clinical features of syphilis.

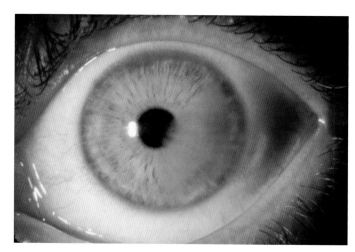

Fig. 4.72 'Salmon patch' in active interstitial keratitis (Courtesy of R Curtis)

Syphilitic

Syphilitic IK is due to the spread of infection from the mother to child during primary, secondary, or early latent phases (i.e. within 2 years of maternal primary infection).

Diagnosis

1. **Presentation** is between 5 and 25 years of age, with acute bilateral pain and severe blurring of vision.

2. **Signs,** in chronological order:

   - Limbitis associated with deep vessels invading the corneal stroma (Fig. 4.71) associated with corneal cellular infiltration and clouding that may obscure the vessels, resulting in the characteristic 'salmon patch' (Fig. 4.72).

   - Anterior uveitis may be obscured by corneal clouding.

   - After several months, the cornea begins to clear and the vessels become non-perfused ('ghost vessels') (Fig. 4.73).

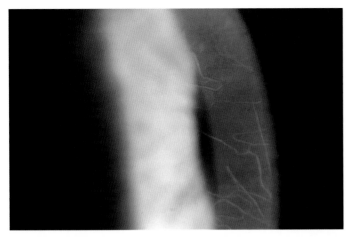

Fig. 4.73 'Ghost vessels' in inactive interstitial keratitis

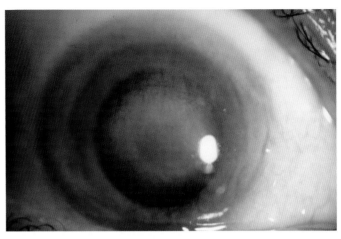

Fig. 4.75 Central corneal scarring in old syphilitic interstitial keratitis

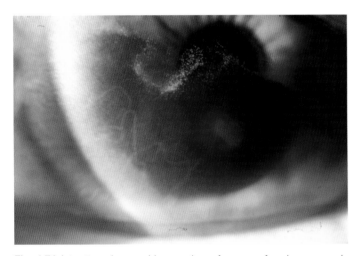

Fig. 4.74 Intrastromal corneal haemorrhage from reperfused new vessels in old interstitial keratitis

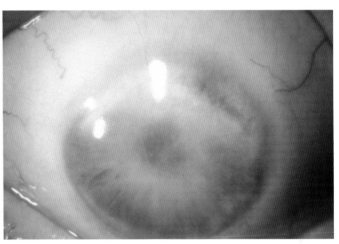

Fig. 4.76 Diffuse corneal scarring in old syphilitic interstitial keratitis

- If the cornea later becomes inflamed, the vessels may refill with blood and, rarely, bleed into the stroma (Fig. 4.74).

- The healed stage is characterised by 'ghost' vessels and deep stromal scarring and thinning (Figs 4.75 and 4.76).

Treatment

- All patients with positive treponemal serology should be referred to a genitourinary medicine specialist for evaluation, treatment (see Ch. 8) and screening of siblings, parents and partners.

- Active IK is treated with systemic penicillin, topical steroids and cycloplegics.

Cogan syndrome

Cogan syndrome is a rare non-syphilitic cause of IK. It is characterised by corneal disease and middle ear symptoms (tinnitus, vertigo, deafness) that develop within months of each other. The disease primarily occurs in young adults, with both sexes affected equally. Organ-specific autoimmunity is the most likely cause, possible precipitated by infection.

Diagnosis

1. Signs

- Redness, pain, photophobia and blurred vision.

- Faint bilateral peripheral anterior stromal opacities.

- Deeper opacities and neovascularisation may ensue (Fig. 4.77).

- Uveitis, scleritis and retinal vasculitis may develop.

- Systemic necrotising vasculitis and aortitis may occur.

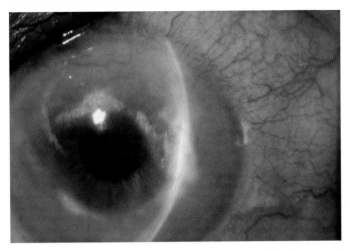

Fig. 4.77 Old interstitial keratitis in Cogan syndrome with clear central cornea (Courtesy of R Curtis)

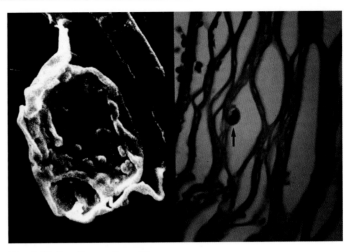

Fig. 4.78 Acanthamoeba cysts

2. **Investigations.** There are no specific investigations. Rheumatoid and antinuclear antibodies are usually negative.

Treatment

Topical steroids are effective for keratitis. Systemic steroids are usually required for scleritis or retinal vasculitis.

NB: Vestibulo-auditory symptoms require immediate treatment with systemic steroid (1–2 g/kg) to prevent hearing loss. Management in conjunction with an otolaryngologist is essential; immunosuppression may also be required.

FURTHER READING

Bergloff J, Gasser R, Feigl B. Ophthalmic manifestations in Lyme borreliosis. *J Neuro-Ophthalmol* 1994;14:15–20.

Cogan DG. Syndrome of nonsyphilitic interstitial keratitis and vestibuloauditory symptoms. *Arch Ophthalmol* 1945;33:144–149.

Grasland A, Pouchot J, Hachulla E, et al. Typical and atypical Cogan's syndrome: 32 cases and review of the literature. *Rheumatology (Oxford)* 2004;43:1007–1015.

Hariprasad SM, Moon SJ, Allen RC, et al. Keratopathy from congenital syphilis. *Cornea* 2002;21:608–609.

Huppertz H-I, Munchmeier D, Lieb W. Ocular manifestations in children and adolescents with Lyme arthritis. *Br J Ophthalmol* 1999;83:1149–1152.

Karma A, Seppala I, Mikkila H, et al. Diagnosis and clinical characteristics of ocular Lyme borreliosis. *Am J Ophthalmol* 1995;119:127–135.

Kornmehl EW, Lesser RL, Jaros P, et al. Bilateral keratitis in Lyme disease. *Ophthalmology* 1989;96:1194–1197.

Krist D, Wenkel H. Posterior scleritis associated with Borrelia burgdorferi (Lyme disease) infection. *Ophthalmology* 2002;109:143–145.

Mikkila HO, Seppala IJT, Viljanen MK, et al. The expanding clinical spectrum of ocular Lyme disease. *Ophthalmology* 2000;107:581–587.

St Claire EW, McCallum RM. Cogan's syndrome. *Curr Opin Rheumatol* 1999;11:47–52.

Zaidman GW. The ocular manifestations of Lyme disease. *Int Ophthalmol Clin* 1997;37:13–28.

PROTOZOAN KERATITIS

Acanthamoeba keratitis

Pathogenesis

Acanthamoeba sp. are ubiquitous free-living protozoa commonly found in soil, fresh or brackish water, and the upper respiratory tract. They exist in both active (trophozoite) and dormant (cystic) forms. The cystic form (Fig. 4.78) is highly resilient and able to survive for prolonged periods under hostile environmental conditions. Under appropriate environmental conditions, the cysts turn into trophozoites, which produce a variety of enzymes that aid tissue penetration and destruction. In developed countries, keratitis is most frequently associated with contact lens wear, and about 10% of cases are associated with injury (e.g. gardening) and contamination with standing water. The incidence in the UK is high compared with in other developed countries, due to contamination of header water tanks in most houses.

Diagnosis

1. **Symptoms** are pain, which may be severe and disproportionate to the clinical signs, and blurred vision.

2. **Signs**

- In early disease, the epithelial surface is irregular and greyish (Fig. 4.79).

- Epithelial changes may have a dendritic configuration and may be mistaken for herpes simplex keratitis (Fig. 4.80).

- Limbitis with diffuse or focal anterior stromal infiltrates (Fig. 4.81).

- Perineural infiltrates (radial keratoneuritis) (Fig. 4.82) are seen during the first 1–4 weeks and are pathognomonic (pseudomonal infection may be an exception).

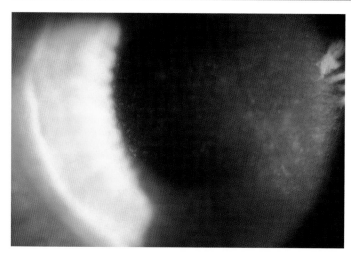

Fig. 4.79 Epithelial keratitis in early acanthamoeba infection

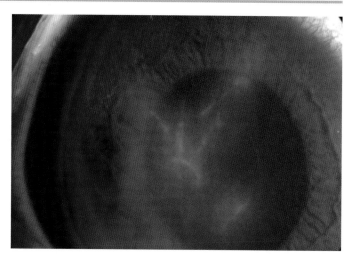

Fig. 4.82 Radial perineuritis in acanthamoeba keratitis

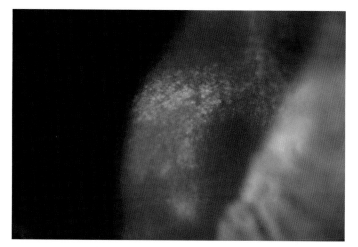

Fig. 4.80 Epithelial pseudodendrites in early acanthamoeba infection

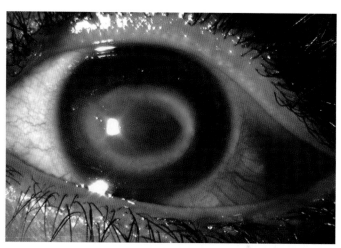

Fig. 4.83 Ring abscess in acanthamoeba keratitis

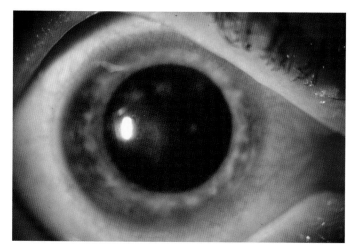

Fig. 4.81 Focal anterior stromal infiltrates in acanthamoeba keratitis

- Gradual enlargement and coalescence of the infiltrates to form a ring abscess with a relatively clear axial zone (Fig. 4.83).

- Scleritis may develop without obvious extension of the infection (Fig. 4.84).

- Enlargement of the abscess (Fig. 4.85).

- Slowly progressive stromal opacification and vascularisation (Fig. 4.86).

- Corneal melting (Fig. 4.87) may occur at any stage when there is stromal disease and often develops at the periphery of the area of infiltrate.

- Secondary closed-angle glaucoma and cataract are common in advanced cases.

3. Investigations

- Epithelial biopsy should be performed in early disease. If there is stromal involvement a sample can be taken with

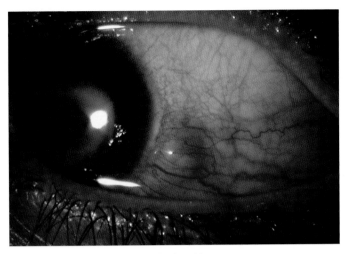

Fig. 4.84 Scleritis in acanthamoeba keratitis

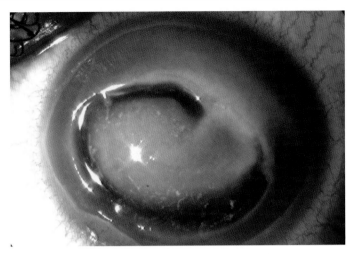

Fig. 4.87 Severe corneal melting in acanthamoeba keratitis

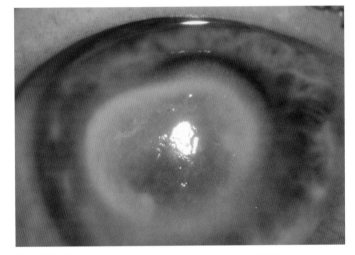

Fig. 4.85 Enlarging ring abscess in acanthamoeba keratitis

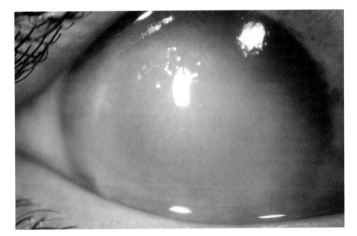

Fig. 4.86 Severe opacification in acanthamoeba keratitis

the tip of a needle. If there is a high index of suspicion and cultures are negative, a stromal biopsy should be taken.

- Cultures are performed by placing the sample on non-nutrient agar which is later seeded with killed *E. coli*. Culture of the contact lens case will often yield acanthamoeba and Gram-negative organisms.

- Immunohistochemistry is the most sensitive test.

- Staining using periodic acid–Schiff or calcofluor white (a fluorescent dye with an affinity for amoebic cysts and fungi) are alternatives.

NB: About 30% of patients are culture-negative. If there is a high index of suspicion (non-suppurative keratitis in a contact lens wearer), treatment should be as for acanthamoeba infection.

Treatment

It is important to have a high index of suspicion. The outcome is very much better if treatment is started within 4 weeks of onset of symptoms.

1. **Debridement** to remove infected epithelium is important for early disease (Fig 4.88).

2. **Topical amoebicides** given as dual therapy involving either propamidine isethionate 0.1% (Brolene) and poly-hexamethylene biguanide 0.02% drops, or hexamidine and chlorhexidine 0.02%. An antibiotic such as cipro-floxacin should be added if there is ulceration, to cover potential Gram-negative co-infection. Because cysts are difficult to eradicate, stromal relapses are common as treatment is tapered. In these cases, treatment should be increased and the tapering process restarted.

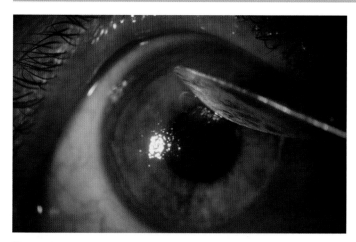

Fig. 4.88 Debridement of infected epithelium in acanthamoeba keratitis

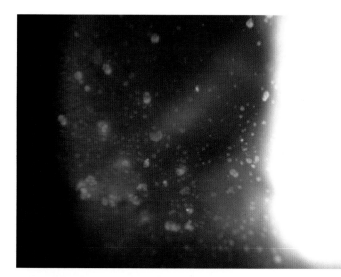

Fig. 4.89 Diffuse punctate epithelial lesions in microsporidial keratitis (Courtesy of D Tan)

Table 4.4 Topical amoebicides for acanthamoeba keratitis

Diamidines	Biguanides	Aminoglycosides	Imidazoles
Propamidine	PHMB	Neomycin	Miconazole
Hexamidine	Chlorhexidine	Paromomycin	Clotrimazole
			Ketaconazole
			Itraconazole

PHMB, polyhexamethylene biguanide.

3. **Topical steroids** should be avoided if possible. However, low-dose therapy may be useful for persistent inflammation which may be due to acanthamoeba antigen rather than viable organisms. The frequency of steroid administration should be tapered in parallel with anti-amoebic therapy.

4. **Pain control** for corneal disease or scleritis is with an oral non-steroidal anti-inflammatory agent such as flurbiprofen 100 mg t.i.d. Occasionally, oral ciclosporin may be required to control pain and inflammation. Even with maximum therapy, patients with advanced disease occasionally elect to have a persistently painful eye removed.

5. **Keratoplasty** is seldom necessary, because of effective medical therapy. Therapeutic keratoplasty should be avoided in inflamed eyes or if there is uncontrolled infection, because of the risk of recurrence in the graft, but may be necessary in severe cases to preserve the globe. When the infection has resolved, a lamellar or penetrating graft may be necessary to restore vision.

Differential diagnosis

In early disease, this includes herpetic keratitis and adenoviral keratoconjunctivitis. In advanced disease, fungal keratitis should be considered.

Microsporidial keratitis

Pathogenesis

Microsporidia are small, obligate, intracellular, spore-forming protozoa that are opportunistic pathogens in many animals. Over 14 species infect man. Infection occurs when the spores are injected into the host cell by the characteristic polar tube of the spore. Until the advent of AIDS, Microsporidia were rare human pathogens. The most common infection is enteritis associated with HIV infection. The most common ocular presentation is keratoconjunctivitis in immunocompromised patients (usually *Encephalitozoon* species). A slowly progressive stromal disease in immunocompetent patients is very rare (usually *Nosema* sp.).

Diagnosis

1. **Signs**

* Bilateral chronic diffuse punctate epithelial keratoconjunctivitis (Fig. 4.89).

* Unilateral slowly progressive deep stromal keratitis may rarely affect immunocompetent patients (Fig. 4.90).

* Sclerokeratitis and endophthalmitis are rare.

2. **Histology**

* Characteristic appearance of spores and intracellular parasites on biopsy.

* Electron microscopy for confirmation and speciation.

* Culture requires injection in rodents and is not usually performed.

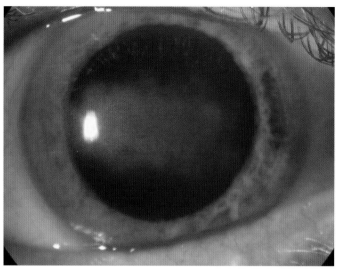

Fig. 4.90 Deep stromal infiltrates in microsporidial keratitis

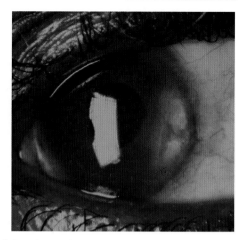

Fig. 4.91 Sclerosing onchocercal keratitis (Courtesy of I Murdoch)

Treatment

1. **Medical** therapy of epithelial disease is with topical fumagillin. Highly active antiretroviral therapy (HAART) for AIDS may also help resolution. Stromal disease is treated with a combination of topical fumagillin and oral albendazole (400 mg daily for 2 weeks, repeated two weeks later with a second course). Patients should be closely monitored for hepatic toxicity.

2. **Keratoplasty** may be indicated, although recurrence of disease can occur in the graft periphery; cryotherapy to the residual tissue may reduce this risk.

Onchocercal keratitis

Onchocerciasis or river blindness is caused by infestation with the parasitic helminth *Onchocerca volvulus* (see Ch. 8).

Clinical features

1. **Punctate keratitis** (0.5 mm diameter) represents white cell infiltrate surrounding dead microfilariae in the cornea. The lesions are most commonly at the 3 o'clock and 9 o'clock positions in the anterior third of the stroma.

2. **Sclerosing keratitis** represents permanent scarring of the cornea.

- Opacification is continuous with the limbus, usually at the 3 o'clock and 9 o'clock positions (Fig. 4.91).

- Slow progression of opacification occurs, to eventually involve the entire cornea. Full-thickness scarring has superficial and deep vessels with pigment migration over the surface (Fig. 4.92).

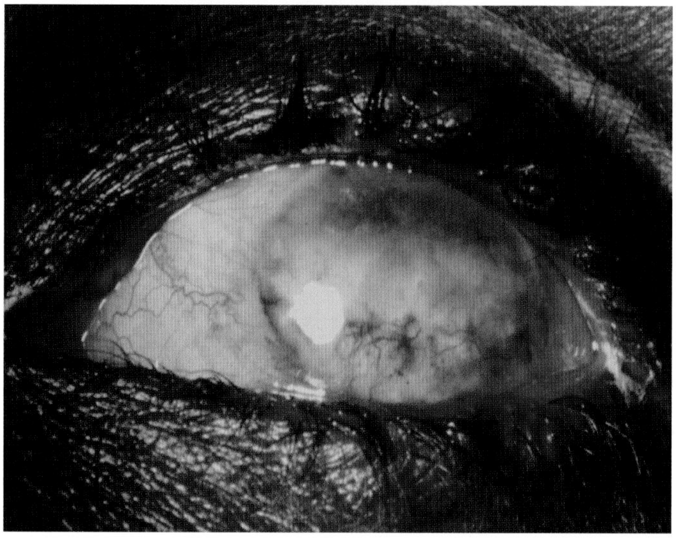

Fig. 4.92 Advanced sclerosing onchocercal keratitis

Treatment

Topical steroids are used for acute corneal inflammation. Systemic therapy is described in Chapter 8.

FURTHER READING

Bacon AS, Dart JK, Ficker LA, et al. Acanthamoeba keratitis. The value of early diagnosis. *Ophthalmology* 1993;100:1238–1243.

Bacon AS, Frazer DG, Dart JK, et al. A review of 72 consecutive cases of Acanthamoeba keratitis, 1984–1992. *Eye* 1993;7:719–725.

Font RL, Su GW, Matoba AY. Microsporidial stromal keratitis. *Arch Ophthalmol* 2003;121:1045–1047.

Friedberg DN, Stenson SM, Orenstein JM, et al. Microsporidian keratoconjunctivitis in acquired immunodeficiency syndrome. *Arch Ophthalmol* 1990;108:504–508.

Illingworth CD, Cook SD. Acanthamoeba keratitis. *Surv Ophthalmol* 1998;42:493–508.

Lee GA, Gray TB, Dart JK, et al. Acanthamoeba sclerokeratitis: treatment with systemic immunosuppression. *Ophthalmology* 2002;109:1178–1182.

O'Day DM, Head WS. Advances in the management of keratomycosis and Acanthamoeba keratitis. *Cornea* 2000;19:681–687.

Radford CF, Bacon AS, Dart JK, et al. Risk factors for acanthamoeba keratitis in contact lens users: a case-control study. *BMJ* 1995;310:1567–1570.

Radford CF, Minassian DC, Dart JK. Acanthamoeba keratitis in England and Wales: incidence, outcome, and risk factors. *Br J Ophthalmol* 2002;86:536–542.

Rauz S, Tuft S, Dart JKG, et al. Ultrastructural examination of two cases of stromal microsporidial keratitis. *J Med Microbiol* 2004;53:775–781.

Rosberger DF, Serdarevic ON, Erlandson RA, et al. Successful treatment of microsporidial keratoconjunctivitis with topical fumagillin in a patient with AIDS. *Cornea* 1993;12:261–265.

Sharma S, Garg P, Rao GN. Patient characteristics, diagnosis, and treatment of non-contact lens related Acanthamoeba keratitis. *Br J Ophthalmol* 2000;84:1103–1108.

Theng J, Chan C, Ling ML, et al. Microsporidia keratoconjunctivitis in a healthy contact lens wearer without human immunodeficiency virus infection. *Ophthalmology* 2001;108:976–978.

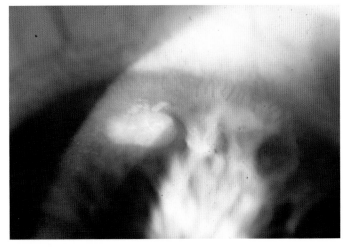

Fig. 4.93 Early marginal keratitis

BACTERIAL HYPERSENSITIVITY-MEDIATED CORNEAL DISEASE

Marginal keratitis

Pathogenesis

Marginal keratitis is thought to be the result of a reaction against staphylococcal exotoxins and cell wall proteins, with deposition of antigen–antibody complexes in the peripheral cornea (antigen diffusing from the tear film, antibody from the blood vessels) and a secondary lymphocytic infiltration. The lesions are culture-negative but *Staph. aureus* can frequently be isolated from the lid margins.

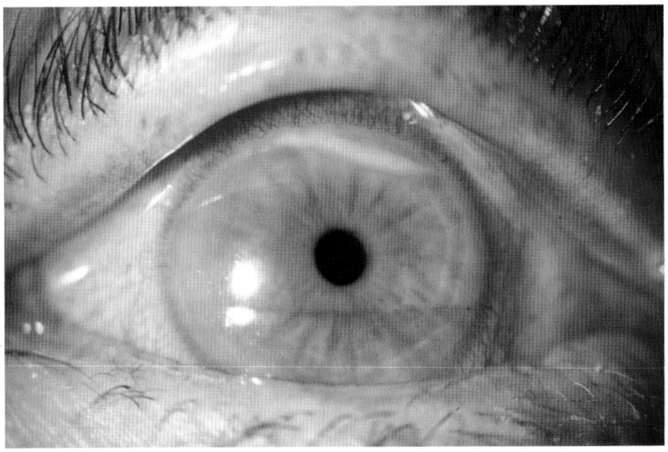

Diagnosis

1. **Presentation** is with mild irritation, lacrimation and discomfort.

2. **Signs**

- A subepithelial marginal infiltrate separated from the limbus by a clear zone, often associated with a focal adjacent area of conjunctivitis and episcleritis (Fig. 4.93).

- Circumferential spread accompanied by staining of the overlying epithelium with fluorescein (Fig. 4.94).

- Ulceration may occur if left untreated, but may also indicate secondary infection.

- Without treatment, resolution occurs in 3–4 weeks, leaving slight thinning and a superficial scar, usually without vascularisation.

- Gross corneal infiltration (Fig. 4.95) can occur in the presence of modifying factors such as recurrent epithelial erosion or recent laser in-situ keratomileusis (LASIK) surgery. Large infiltrates, corneal oedema and hypopyon can occur.

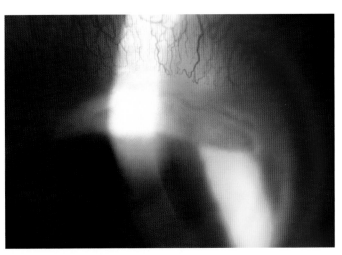

Fig. 4.94 Circumferential spread of marginal keratitis

Fig. 4.95 Gross marginal keratitis

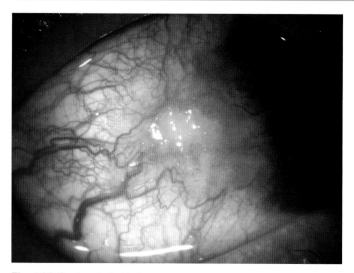

Fig. 4.96 Conjunctival phlycten

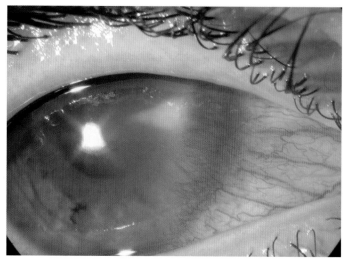

Fig. 4.97 Corneal phlycten

Treatment

- Coexisting lid margin disease should be treated with hygiene and topical antibiotics (see Ch. 1).

- Topical fluorometholone 0.1% q.i.d for 1 week, if symptoms dictate.

- The frequency of recurrences may be reduced with oral tetracycline.

> **NB:** If there is a significant epithelial defect (>1 mm), treatment is that of suspected bacterial keratitis.

Phlyctenulosis

Pathogenesis

Phlyctenulosis is usually a self-limiting disease although rarely it may be severe and even blinding. Most cases seen in developed countries are the result of a presumed delayed hypersensitivity reaction to staphylococcal cell wall antigen. However, in developing countries, the majority are associated with tuberculosis or helminth infestation. The most common systemic association is rosacea.

Diagnosis

1. **Presentation** is usually in children or young adults, with photophobia, lacrimation and blepharospasm.

2. **Signs**

- A small white nodule associated with intense local hyperaemia on the conjunctiva or limbus (Fig. 4.96).

- A limbal phlycten may then extend (wander) progressively onto the cornea (Fig. 4.97).

- A healed corneal phlycten usually leaves a triangular limbal-based scar associated with superficial vascularisation and thinning.

- Spontaneous resolution usually occurs in 2–3 weeks, but severe thinning and even perforation can occur.

3. **Treatment**

- A short course of topical steroids will accelerate healing.

- Associated chronic staphylococcal blepharitis, which is frequent, should also be treated.

- Recurrent disease is treated with oral tetracycline.

> **NB:** A Mantoux test and chest X-ray is only indicated in tuberculosis-endemic areas.

FURTHER READING

Beauchamp GR, Gillette TE, Friendly DS. Phlyctenular keratoconjunctivitis. *J Pediatr Ophthalmol Strabismus* 1981;18:22–28.

Chignell AH, Easty DL, Chesterton JR, et al. Marginal ulceration of the cornea. *Br J Ophthalmol* 1970;54:433–440.

Culbertson W, Huang A, Mandelbaum S, et al. Effective treatment of phlyctenular keratoconjunctivitis with oral tetracycline. *Ophthalmology* 1993;100:1358–1366.

Hussein AA, Nasr ME. The role of parasitic infection in the aetiology of phlyctenular eye disease. *J Egypt Soc Parasitol* 1991;21:865–868.

Ionides AC, Tuft SJ, Ferguson VM, et al. Corneal infiltration after recurrent corneal epithelial erosion. *Br J Ophthalmol* 1997;81:537–540.

Mondino BJ, Kowalski RP. Phlyctenulae and catarrhal infiltrates. Occurrence in rabbits immunized with staphylococcal cell walls. *Arch Ophthalmol* 1982;100:1968–1971.

Rohatgi J, Dhaliwal U. Phlyctenular eye disease: a reappraisal. *Jpn J Ophthalmol* 2000;44:146–150.

Zaidman G, Brown S. Orally administered tetracycline for phlyctenular keratoconjunctivitis. *Am J Ophthalmol* 1981;92:173–182.

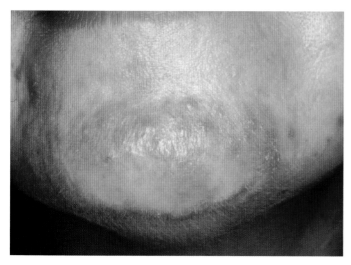

Fig. 4.98 Erythema and telangiectasis in acne rosacea

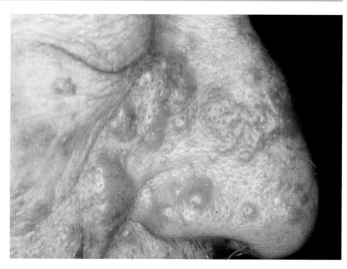

Fig. 4.100 Sebaceous gland hypertrophy in rosacea

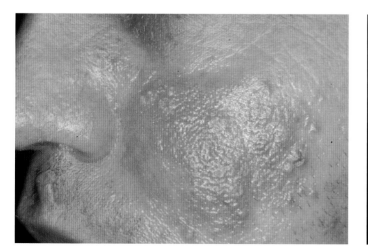

Fig. 4.99 Erythema and small pustules in acne rosacea

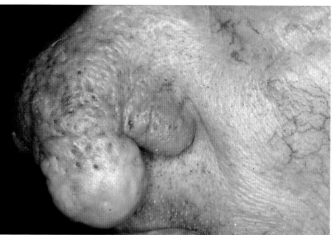

Fig. 4.101 Rhinophyma in advanced acne rosacea

ROSACEA KERATITIS

Acne rosacea

Acne rosacea is a common, idiopathic, chronic dermatosis involving the sun-exposed skin of the face and upper neck. The condition affects all races but may be missed in black patients if facial skin is not examined specifically.

Pathogenesis

The papules and pustules may be precipitated by lipases secreted by *Staph. epidermidis*. Lipases may break down the wax and sterol esters of the meibomian glands to release inflammatory free fatty acids. Co-infection with *Helicobacter pylori* has been implicated as an aggravating factor. Tetracyclines reduce the bacterial flora on the lids, and thereby decrease lipase production. They also non-specifically block matrix metalloproteinases in tears.

Diagnosis

1. **Presentation** is in adult life with itching and flushing of facial skin, principally the forehead, cheeks, nose and chin. Symptoms are often precipitated by ingestion of alcohol, hot drinks or spicy food.

2. **Signs**

- Erythema progressing to telangiectasis (Fig. 4.98).

- Papules and pustules (Fig. 4.99).

- Sebaceous gland hypertrophy (Fig. 4.100).

- Rhinophyma (Fig. 4.101).

NB: In contrast to acne vulgaris, comedones (blackheads or whiteheads) are absent.

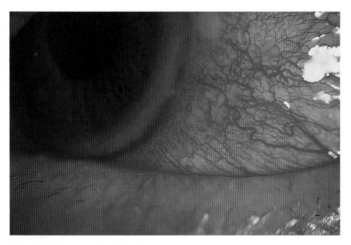

Fig. 4.102 Conjunctival injection in acne rosacea

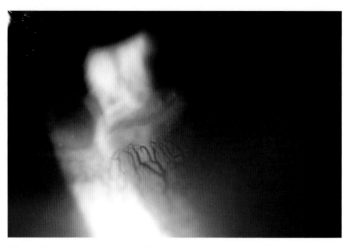

Fig. 4.103 Inferior marginal infiltrate in early rosacea keratitis

Treatment

- Topical metronidazole gel, azelaic acid cream and oral tetracycline; the comparative benefits of the different tetracyclines have not been established.

- Other measures include oral isotretinoin and laser therapy.

Ocular rosacea

Between 6% and 18% of patients with acne rosacea develop ocular complications. Ocular rosacea is a term used to define a spectrum of eye findings in the presence of lid margin telangiectasia, often without significant involvement of the rest of the face.

Pathogenesis

Ocular rosacea probably represents a type IV hypersensitivity response to an unidentified antigen, although some of the corneal changes may be the result of released inflammatory mediators such as interleukin 1 and matrix metalloproteinase 9.

Diagnosis

1. **Presentation** is with non-specific irritation, burning, tearing and redness.

2. **Lid** signs include margin telangiectasia and intractable posterior blepharitis, often associated with recurrent meibomian cyst formation.

3. **Conjunctiva**

- Conjunctival hyperaemia, especially bulbar (Fig. 4.102).

- Other signs include episcleritis, tear film dysfunction and, rarely, cicatricial conjunctivitis, conjunctival granulomas and phlyctenulosis.

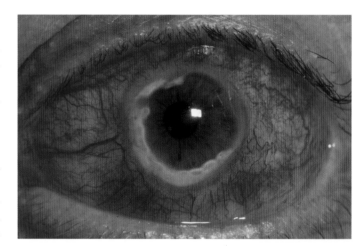

Fig. 4.104 Extensive peripheral marginal infiltration in rosacea keratitis

4. **Cornea**

- Inferior punctate erosions.

- Marginal keratitis and peripheral neovascularisation, especially involving the inferonasal and inferotemporal cornea (Fig. 4.103).

- Circumferential spread (Fig. 4.104).

- Corneal thinning in severe cases (Figs 4.105 and 4.106).

- Perforation (Fig. 4.107) may occur as a result of severe peripheral or central melting, which may be precipitated by secondary bacterial infection.

- Corneal scarring and vascularisation (Figs 4.108 and 4.109).

Treatment

1. **Topical**

- Hot compresses and lid hygiene.

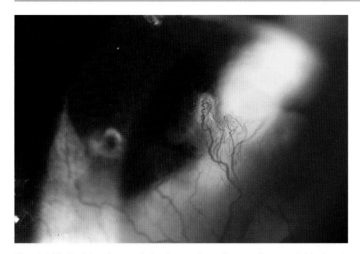

Fig. 4.105 Peripheral vascularisation and small area of corneal thinning in rosacea keratitis

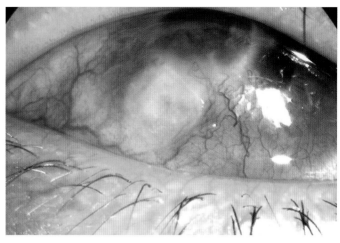

Fig. 4.108 Peripheral scarring and vascularisation in rosacea keratitis

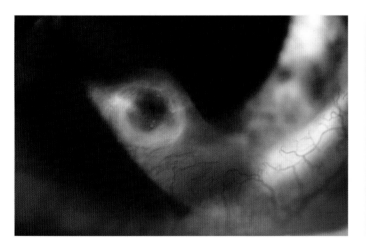

Fig. 4.106 More severe corneal thinning in rosacea keratitis

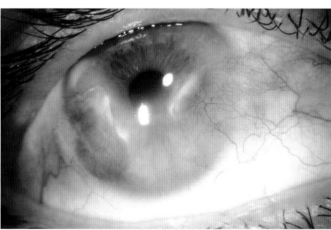

Fig. 4.109 Severe scarring and vascularisation in rosacea keratitis

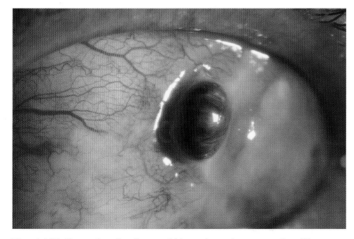

Fig. 4.107 Corneal perforation and iris prolapse in rosacea keratitis

- Fusidic acid ointment at bedtime for 4 weeks.
- Fluorometholone 0.1% as a short-term measure.
- Lubricants for symptomatic relief.
- The role of topical ciclosporin is uncertain.

2. Systemic

- Oxytetracycline 500 mg b.d. suppresses but does not cure the disease; improvement usually lasts for 6 months after cessation of therapy. The therapeutic effect of tetracycline is not related to its antibacterial action.
- Doxycycline 100 mg once daily is an alternative.
- Minocycline may cause facial pigmentation with prolonged use (see Fig. 1.26).
- Severe disease with corneal melt may require immunosuppression (azathioprine).

NB: Systemic tetracyclines should not be used in children under the age of 12 years or in pregnant or breastfeeding women because the antibiotic is deposited in teeth (being bound to calcium), and may cause dental hypoplasia and discoloration. Erythromycin can be used in children.

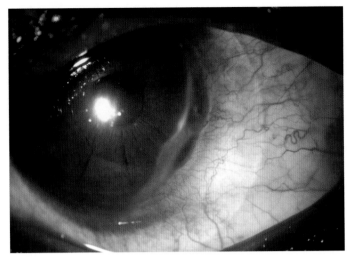

Fig. 4.110 Early peripheral ulcerative keratitis

FURTHER READING

Akpek EK, Merchant A, Pinar V, et al. Ocular rosacea patients characteristics and follow-up. *Ophthalmology* 1997;104:1863–1867.

Browning D, Proia A. Ocular rosacea. *Surv Ophthalmol* 1986;31:145–158.

Erzurum S, Feder R, Greenwald M. Acne rosacea with keratitis in childhood. *Arch Ophthalmol* 1993;111:228–230.

Ghanem VC, Mehra N, Wong S, et al. The prevalence of ocular signs in acne rosacea. Cornea 2003;22:230–233.

Knox CM, Smolin G. Rosacea. *Ophthalmol Clin* 1997;37:29–40.

Michel JL, Cabibel F. Frequency, severity and treatment of ocular rosacea during cutaneous rosacea. *Ann Dermatol Venereol* 2003;130:20–24.

Nazir SA, Murphy S, Siatkowski RM, et al. Ocular rosacea in childhood. *Am J Ophthalmol* 2004;137:138–144.

Stone DU, Chodosh J. Oral tetracyclines for ocular rosacea: an evidence-based review of the literature. *Cornea* 2004;23:106–109.

SEVERE PERIPHERAL CORNEAL MELTING

Peripheral ulcerative keratitis (PUK)

PUK is a severe condition that may precede or follow the onset of systemic disease. Severe, persistent, peripheral corneal infiltration, ulceration or thinning unexplained by coexistent ocular disease should therefore prompt a search for an associated systemic collagen vascular disorder which may be life-threatening (see below).

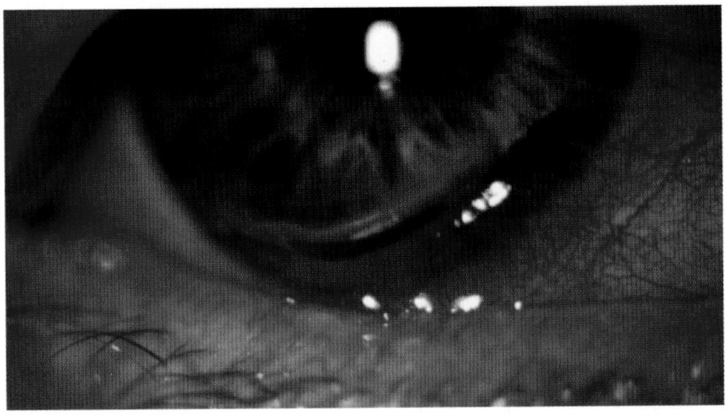

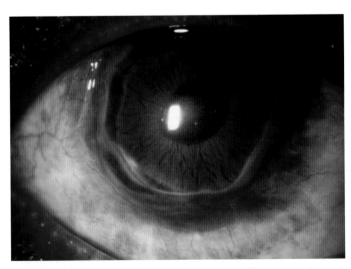

Fig. 4.111 Circumferential spread of peripheral ulcerative keratitis

Pathogenesis

In patients with an underlying autoimmune disease, there is immune complex deposition in peripheral cornea. Diseased epithelium, keratocytes and recruited inflammatory cells may result in release of matrix metalloproteinases that degrade collagen and the extracellular matrix. Autoantibodies may target sites in the corneal epithelium.

Signs

- Crescent-shaped ulceration and stromal infiltration at the limbus (Fig. 4.110).

- Limbitis, episcleritis or scleritis is usually present.

- Circumferential and occasionally central spread (Fig. 4.111).

- End-stage disease may result in a 'contact lens' cornea (Fig. 4.112).

Fig. 4.112 Advanced peripheral ulcerative keratitis giving rise to a 'contact lens' cornea

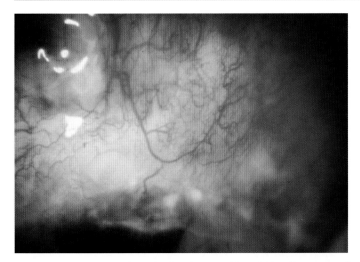

Fig. 4.113 Sclerosing keratitis in rheumatoid arthritis (Courtesy of P Watson)

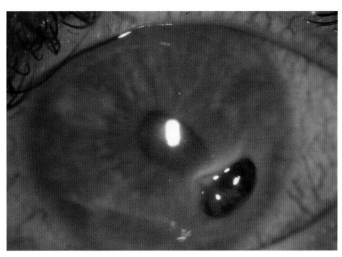

Fig. 4.115 Peripheral perforation melting in rheumatoid arthritis

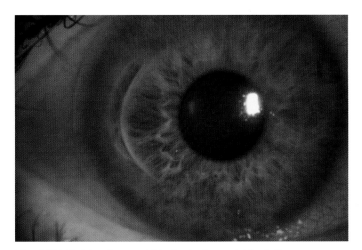

Fig. 4.114 Peripheral corneal thinning in rheumatoid arthritis

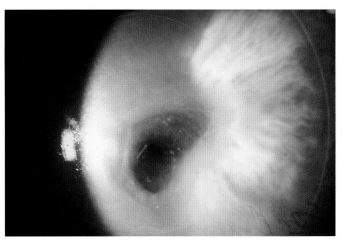

Fig. 4.116 Central corneal melting in rheumatoid arthritis

NB: Unlike Mooren ulcer, the process may also extend to involve the sclera.

Associated systemic diseases

Rheumatoid arthritis and Wegener granulomatosis account for about 95% of associated disease.

1. **Rheumatoid arthritis** (see Ch. 8) is the commonest systemic association. PUK involves both eyes in 30% of cases and tends to affect patients during the late and advanced vasculitic phase of the disease. Patients with rheumatoid arthritis may also develop the following non-ulcerative types of keratitis:

a. **Sclerosing keratitis** is characterised by gradual thickening and opacification of the corneal stroma adjacent to a site of scleritis (Fig. 4.113).

b. **Peripheral corneal thinning** is characterised by gradual resorption of peripheral stroma, leaving the epithelium intact (Fig. 4.114). Perforation may occur in advanced cases (Fig. 4.115). This is distinct from the 'contact lens' cornea following peripheral ulceration.

c. **Acute central corneal melting** may occur in association with inflammation or severe dry eye (Fig. 4.116).

2. **Wegener granulomatosis** (see Ch. 8) is the second most common systemic association. In contrast with rheumatoid arthritis, ocular complications are the initial presentation in 50% of cases. PUK may progress to peripheral corneal melting.

3. **Relapsing polychondritis** (see Ch. 8) is more commonly associated with episcleritis or scleritis than with PUK.

4. **Systemic lupus erythematosus** is a rare association; keratitis is more commonly the result of severe keratoconjunctivitis sicca.

Treatment

PUK associated with a potentially life-threatening systemic vasculitis must be treated with systemic immunosuppressive agents in collaboration with a rheumatologist.

1. Systemic

- High-dose steroids are used to control acute disease.

- Cytotoxic therapy is required for longer-term management to prevent the unacceptable side effects of steroids. Cyclophosphamide is especially useful for Wegener granulomatosis; other options include azathioprine, mycophenolate mofetil and methotrexate.

2. Surgery

- Emergency keratoplasty (preferably lamellar) may be required for peripheral corneal perforation.

- Elective keratoplasty (lamellar or penetrating) may be performed subsequently, to restore vision.

Mooren ulcer

Mooren ulcer is a rare, idiopathic disease characterised by progressive, circumferential, peripheral, stromal ulceration with later central spread. The diagnosis depends upon identification of the clinical features and exclusion of other causes of PUK. Mooren ulcer is rare in the Northern Hemisphere but more common in southern and central Africa, China and the Indian subcontinent. It affects males more commonly than females and is very rare in children. Bilateral disease is present in 30% of cases and is more aggressive than unilateral involvement, which tends to be more slowly progressive and responds better to treatment.

Pathogenesis

The aetiology is uncertain, although the following observations may be significant:

- There is a reduction in the number of CD8 (T suppressor) cells in the blood, and an imbalance between the ratio of CD4 and CD8 cells could lead to overproduction of antibody and immune complex deposition in the peripheral cornea. The conjunctiva adjacent to active lesions contains increased IgA and a B-cell infiltrate. Immunoglobulins and complement are deposited in both the conjunctiva and peripheral cornea.

- The serum of patients with Mooren ulcer contains increased levels of an antibody against a corneal stromal antigen (COAg). It has been proposed that trauma or inflammation may induce autoimmunity to this previously hidden antigen. The resulting inflammation then releases tissue matrix metalloproteinases from the conjunctiva or cornea that cause corneal ulceration. The presence of corneal autoantibodies could be the result rather than the cause of corneal destruction.

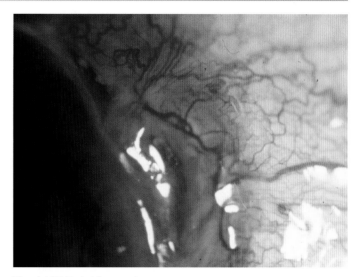

Fig. 4.117 Early Mooren ulcer

- An autoimmune process may be present that is directed against a specific target antigen in the corneal stroma, possibly triggered in genetically susceptible individuals by trauma. The reported rate of previous trauma, surgery or infection in eyes with Mooren ulcer varies between 11% and 68%.

- It has been suggested that genetic and environmental factors may also confer susceptibility to Mooren ulcer.

Diagnosis

1. Symptoms include severe pain, photophobia and blurred vision due to astigmatism.

2. Signs

- Greyish patch of corneal swelling 2–3 mm from the limbus, often in the interpalpebral zone, quickly followed by ulceration affecting the superficial one-third of the cornea (Fig. 4.117).

- Progressive circumferential and central stromal thinning with an undermined and infiltrated leading edge (Fig. 4.118).

- Vascularisation involving the bed of the ulcer up to its leading edge but not beyond (Fig. 4.119).

- Corneal swelling central to the ulcer, with intact epithelium over the base and adjacent cornea (Fig. 4.120).

- The healing stage is characterised by thinning, vascularisation and scarring (Fig. 4.121).

3. Fluorescein angiography initially shows capillary closure at the limbus and then leakage from vascularisation extending into the base of the ulcer.

4. Complications include severe astigmatism, perforation following minor trauma (spontaneous perforation is rare), secondary bacterial infection, cataract and glaucoma.

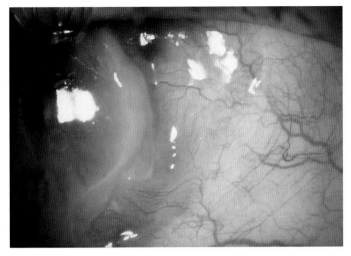

Fig. 4.118 Circumferential and central spread of Mooren ulcer

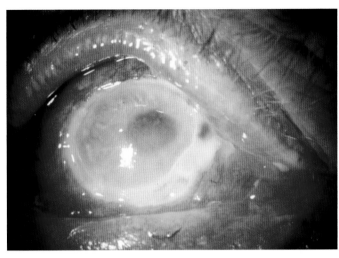

Fig. 4.120 Very advanced Mooren ulcer with central corneal swelling

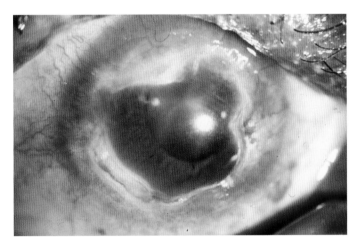

Fig. 4.119 Advanced Mooren ulcer with vascularisation

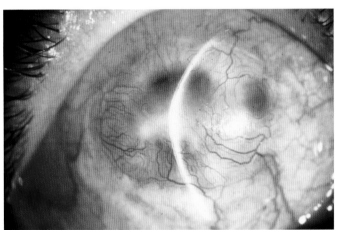

Fig. 4.121 Healed Mooren ulcer

Management

There is no single effective treatment for Mooren ulcer. Untreated, the disease eventually burns itself out over 6 to 18 months, with blindness from a thinned and vascularised cornea. Even with treatment, vision is reduced to light perception in about 18% of eyes. The response to both topical and systemic immunotherapy is poor. The results of corneal grafting are also unsatisfactory, with recurrence of ulceration in the graft. A wide range of therapies has been reported. The following graded therapeutic strategy according to the severity of the disease and the response to initial treatment is recommended.

1. **Topical** treatment initially involves steroids or ciclosporin 1.0%. Other topical treatments include artificial tears and collagenase inhibitors (acetylcysteine 10%, L-cysteine 0.2 Molar).

2. **Conjunctival resection or cryotherapy**, which may be combined with excision of necrotic tissue, may be effective for unilateral but not bilateral disease. Treatment should extend 4 mm back from the limbus and 2 mm beyond the margins of the lesion. Conjunctival resection may be combined with keratoepithelioplasty to produce a physical barrier against conjunctival regrowth and further melting.

3. **Systemic** immunosuppression should be instituted earlier for bilateral disease, or if involvement is advanced at first examination. Traditionally, treatment has been with cyclophosphamide, but more recently, ciclosporin (5 mg/kg) has also been shown to be effective.

4. **Surgery**

- Primary lamellar keratoplasty is generally contraindicated, although there have been some good reports when it is combined with topical ciclosporin.

- Lamellar dissection of the residual central island in advanced disease may remove the stimulus for further inflammation.

- Cyanoacrylate glue may be used to treat perforations.

- Reconstruction should ideally involve lamellar surgery with systemic immunosuppression cover to reduce the risk of recurrence; without systemic cover, the recurrence rate is about 25%.

FURTHER READING

Bernauer W, Ficker LA, Watson PG, et al. The management of corneal perforations associated with rheumatoid arthritis. *Ophthalmology* 1995;102:1325–1327.

Chen J, Xie H, Wang Z, et al. Mooren's ulcer in China: a study of clinical characteristics and treatment. *Br J Ophthalmol* 2000;84:1244–1249.

Chow CYC, Foster CS. Mooren's ulcer. *Int Ophthalmol Clin* 1996;36:1–13.

Foster CS. Systemic immunosuppressive therapy for progressive bilateral Mooren's ulcer. *Ophthalmology* 1985;92:1436–1439.

Geerling G, Joussen AM, Daniels JT, et al. Matrix metalloproteinases in sterile corneal melts. *Ann N Y Acad Sci* 1999;878;571–574.

Ladas JG, Mondino BJ. Systemic disorders associated with peripheral corneal ulceration. *Curr Opin Ophthalmol* 2000;11:468–471.

Lewallen S, Courtright P. Problems with current concepts of the epidemiology of Mooren's corneal ulcer. *Ann Ophthalmol* 1990;22:52–55.

McKibben M, Isaacs JD, Morrell AJ. Incidence of corneal melting in association with systemic disease in the Yorkshire region, 1995–7. *Br J Ophthalmol* 1999;83:941–943.

Messmer EM, Foster CS. Vasculitic peripheral ulcerative keratitis. *Surv Ophthalmol* 1999;43:379–396.

Moazami G, Auran JD, Florakis GJ, et al. Interferon treatment of Mooren's ulcers associated with hepatitis C. *Am J Ophthalmol* 1995;119:365–366.

Reynolds I, Tullo AB, John SL, et al. Corneal epithelial-specific cytokeratin 3 is an autoantigen in Wegener's granulomatosis-associated peripheral ulcerative keratitis. *Invest Ophthalmol Vis Sci* 1999;40:2147–2151.

Tauber J, Saunz de la Maza M, Hoang-Xuan T, et al. An analysis of therapeutic decision making regarding immunosuppressive chemotherapy for peripheral ulcerative keratitis. *Cornea* 1990;9:66–73.

Taylor CJ, Smith SI, Morgan CH, et al. HLA and Mooren's ulceration. *Br J Ophthalmol* 2000;84:72–75.

Watson PG. Management of Mooren's ulceration. *Eye* 1997;11:349–356.

Zegans ME, Srinivasan M. Mooren's ulcer. *Int Ophthalmol Clin* 1998;38:81–88.

NEUROTROPHIC AND EXPOSURE KERATITIS

Neurotrophic keratitis

Neurotrophic keratopathy occurs when there is loss of the trigeminal innervation to the cornea, resulting in partial or complete anaesthesia.

Pathogenesis

Sensory innervation is vital to the health of the corneal epithelium and stroma. The loss of neural influences results in intracellular oedema, exfoliation of the epithelial cells, impairment of epithelial healing and loss of goblet cells, culminating in epithelial breakdown and persistent ulceration. Loss of acetylcholine, substance P and growth factors from the epithelium appears to be important.

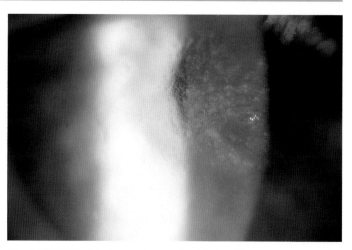

Fig. 4.122 Epithelial changes in neurotrophic keratitis

Causes

1. **Acquired damage** to the fifth cranial nerve or trigeminal ganglion following surgical ablation for trigeminal neuralgia (tic douloureux), stroke, aneurysm, multiple sclerosis or tumour (acoustic neuroma or neurofibroma).

2. **Systemic diseases** such as diabetes and leprosy.

3. **Ocular disease** such as herpes simplex and herpes zoster keratitis, abuse of topical anaesthetic, chemical burn and refractive corneal surgery.

4. **Congenital** causes include familial dysautonomia (Riley–Day syndrome), Möbius syndrome, Goldenhar–Gorlin syndrome, anhidrotic ectodermal dysplasia and hereditary sensory neuropathy.

Diagnosis

The severity of signs can vary during the course of disease. Some patients develop serious lesions early while others only develop problems after many years.

1. **Examination**

- Corneal sensation should be evaluated with a wisp of cotton or an anaesthesiometer (<5 mm is clinically significant).

- The blink rate, Bell's phenomenon, tear film and lid position should be evaluated.

2. **Signs**

- Punctate keratopathy in the interpalpebral zone in which the epithelium appears irregular, slightly opaque and oedematous (Fig. 4.122).

- Persistent epithelial defect in which the epithelium at the edge of the lesion appears rolled and thickened, and is poorly attached (Figs 4.123 and 4.124).

- Superficial neovascularisation, stromal oedema and sterile hypopyon.

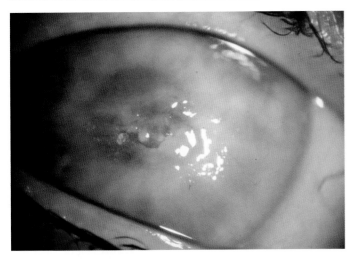

Fig. 4.123 Early epithelial defect in neurotrophic keratitis

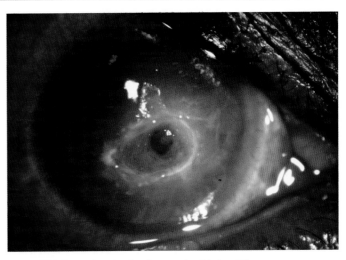

Fig. 4.125 Corneal perforation in neurotrophic keratitis

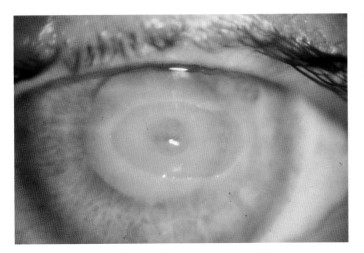

Fig. 4.124 Large epithelial defect in neurotrophic keratitis

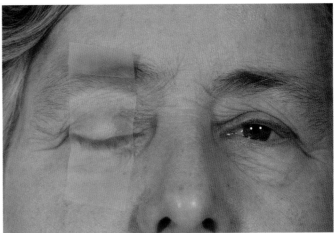

Fig. 4.126 Taping of the lids in neurotrophic keratitis

- Stromal corneal melting and perforation (Fig. 4.125) are uncommon but can occur rapidly if there is secondary infection.

> **NB:** Progression to ulceration may be virtually asymptomatic.

Management

1. **Topical** lubricants (non-preserved) for associated dry eye or corneal exposure. Topical insulin-like growth factor-1, substance P and neurogenic growth factor have been evaluated but are not commercially available.

> **NB:** It is also important to eliminate potentially toxic medications already in use.

2. **Protection of the ocular surface**

- Simple taping of the lids may provide temporary protection (Fig. 4.126).

- Botulinum toxin injection to induce protective ptosis (Fig. 4.127).

- Temporary central tarsorrhaphy tied with a bow or a Frost suture (Fig. 4.128).

- Permanent tarsorrhaphy (Fig. 4.129) may help prevent drying and reduce exposure.

- Therapeutic silicone rubber contact lens, provided the eye is carefully monitored for infection.

- Amniotic membrane onlay with temporary central tarsorrhaphy, or a limbal sparing conjunctival flap if other treatments fail.

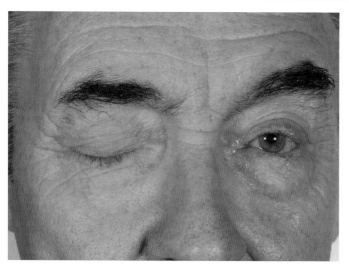

Fig. 4.127 Ptosis induced by botulinum toxin injection into the levator muscle

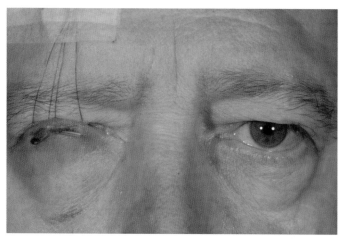

Fig. 4.128 Frost suture in neurotrophic keratitis

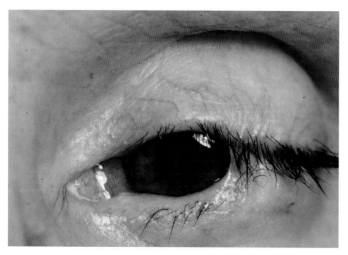

Fig. 4.129 Permanent lateral tarsorrhaphy in neurotrophic keratitis

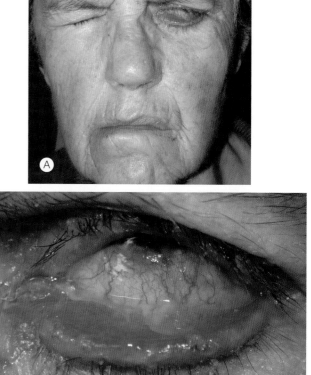

Fig. 4.130 (a) Left lagophthalmos due to facial palsy; (b) paralytic ectropion and exposure keratitis

Exposure keratitis

Pathogenesis

Exposure keratopathy is the result of incomplete lid closure (lagophthalmos) during blinking. Mild exposure during sleep is normal in some individuals but may become symptomatic if there is a poor Bell's phenomenon. Lagophthalmos may be present only on blinking or gentle lid closure, but absent on forced lid closure. The result is drying of the cornea despite normal tear production.

Causes

1. **Neuroparalytic**, especially facial nerve palsy (Fig. 4.130), which may be idiopathic or the result of surgery for acoustic neuroma or parotid tumour.

2. **Reduced muscle tone** as in coma or parkinsonism.

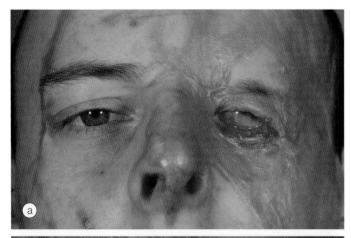

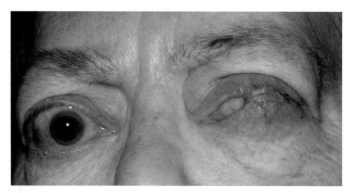

Fig. 4.133 Proptosis due to thyroid ophthalmopathy requiring tarsorrhaphy for exposure keratitis

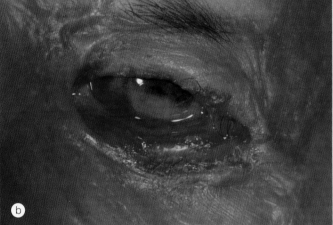

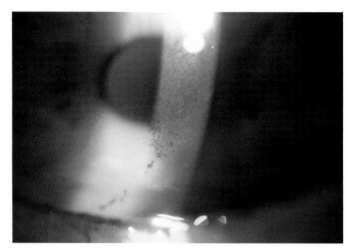

Fig. 4.131 (a) Left lagophthalmos due to severe burns; (b) cicatricial ectropion and exposure keratitis

Fig. 4.134 Inferior epithelial changes in early exposure keratitis

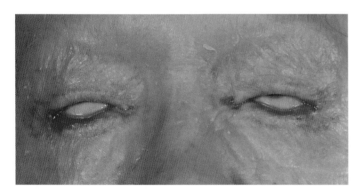

Fig. 4.132 Bilateral lagophthalmos due to tight facial skin

3. Mechanical

- Eyelid scarring associated with cicatricial pemphigoid, burns (Fig. 4.131) and trauma.

- Tight facial skin due to severe eczema (Fig. 4.132), solar keratosis, xeroderma pigmentosa and following blepharoplasty.

4. Abnormality of globe position

- Severe proptosis resulting in lagophthalmos due to thyroid ophthalmopathy (Fig. 4.133) or orbital tumour.

- Severe enophthalmos.

Diagnosis

1. **Symptoms** are those of a dry eye.

2. **Signs**

- Mild punctate epithelial changes involving the inferior third of the cornea (Fig. 4.134), particularly with nocturnal lagophthalmos.

- Epithelial breakdown (Fig. 4.135).

- Stromal melting, which may result in perforation (Figs 4.136 and 4.137).

- Secondary infection may supervene at any stage (Fig. 4.138).

- Inferior fibrovascular change with Salzmann degeneration may develop over time.

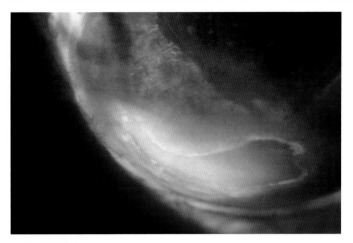

Fig. 4.135 Inferior epithelial defect in exposure keratopathy

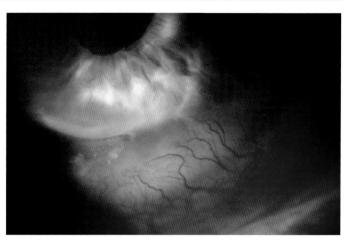

Fig. 4.137 Advanced stromal melting in exposure keratitis

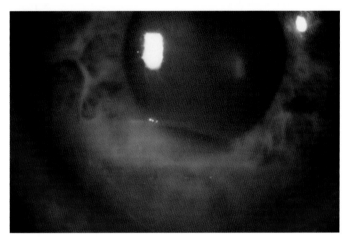

Fig. 4.136 Early stromal melting in exposure keratitis

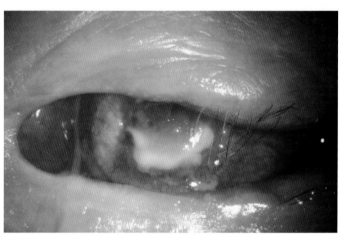

Fig. 4.138 Secondary bacterial keratitis in exposure keratitis

Management

Management is dependent on the severity of exposure and whether recovery is anticipated.

1. Reversible exposure

- Artificial tears (non-preserved) during the day and ointment at night.

- Taping the lid closed at night may be an alternative to ointment. Taping or antibiotic ointment are essential for ventilated patients.

- Bandage silicone rubber or scleral contact lenses.

- Temporary tarsorrhaphy or Frost suture.

2. Permanent exposure

- Permanent lateral or median tarsorrhaphy.

- Gold weights inserted in the upper lid for seventh nerve palsy.

- Permanent central tarsorrhaphy and conjunctival flap may be required for severe cases.

- Management of proptosis by orbital decompression if necessary.

> **NB:** Combined neuroparalytic and neurotrophic keratopathy is particularly difficult to manage.

FURTHER READING

Bonini S, Rama P, Olzi D, et al. Neurotrophic keratitis. *Eye* 2003;17:989–995.

Chikama T, Fukuda K, Morishige N, et al. Treatment of neurotrophic keratopathy with substance-P-derived peptide (FGLM) and insulin growth factor 1. *Lancet* 1998;351:1783–1784.

Donzis PB, Mondino BJ. Management of noninfectious corneal ulcers. *Surv Ophthalmol* 1987;32:94–110.

Lambiase A, Rama P, Bonini S, et al. Topical treatment with nerve growth factor for neurotrophic keratitis. *N Engl J Med* 1998;338:1174–1180.

Lambiase A, Rama P, Aloe L, et al. Management of neurotrophic keratopathy. *Curr Opin Ophthalmol* 1999;10:270–276.

Lee SH, Tseng SC. Amniotic membrane transplantation for persistent epithelial defects with ulceration. *Am J Ophthalmol* 1997;123:303–312.

CONTACT LENS-RELATED KERATITIS

Most of the oxygen for corneal metabolism is supplied from the atmosphere and diffuses from the tear film. The endothelium is supplied from the aqueous. A contact lens lies within the tear film and is a barrier to the diffusion of oxygen to the cornea. Lens movement and circulation of oxygenated tears behind the lens is an important mechanism of providing oxygen to the cornea. The presence of a contact lens may modify the normal circulation of tears, cause mechanical and hypoxic damage to the tissues, and bind proteins and debris that are then kept in contact with the ocular surface. Contact lens care products can be associated with both acute and chronic keratopathy. Extended-wear contact lenses, poor lens hygiene and poor lens fit are particular risk factors for complications. After long-term contact lens wear, the epithelium becomes thinner and less sensitive to touch. The wearing of contact lenses may also exacerbate pre-existing disease. Contact lens-associated giant papillary conjunctivitis is described in Chapter 3.

Mechanical and hypoxic keratitis

Pathogenesis

The oxygen transmission through the lens (Dk/t value) may be insufficient. A tightly fitting contact lens, which does not move with blinking, will impair tear circulation under the lens. This is exacerbated by lid closure if the lens is worn during sleep. Hypoxia leads to anaerobic metabolism and lactic acidosis that inhibits the normal barrier and pump mechanisms of the cornea. The cornea may be abraded by the contact lens or by a foreign body trapped by the lens.

Diagnosis

- Superficial punctate keratopathy is the most common complication. The pattern may give a clue as to the aetiology. For example, staining at 3 o'clock and 9 o'clock (Fig. 4.139) is associated with incomplete blinking and drying in rigid lens wearers.

- The tight lens syndrome is characterised by indentation and staining of the conjunctival epithelium in a ring around the cornea.

- Acute hypoxia is characterised by epithelial microcysts (Fig. 4.140) and necrosis, and endothelial blebs. Very painful macroerosions may develop only several hours after lenses are removed following a period of overwear.

- Chronic hypoxia may result in neovascularisation (Fig. 4.141) and lipid deposition (Fig. 4.142).

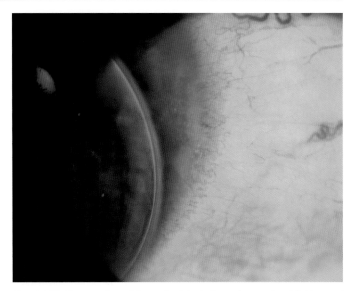

Fig. 4.139 Fluorescein staining at 3 o'clock due to incomplete blinking and drying

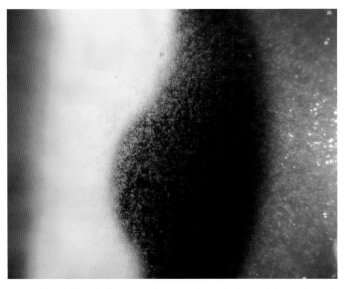

Fig. 4.140 Epithelial microcysts due to acute contact lens-induced hypoxia

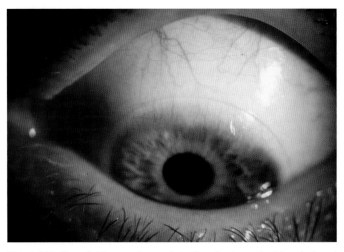

Fig. 4.141 Superficial corneal vascularisation due to contact lens-induced chronic hypoxia

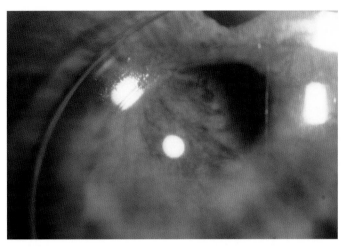

Fig. 4.142 Lipid deposition due to contact lens-induced chronic hypoxia

- After decades of hard contact lens wear, the endothelial cell count may be slightly reduced.

Management

Management depends on the cause and may involve the following:

- Oxygen permeability can be increased by refitting with a thinner lens or one with a higher Dk/t value such as a gas-permeable rigid lens or silicone hydrogel soft lens.

- Modifying lens fit to increase movement.

- Reducing lens wearing time.

> **NB:** Superficial peripheral neovascularisation of <1.5 mm is common in myopic contact lens wearers and can be monitored.

Immune response keratitis

Pathogenesis

Contact lens acute red eye (CLARE) may be associated with marginal corneal infiltrates which are thought to be the result of sensitisation to bacterial toxins. The mechanism is similar to the development of marginal infiltrates associated with blepharitis.

Diagnosis

- Red eye associated with marginal infiltrates with no or minimal epithelial defects (Fig. 4.143).

Management

Contact lens wear should be stopped until resolution occurs. Topical antibiotic and steroid may be used in severe cases, but if the diagnosis is uncertain, treatment should be that of sup-

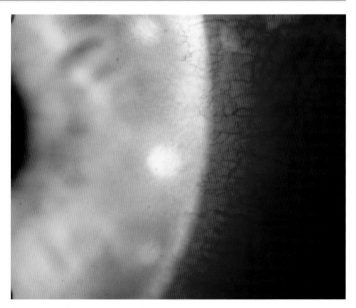

Fig. 4.143 Sterile marginal infiltrates in immune-response contact lens-related keratitis

purative keratitis. It is also important to review lens fit and hygiene.

Toxic keratitis

Pathogenesis

Acute chemical injury may be caused by placing a contact lens on the eye without neutralising hydrogen peroxide or surfactant cleaners. Chronic toxicity can result from long-term exposure to disinfecting agents such as thiomersal or benzalkonium chloride. The mechanism of thiomersal keratopathy may have been partly an induced hypersensitivity response resulting in apparent corneal epithelial stem cell failure. Thiomersal has been withdrawn from lens care products, but established cases are still seen.

Diagnosis

- Acute pain, redness and chemosis on lens insertion, which may take 48 hours to resolve completely.

- Vascularisation and conjunctivalisation of the cornea (Fig. 4.144).

- Scarring of the limbal conjunctiva.

Management

Daily disposable contact lenses should be fitted and a non-preserved disinfectant used, such as hydrogen peroxide or heat.

> **NB:** In some patients with persistent problems associated with contact lens wear, refractive corneal surgery is an alternative for visual correction.

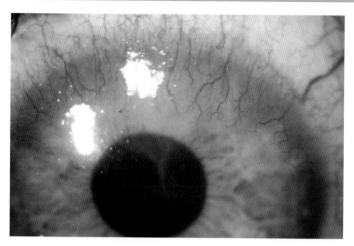

Fig. 4.144 Corneal vascularisation due to thiomersal toxicity (Courtesy of J Dart)

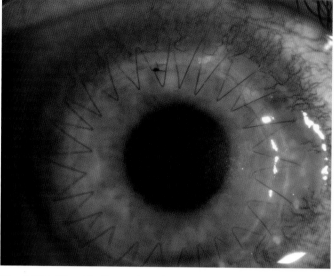

Fig. 4.145 Ciliary injection and anterior uveitis in pre-rejection

Suppurative keratitis

Contact lens wear is the greatest risk factor for the development of bacterial keratitis. The risk is least for rigid contact lenses. Bacteria in the tear film are normally unable to bind to the corneal epithelium. Following an abrasion and hypoxia, bacteria can attach and penetrate the epithelium, with the potential to cause infection. Bacteria and amoeba may also be introduced onto the corneal surface by poor lens hygiene or the use of tap water. *Pseudomonas aeruginosa* and *Acanthamoeba* species are significantly more associated with soft contact lens wear.

FURTHER READING

Bates AK, Morris RJ, Stapleton F, et al. 'Sterile' corneal infiltrates in contact lens wearers. *Eye* 1989;3:803–810.

MacRae SM, Matsuda M, Phillips DS. The long-term effects of polymethylmethacrylate contact lens wear on the corneal endothelium. *Ophthalmology* 1994;101:365–370.

Schein OD, Buehler PO, Stamler JF, et al. The impact of overnight wear on the risk of contact lens-associated ulcerative keratitis. *Arch Ophthalmol* 1994;112:186–189.

Stamler JF. The complications of contact lens wear. *Curr Opin Ophthalmol* 1998;9:66–71.

Suchecki JK, Donshik P, Ehlers WH. Contact lens complications. *Ophthalmol Clin North Am* 2003;16:471–484.

Wilson-Holt N, Dart JK. Thiomersal keratoconjunctivitis, frequency, clinical spectrum and diagnosis. *Eye* 1989;3:581–587.

CORNEAL ALLOGRAFT REJECTION AND DIFFUSE LAMELLAR KERATITIS

Corneal allograft rejection

Approximately 40 000 corneal grafts are performed each year in the USA (2300 in the UK). Allograft rejection can occur following penetrating keratoplasty and, less commonly, lamellar grafts. Rejection of any layer of the cornea can occur. Endothelial rejection is the most common and most severe, as it can lead to severe endothelial cell loss and decompensation. Late graft failure through decompensation can also occur in the absence of further rejection episodes. Stromal rejection and epithelial rejection are less frequent and respond readily to topical steroid treatment, with few long-term consequences. Elements of the different types of rejection can coexist.

Pathogenesis

The cornea is immunologically privileged and a normal cornea will usually not reject. However, if there is inflammation, this privilege is lost and rejection may occur. Other important predisposition for rejection includes corneal vascularisation, grafts over 8 mm in diameter, eccentric grafts, infection, glaucoma and previous keratoplasty. If the host becomes sensitised to the major or minor histocompatibility antigens present in the donor cornea, a type IV hypersensitivity can develop against the graft, and rejection and graft failure may result. Antigen-presenting cells in the donor cornea may initiate this process. HLA class I matching has a small beneficial effect on graft survival.

Diagnosis

1. **Symptoms** of graft rejection include blurred vision, photophobia and a dull periocular ache. However, many cases are asymptomatic until advanced rejection is established.

2. **Signs**

- Ciliary injection and anterior uveitis is a pre-rejection manifestation (Fig. 4.145).

- Epithelial rejection may be accompanied by an elevated line of abnormal epithelium (Fig. 4.146).

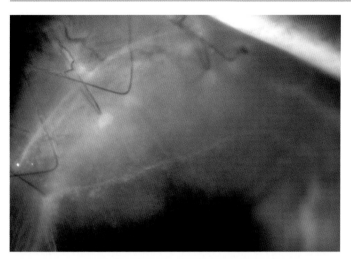

Fig. 4.146 Elevated epithelial line in epithelial rejection

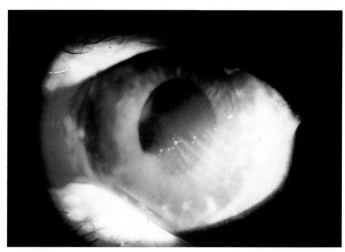

Fig. 4.148 Endothelial line of keratic precipitates (Khodadoust line) in endothelial rejection (Courtesy of D Easty)

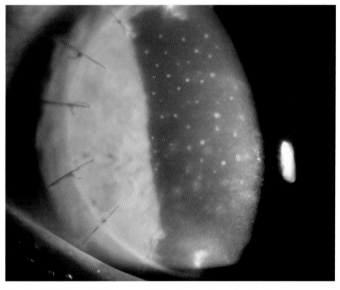

Fig. 4.147 Subepithelial corneal infiltrates in stromal rejection

- Subepithelial infiltrates limited to donor cornea occur in stromal rejection (Fig. 4.147).

- A linear pattern of keratic precipitates may form (endothelial rejection line), usually from an area of inflammation at the graft margin (Fig. 4.148).

- Stromal oedema is indicative of endothelial failure.

Management

Early treatment is essential, as this greatly improves the chances of reversing the rejection episode.

1. **Topical steroids** (dexamethasone phosphate 0.1% or prednisolone acetate 1%) hourly for 24 hours are the mainstay of therapy. The frequency is reduced gradually over several weeks. High-risk patients should be maintained on the highest tolerated topical dose (e.g. prednisolone acetate 1% q.i.d.).

2. **Systemic steroids** (oral prednisolone 1 mg/kg/day in divided doses, or a single intravenous dose of methylprednisolone 500 mg) may help to reverse rejection and prevent further rejection episodes, but only if given within 8 days of onset of rejection.

3. **Subconjunctival steroids** (betamethasone 2 mg) may be useful if compliance to topical therapy is poor.

Failure to reverse rejection occurs in about 10–60% of cases, depending on associated risk factors described above.

Differential diagnosis

Rejection must be distinguished from graft exhaustion, reactivation of HSV, uveitis and epithelial downgrowth.

Diffuse lamellar keratitis

Pathogenesis

Diffuse lamellar keratitis (sands of Sahara) may develop 1 to 7 days following laser in-situ keratomileusis (LASIK). It is characterised by infiltration at the flap interface with mononuclear cells and granulocytes without evidence of infection. Risk factors are meibomian gland disease, epithelial loss and secondary abrasion. Gram-negative endotoxins from water used for sterilising instruments and diffusion of toxins from the tear film are potential stimuli. Dense focal infiltrates can develop at the flap margin in patients with blepharitis.

Diagnosis

1. **Symptoms** are photophobia and blurred vision, although patients with mild cases may be asymptomatic.

2. **Signs**

- Stage 1: granular peripheral deposits.

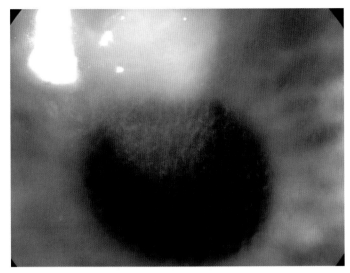

Fig. 4.149 Stage 2 diffuse lamellar keratitis and peripheral bacterial infection following LASIK

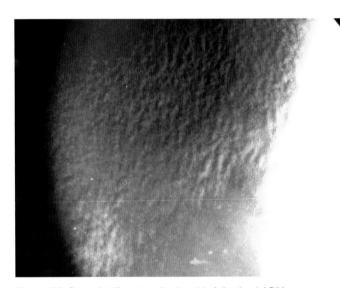

Fig. 4.150 Stage 2 diffuse lamellar keratitis following LASIK

- Stage 2: granular central deposits in the visual axis (Figs 4.149 and 4.150).

- Stage 3: dense central clumps of cells.

- Stage 4: severe keratitis with melting.

Treatment

1. **Topical** intensive antibiotics (fluoroquinolone) and steroids (prednisolone acetate 1%) that will penetrate the epithelium. Treatment is gradually tapered after 48 hours.

2. **Irrigation** of the interface to remove inflammatory material is indicated only in severe cases that do not have flap melting (stage 3).

FURTHER READING

Buhren J, Baumeister M, Kohnen T. Diffuse lamellar keratitis after laser in situ keratomileusis imaged by confocal microscopy. *Ophthalmology* 2001;108:1075–1081.

Coster DJ, Williams KA. Management of high-risk corneal grafts. *Eye* 2003;17:996–1002.

Hill JC, Ivey A. Corticosteroids in corneal graft rejection: double versus single pulse therapy. *Cornea* 1994;13:383–388.

Hill JC, Maske R, Watson P. Corticosteroids in corneal graft rejection. Oral versus single pulse therapy. *Ophthalmology* 1991;98:329–333.

Hudde T, Minassian DC, Larkin DF. Randomised controlled trial of corticosteroid regimens in endothelial corneal allograft rejection. *Br J Ophthalmol* 1999;83:1348–1352.

Knorz MC. Flap and interface complications in LASIK. *Curr Opin Ophthalmol* 2002;13:242–245.

Linebarger EJ, Hardten DR, Lindstrom RL. Diffuse lamellar keratitis: diagnosis and management. *J Cataract Refract Surg* 2000;26:1072–1077.

Melki SA, Azar DT. LASIK complications: etiology, management, and prevention. *Surv Ophthalmol* 2001;46:95–116.

Musch DC, Schwartz AE, Fitzgerald-Shelton K, et al. The effect of allograft rejection after penetrating keratoplasty on central endothelial cell density. *Am J Ophthalmol* 1991;111:739–742.

Perez-Santonja JJ, Sakla HF, Cardona C, et al. Corneal sensitivity after photorefractive keratectomy and laser in situ keratomileusis for low myopia. *Am J Ophthalmol* 1999;127:497–504.

Peters NT, Iskander NG, Anderson Penno EE, et al. Diffuse lamellar keratitis: isolation of endotoxin and demonstration of the inflammatory potential in a rabbit laser in situ keratomileusis model. *J Cataract Refract Surg* 2001;27:917–923.

Rinne JR, Stulting RD. Current practices in the prevention and treatment of corneal graft rejection. *Cornea* 1992;11:326–328.

Smith RJ, Maloney RK. Diffuse lamellar keratitis: a new syndrome in lamellar refractive surgery. *Ophthalmology* 1998;105:1721–1726.

Solomon A, Karp CL, Miller D, et al. Mycobacterium interface keratitis after laser in situ keratomileusis. *Ophthalmology* 2001;108:2201–2208.

MISCELLANEOUS KERATITIS

Infectious crystalline keratitis

Pathogenesis

Infectious crystalline keratitis is a rare, indolent infection usually associated with long-term topical steroid therapy where there has been an epithelial defect. It is most frequently seen following treatment after penetrating keratoplasty, chronic ocular surface disease, herpes simplex keratitis or atopic keratoconjunctivitis. *Strep. viridans* is most commonly isolated, although numerous other bacteria and fungi have been implicated. The mechanism appears to be slow proliferation of low-virulence organisms along the plane of stromal lamellae when the inflammatory response has been suppressed. Bacteria may also grow within a protective biofilm (bacterial extracellular matrix), which could explain the lack of inflammation and the relative resistance to therapy.

Diagnosis

- Slowly progressive, grey–white, branching opacities in the anterior or mid stroma, with minimal inflammation and usually intact overlying epithelium (Figs 4.151–4.153).

- Corneal culture or corneal biopsy to determine the organism.

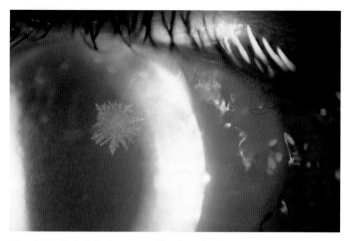

Fig. 4.151 Early infectious crystalline keratitis (Courtesy of M Kerr-Muir)

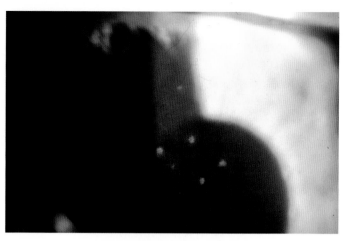

Fig. 4.154 Thygeson superficial punctate keratitis

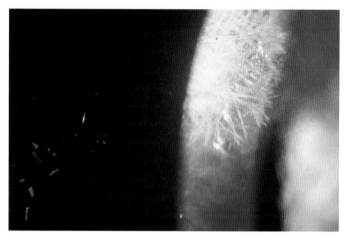

Fig. 4.152 Advanced infectious crystalline keratitis (Courtesy of M Kerr-Muir)

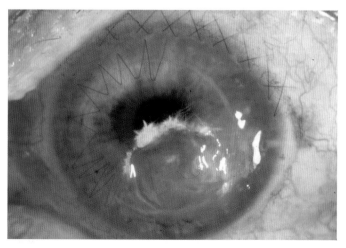

Fig. 4.153 Infectious crystalline keratitis on a corneal graft

Treatment

* Topical antibiotics are effective but have to be used for several weeks.

* Stopping topical steroid without adequate antibiotic cover can precipitate a rapid increase in inflammation and even suppuration.

* Management of associated disease such as ocular allergy is important.

Thygeson superficial punctate keratitis

Thygeson disease is an uncommon, usually bilateral condition of unknown aetiology, characterised by exacerbations and remissions. It most commonly affects young adults but may occur at any age and recurrences can continue for decades. Although reports of virus isolation exist, these have not been repeatable, and examination for HZV antigen by PCR has been negative. It has been linked to HLA-DR3.

Diagnosis

1. **Presentation** is with ocular irritation, photophobia and blurred vision.

2. **Signs**

* Coarse, distinct, granular, greyish, elevated epithelial lesions (Figs 4.154 and 4.155).

* A mild subepithelial haze may be present (Fig. 4.156), especially if topical idoxuridine has been used.

NB: The conjunctiva is uninvolved and vascularisation is not a feature. The most common differential diagnosis is staphylococcal hypersensitivity punctate epitheliopathy and post-adenoviral keratitis.

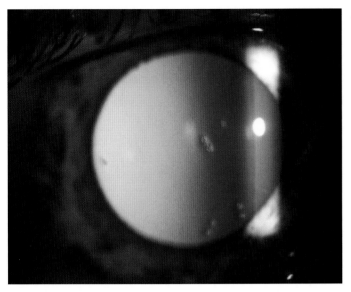

Fig. 4.155 Thygeson superficial punctate keratitis on retroillumination

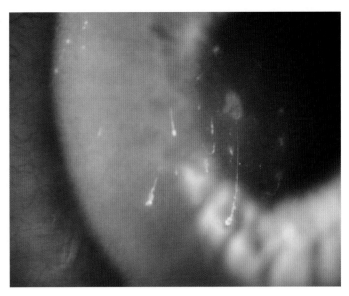

Fig. 4.157 Fine corneal filaments

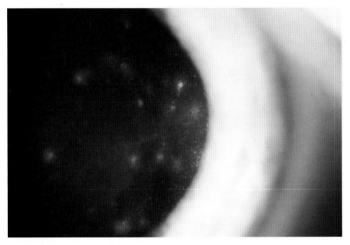

Fig. 4.156 Thygeson superficial punctate keratitis with mild subepithelial haze (Courtesy of R Curtis)

Treatment

1. Topical

- Lubricants may suffice in mild cases.

- Steroids (fluorometholone 0.1% b.d) initially, with gradual tapering. In some cases, long-term low-dose therapy (one drop weekly) may be required.

- Ciclosporin 2% may be effective in steroid-resistant cases.

2. Contact lenses (extended wear or daily disposable soft) may be considered if steroids are contraindicated. Most patients can be instructed to manage these themselves.

3. Phototherapeutic keratectomy brings short-term relief but eventual recurrence is likely.

NB: Topical steroids may delay eventual resolution.

Filamentary keratitis

Pathogenesis

Filamentary keratitis is a common condition that can cause considerable discomfort. A loose area of epithelium acts as a focus for deposition of mucus and cellular debris. Causes include the following:

- Aqueous deficiency dry eye (keratoconjunctivitis sicca) is the most common.

- Corneal epithelial instability (recurrent erosion syndrome, corneal graft, cataract surgery, refractive surgery and drug toxicity).

- Superior limbic keratoconjunctivitis.

- Neurotrophic keratitis.

- Prolonged occlusion as from patching or associated with essential blepharospasm.

Diagnosis

1. Symptoms are discomfort and foreign body sensation.

2. Signs

- Strands of degenerating epithelial cells and mucus attached at one end to the cornea that move with blinking (Figs 4.157 and 4.158).

- Filaments stain with fluorescein (Fig. 4.159) and rose bengal.

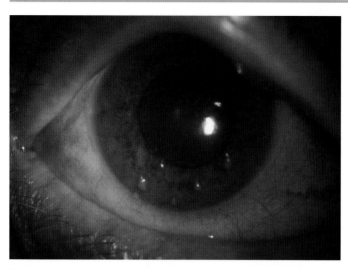

Fig. 4.158 Coarse corneal filaments

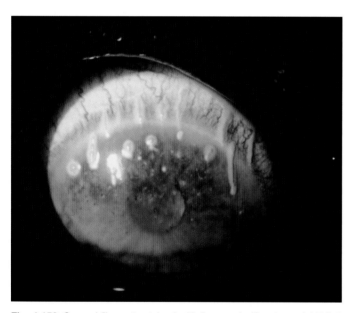

Fig. 4.159 Corneal filaments stained with fluorescein (Courtesy of J Talks)

- A small epithelial defect may be present at the base of a filament.

Management

1. General

- Underlying cause such as dry eye should be treated (see Ch. 2).

- All unnecessary medications should be stopped.

- Short-term topical steroids.

- Non-steroidal anti-inflammatory drops such as diclofenac may also be used and they also seem to have an anaesthetic effect.

2. Specific treatment for filaments

- Mechanical removal of filaments for short-term symptomatic relief.

- Hypertonic 5% saline to encourage adhesion of loose epithelium.

- Mucolytic agents such as 5% or 10% acetylcysteine.

- Bandage contact lenses to protect the surface of the eye from the shearing action of the lids. They are justified only for short-term use because of the risk of infection.

Xerophthalmia

Pathogenesis

Ascorbic acid is an essential fat-soluble vitamin in humans as it cannot be synthesised. In the eye, it is essential for the synthesis of retinal photopigments and conjunctival glycoproteins. It is also essential for normal immunity, and deficiency leads to susceptibility to respiratory, intestinal and genitourinary infection. Lack of vitamin A in the diet may be caused by malnutrition, malabsorption (coeliac disease, cystic fibrosis, small bowel resection), chronic alcoholism or highly selective dieting. Xerophthalmia is a spectrum of ocular disease caused by vitamin A deficiency. It is responsible for up to 100 000 new cases of blindness worldwide each year and is the leading cause of childhood blindness. The risk in infants is increased if their mothers are malnourished and by coexisting diarrhoea or measles (see below).

Diagnosis

1. Symptoms are night blindness (nyctalopia) and ocular irritation due to dryness.

2. Conjunctiva

- Xerosis is characterised by dryness of the conjunctiva in the interpalpebral zone, with loss of goblet cells, squamous metaplasia and keratinisation.

- Bitot spots are triangular patches of foamy keratinised epithelium in the interpalpebral zone (Fig. 4.160) thought to be caused by infection with *Corynebacterium xerosis*.

Table 4.5 WHO grading of xerophthalmia
XN = night blindness
X1 = conjunctival xerosis (X1A) with Bitot spot (X1B)
X2 = corneal xerosis
X3 = corneal ulceration, less than one-third (X3A); more than one-third (X3B)
XS = corneal scar
XF = xerophthalmic fundus

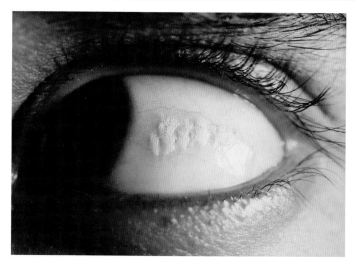

Fig. 4.160 Bitot spot (Courtesy of U Raina)

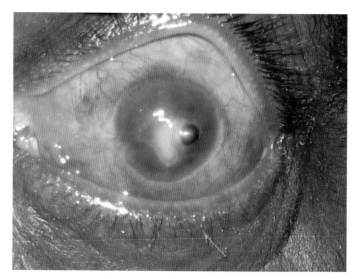

Fig. 4.161 Keratomalacia with perforation (Courtesy of S Kumar Puri)

3. Cornea

- Lustreless appearance due to secondary xerosis.

- Bilateral punctate corneal epithelial erosions in the interpalpebral zone which can progress to epithelial defect but are reversible with treatment.

- Sterile corneal melting by colliquative necrosis (keratomalacia) which may result in perforation (Fig. 4.161).

4. Retinopathy characterised by yellowish peripheral dots may occur in advanced cases and is associated with decreased electroretinogram amplitude.

Investigations

Investigations are not generally required and the diagnosis is usually confirmed by response to treatment. Impression cytology shows loss of goblet cells and squamous metaplasia which may detect preclinical xerosis. Serum shows reduced vitamin A and retinol binding proteins.

Management

Keratomalacia is a medical emergency associated with significant mortality.

1. Systemic

- Oral (oil based 200 000 IU) or intramuscular vitamin A (aqueous based 100 000 IU); the latter is indicated for keratomalacia.

- Multivitamin and protein/carbohydrate supplements.

- Dietary sources of vitamin A include milk, meat, eggs and fish (retinol), or green leaf vegetables, yellow fruit and red palm oil (carotene).

2. Local

- Intense lubrication.

- Topical retinoic acid may promote healing but is not sufficient without systemic supplements.

- Emergency surgery for corneal perforation may be necessary.

NB: Children with keratomalacia and perforation usually cannot tolerate general anaesthesia due to general debility, and are thus untreatable.

Measles keratitis

Measles (rubeola) is a highly infectious acute exanthematous disease of childhood transmitted by droplets. Although it has been largely eradicated in developed countries as a result of mass vaccination and good diet, it still remains a major cause of preventable blindness in developing countries. There is a close association between visual loss from measles and vitamin A deficiency (see above). An attack of measles may also precipitate keratomalacia in borderline cases of vitamin A deficiency. Innocuous ocular manifestations of measles include conjunctivitis, subconjunctival haemorrhage and punctate epithelial keratitis.

FURTHER READING

Avisar R, Robinson A, Appel I, et al. Diclofenac sodium, 0.1% (Voltaren Ophtha), versus sodium chloride, 5%, in the treatment of filamentary keratitis. *Cornea* 2000;19:145–147.

Del Castillo JM, Del Castillo JB, Garcia-Sanchez J. Effect of topical cyclosporin A on Thygeson's superficial punctate keratitis. *Doc Ophthalmol* 1996–97;93:193–198.

Fulcher TP, Dart JK, McLaughlin-Borlace L, et al. Demonstration of biofilm in infectious crystalline keratopathy using ruthenium red and electron microscopy. *Ophthalmology* 2001;108:1088–1092.

Grinbaum A, Yassur I, Avni I. The beneficial effect of diclofenac sodium in the treatment of filamentary keratitis. *Arch Ophthalmol* 2001;119:926–927.

Harris EW, Loewenstein JI, Azar D. Vitamin A deficiency and its effects on the eye. *Int Ophthalmol Clin* 1998;38:155–161.

Hunts JH, Matoba AY, Osato MS, et al. Infectious crystalline keratopathy. The role of bacterial exopolysaccharide. *Arch Ophthalmol* 1993;111:528–530.

Nagra PK, Rapuano CJ, Cohen EJ, et al. Thygeson's superficial punctate keratitis: ten years' experience. *Ophthalmology* 2004;111:34–37.

Nelson JD. Superior limbic keratoconjunctivitis (SLK). *Eye* 1989;3:1:80–89.

Reinhard T, Sundmacher R. Topical cyclosporine A in Thygeson's superficial punctate keratitis. *Graefes Arch Clin Exp Ophthalmol* 1999;237:109–112.

Reiss GR, Campbell RJ, Bourne WM. Infectious crystalline keratopathy. *Surv Ophthalmol* 1986;31:69–72.

Semba RD, Bloem MW. Measles blindness. *Surv Ophthalmol* 2004;49:243–255.

Smith J, Steinemann TL. Vitamin A deficiency and the eye. *Int Ophthamol Clin* 2000;40:83–91.

Thygeson P. Superficial punctate keratitis. *JAMA* 1950;144:1544–1549.

Chapter 5

Episcleritis and scleritis

APPLIED ANATOMY

The scleral stroma is composed of collagen bundles of varying size and shape that are not as uniformly orientated as in the cornea. The inner layer of the sclera (lamina fusca) blends with the suprachoroidal and supraciliary lamellae of the uveal tract. Anteriorly, the episclera consists of a dense, vascular connective tissue which lies between the superficial scleral stroma and Tenon capsule. The three vascular layers that cover the anterior sclera are as follows:

1. **The conjunctival vessels** are the most superficial; arteries are tortuous and veins straight.

2. **The superficial episcleral plexus** vessels are straight with a radial configuration.

- In episcleritis, maximal congestion occurs within this vascular plexus (Fig. 5.1). Tenon capsule and the episclera are infiltrated with inflammatory cells, but the sclera itself is not swollen.

- Instillation of topical phenylephrine will cause blanching of the conjunctival and, to a certain extent, the superficial episcleral vessels, allowing visualisation of the underlying sclera.

3. **The deep vascular plexus** lies in the superficial part of the sclera and shows maximal congestion in scleritis (Fig. 5.2). There is also inevitably some engorgement of the superficial vessels, but this should be ignored. Topical phenylephrine has no effect on the engorgement of deep vessels. Examination in daylight is important to localise the level of maximal injection. The scleral stroma is largely avascular.

EPISCLERITIS

Episcleritis is a common benign, recurrent, self-limiting and frequently bilateral condition. The cause of episcleritis is still far from clear. Very occasionally a history of exogenous sen-sitisation is given, e.g. house dust mites or history of atopy. Sometimes there is a definite psychogenic background. Association with systemic disease is present in about 30% of patients, particularly in those with frequent recurrences.

Simple episcleritis

Simple episcleritis accounts for three-quarters of all cases and predominantly affects females. It has a great tendency to recur either in the same eye, or sometimes in both eyes together. The attacks become less frequent and after many years disappear completely.

Diagnosis

1. **Presentation** is almost always sudden, the eye becoming red and uncomfortable within an hour of the start of an attack. The most common sensations described are hotness, pricking or generalised discomfort. Pain is

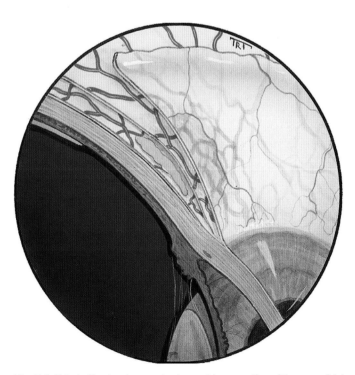

Fig. 5.1 Episcleritis showing maximal vascular congestion of the superficial episcleral plexus

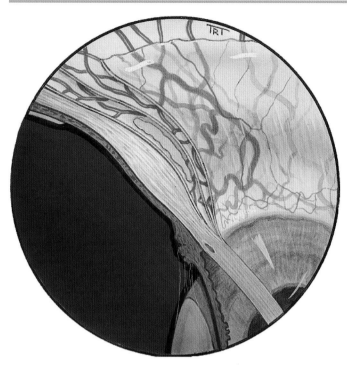

Fig. 5.2 Scleritis showing scleral thickening and maximal vascular congestion of the deep vascular plexus

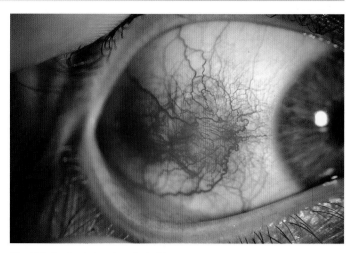

Fig. 5.3 Sectoral simple episcleritis

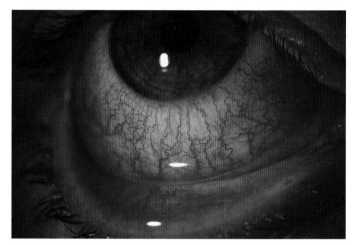

Fig. 5.4 Diffuse simple episcleritis

unusual but if it occurs it is localised to the eye itself and does not radiate to the face or temple.

2. Signs

- Redness may vary from a mild red flush to fiery, and may be sectoral (Fig. 5.3) or diffuse (Fig. 5.4). Often it has an interpalpebral distribution, in contrast with scleral disease, which most commonly starts in the upper temporal or upper nasal quadrants.

- The attack reaches its peak within 12 hours and then gradually fades over the next 10 to 21 days.

- The episcleritis usually flits from one eye to the other or may be bilateral. Some patients always have attacks in the same place.

3. Fluorescein angiography (FA) of the anterior segment, not necessary for diagnosis, typically shows rapid filling and extensive leakage; the vascular pattern is undisturbed (Fig. 5.5).

Treatment

1. First attack. If the patient is seen within 48 hours of onset, topical steroids may be used half-hourly during the day for 2 days, then q.i.d. for 1 day, b.d. for 1 day, and daily for 2 days. The regressive phase requires no treatment other than cold artificial tears for symptomatic relief.

2. Recurrent attacks, if mild, require no treatment other than cold artificial tears. Treatment of extremely frequent or disabling attacks involves a systemic non-steroidal anti-inflammatory drug (NSAID) such as flurbiprofen 100 mg t.i.d. for 10 days. If recurrences occur thereafter, long-term treatment or a change of drug may be necessary.

Nodular episcleritis

Nodular episcleritis also tends to affect young females but has a less acute onset and a more prolonged course than simple episcleritis.

Diagnosis

1. Presentation is with a red eye, typically first noted on waking.

- Over the next 2 to 3 days, the area of redness increases in size but remains in the same position.

- During the same period, the eye becomes more uncomfortable, and by the time the disease is at its height, is very tender.

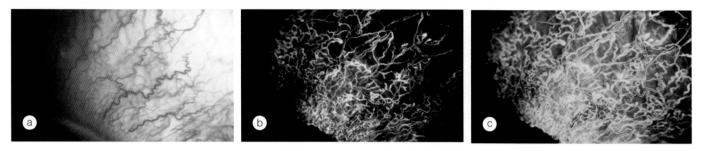

Fig. 5.5 (a) Simple episcleritis; (b) fluorescein angiogram, after 15 seconds, shows filling of the capillaries but not the large veins; (c) thereafter, there is rapid leakage, but the vascular pattern remains normal (Courtesy of Watson, Hazleman, Pavésio and Green, from *The Sclera and Systemic Disorders*, 2nd edition, Butterworth-Heinemann, 2004)

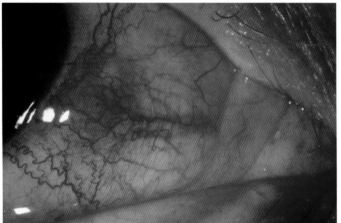

Fig. 5.6 Nodular episcleritis

2. Signs

- One or more tender nodules, almost always within the interpalpebral fissure (Fig. 5.6).

- A thin slit-lamp section shows that the anterior scleral surface is flat, indicating absence of scleral involvement (Fig. 5.7).

- Instillation of 10% phenylephrine drops will decongest the conjunctival and episcleral vessels, allowing better visualisation of underlying sclera.

- Each attack is self-limiting and usually clears without treatment but lasts longer than simple episcleritis.

- After several attacks, the vessels surrounding the inflamed area become permanently dilated.

- Scleral translucency may occur following multiple attacks involving the same location (Fig. 5.8).

3. FA shows rapid filling and hyperfluorescence of the nodule due to leakage but the vascular pattern is undisturbed (Fig. 5.9).

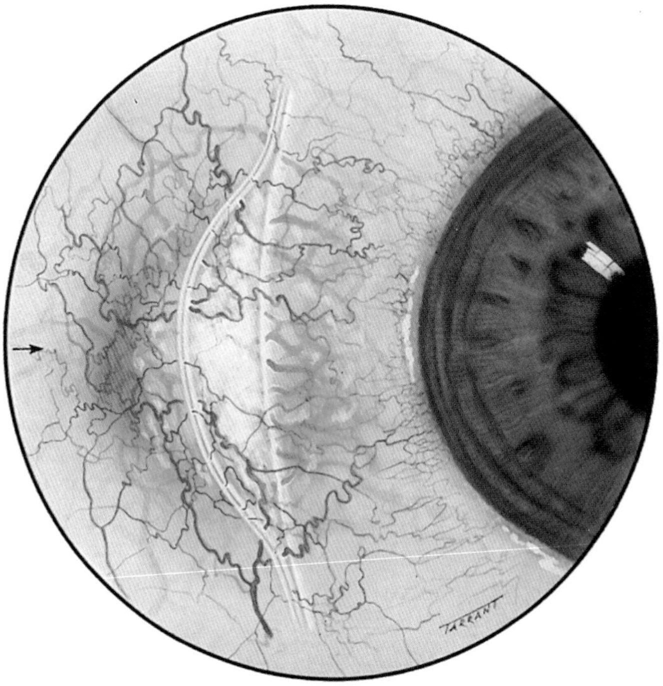

Fig. 5.7 Slit-lamp examination of an episcleral nodule shows that the deep beam is not displaced above the scleral surface (Courtesy of P Watson)

Treatment

1. **First attack.** Patients seen within 48 hours of onset should be treated with intensive topical steroids.

2. **Recurrent attacks** unusual require no treatment, but, if necessary, an NSAID can be used for 2–3 months.

> **NB:** It is important to exclude a local cause for an episcleral nodule, such as a foreign body or granuloma.

SCLERITIS

Scleritis is an uncommon condition characterised by oedema and cellular infiltration of the entire thickness of the sclera.

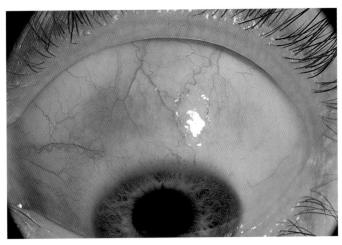

Fig. 5.8 Slight scleral transparency following recurrent nodular episcleritis

Table 5.1 Classification of scleritis

Anterior
Non-necrotising
• Diffuse
• Nodular
Necrotising with inflammation
• Vaso-occlusive
• Granulomatous
Scleromalacia performans
Infective

Posterior
• Diffuse
• Nodular
• Necrotising

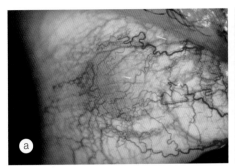
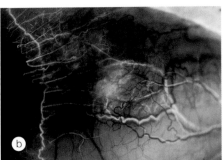
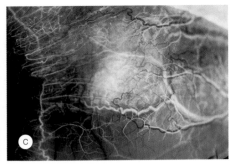

Fig. 5.9 (a) Nodular episcleritis; (b and c) fluorescein angiography shows progressive hyperfluorescence due to leakage, but a normal vascular pattern (Courtesy of Watson, Hazleman, Pavésio and Green, from *The Sclera and Systemic Disorders*, 2nd edition, Butterworth-Heinemann, 2004)

It is much less common than episcleritis and covers a spectrum ranging in severity from trivial self-limiting episodes to a necrotising disease that may involve adjacent tissues and threaten vision.

Classification

The classification shown in Table 5.1 not only facilitates communication regarding the clinical presentation but also has prognostic significance, since patients presenting with one form will usually suffer recurrences of the same form of the disease, with less than 10% progressing to a more aggressive type.

Diffuse anterior non-necrotising scleritis

Diffuse disease is slightly more common in females and usually presents in the fifth decade of life.

Diagnosis

1. **Presentation** is usually with ocular redness followed a few days later by aching and pain which may spread to the face and temple. The pain typically wakes the patient in the early hours of the morning and improves later in the day, but responds poorly to common analgesics.

2. **Signs**

   • Vascular congestion and dilatation associated with oedema. If treatment is started early, which rarely happens, the disease can be completely inhibited.

   • The redness may be generalised (Fig. 5.10) or localised to one quadrant. If confined to the areas under the upper eyelid, the diagnosis may be missed if the eyelid is not elevated.

   • The differential from simple episcleritis is based on history and clinical findings of deep episcleral plexus congestion and scleral oedema, but it can be helped by instilling phenylephrine 10% drops, which will constrict the superficial vessels and allow the deeper tissue to be visualised.

   • As the oedema resolves, these affected areas often take on a slight grey/blue appearance because of increased scleral translucency due to rearrangement of scleral fibres rather than a decrease in scleral thickness (Fig. 5.11).

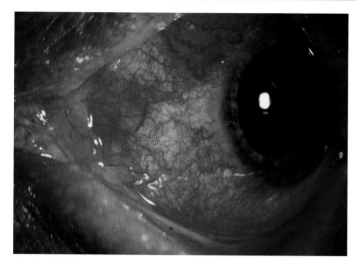

Fig. 5.10 Diffuse anterior non-necrotising scleritis showing intense inflammation of episcleral tissue with disruption of the limbal arcade

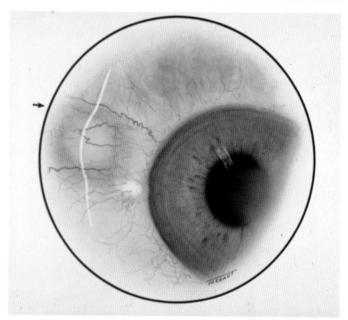

Fig. 5.12 Slit-lamp examination of nodular scleritis shows displacement of the entire beam by the nodule

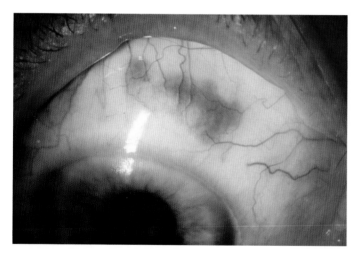

Fig. 5.11 Marked scleral translucency following recurrent diffuse non-necrotising scleritis

- Recurrences at the some location are common unless the underlying cause is eliminated.

- The duration of disease is approximately 6 years and the frequency of recurrences decreases after the first 18 months. The long-term visual prognosis is very good.

3. **FA** shows rapid filling, extensive leakage and a normal vascular pattern.

Nodular anterior non-necrotising scleritis

The incidence of nodular and diffuse anterior scleritis is the same, but a disproportionately large number of those with nodular disease have had a previous attack of herpes zoster ophthalmicus. The age of onset is similar to that of diffuse scleritis.

Diagnosis

1. **Presentation** is with an insidious onset of pain followed by increasing redness, tenderness of the globe and the appearance of a scleral nodule.

2. **Signs**

- Scleral nodules may be single or multiple and most frequently develop in the interpalpebral region, 3–4 mm away from the limbus. They have a deeper blue–red colour than episcleral nodules and are immobile.

- Slit-lamp examination shows that the slit beam is displaced by the scleral nodule (Fig. 5.12).

- Instillation of 10% phenylephrine drops will constrict the conjunctival and superficial episcleral vasculature but not the deep plexus over the nodule (Fig. 5.13).

- Multiple nodules may coalesce, become confluent or expanding, sometimes to an enormous size if treatment is delayed.

- As the inflammation in the nodule subsides, increased translucency of the sclera becomes apparent.

- The duration of the disease is similar to that of diffuse scleritis.

- Because an inflamed scleral nodule may have infective origin, biopsy may be required if the diagnosis is in doubt.

NB: Over 10% of patients with nodular scleritis develop necrotising disease, but if treatment is instituted early, superficial necrosis does not occur and the nodule heals from the centre, leaving a small atrophic scar.

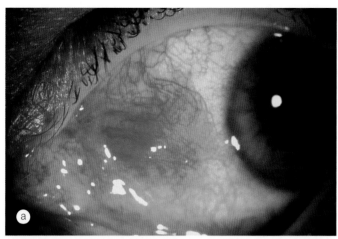

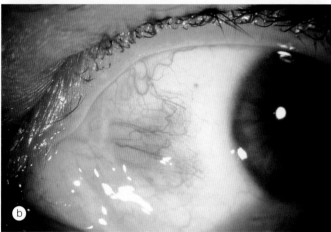

Fig. 5.13 (a) Nodular scleritis in which the conjunctival, superficial and deep episcleral vasculatures are dilated; (b) a few minutes after instillation of 10% phenylephrine, only the deep plexus over the nodule remains dilated (Courtesy of Dr Geux-Crosier, in Watson, Hazleman, Pavésio and Green, *The Sclera and Systemic Disorders*, 2nd edition, Butterworth-Heinemann, 2004)

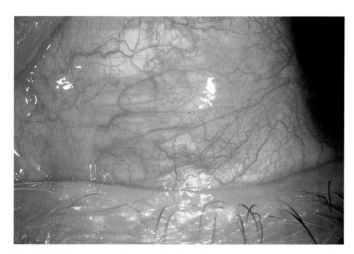

Fig. 5.14 Early necrotising scleritis with deep vascular congestion (Courtesy of Watson, Hazleman, Pavésio and Green, from *The Sclera and Systemic Disorders*, 2nd edition, Butterworth-Heinemann, 2004)

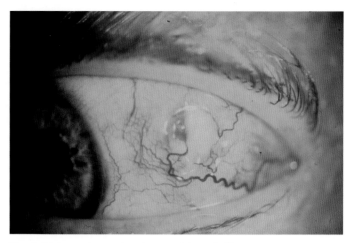

Fig. 5.15 Avascular patches in necrotising scleritis

3. FA usually shows early massive leakage into the nodule.

Necrotising scleritis with inflammation

Necrotising disease is the aggressive form of scleritis. The age at onset is later than that of non-necrotising scleritis, with an average age of 60 years. The condition is bilateral in 60% of patients, and unless appropriately treated, especially in its early stages, it may result in severe visual loss and sometimes loss of the eye itself.

Diagnosis

1. **Presentation** is with gradual onset of pain which becomes severe and persistent and radiates to the temple, brow or jaw; it frequently interferes with sleep and responds poorly to analgesia.

2. **Signs**

- Scleral oedema and congestion of the deep vascular plexus, often confined to one segment of the globe (Fig. 5.14).

- The inflamed area expands around the globe and posteriorly from the site of origin.

- Vascular distortion and occlusion, and the formation of avascular patches (Fig. 5.15).

- The sclera behind the advancing inflammation becomes blue as the choroid shows through the translucent hydrated scar tissue which has replaced normal sclera (Fig. 5.16).

- Progressive scleral thinning and extension of the disease process (Figs 5.17 and 5.18).

- Healing is associated with reduction of vascular congestion and absorption of dead tissue, leaving areas of dark choroid covered only by atrophic conjunctiva (Fig. 5.19).

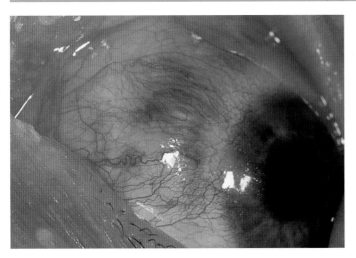

Fig. 5.16 Early scleral thinning in necrotising scleritis (Courtesy of Watson, Hazleman, Pavésio and Green, from *The Sclera and Systemic Disorders*, 2nd edition, Butterworth-Heinemann, 2004)

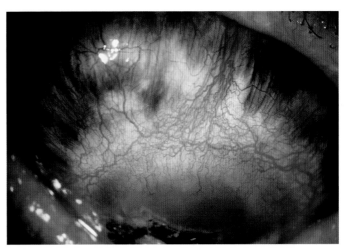

Fig. 5.18 Extension of necrotising scleritis (Courtesy of Watson, Hazleman, Pavésio and Green, from *The Sclera and Systemic Disorders*, 2nd edition, Butterworth-Heinemann, 2004)

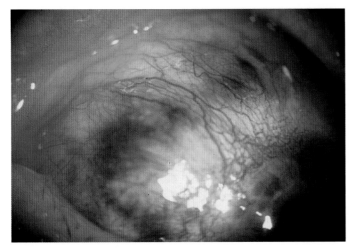

Fig. 5.17 More severe scleral thinning in necrotising scleritis (Courtesy of Watson, Hazleman, Pavésio and Green, from *The Sclera and Systemic Disorders*, 2nd edition, Butterworth-Heinemann, 2004)

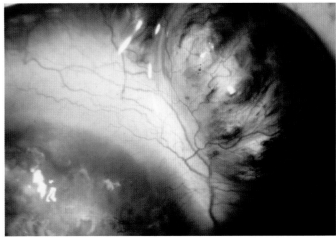

Fig. 5.19 Healed necrotising scleritis

Specific types of necrotising disease

1. **Vaso-occlusive** necrotising scleritis is characterised by areas of congestion which coalesce and become avascular and necrotic (Fig. 5.20). The avascular process also involves overlying episclera and conjunctiva and may result in ulceration.

2. **Granulomatous necrotising scleritis** is often associated with Wegener granulomatosis and polyarteritis nodosa (PAN). The disease typically starts with injection adjacent to the limbus and then extends posteriorly. Within 24 hours, the sclera, episclera, conjunctiva and adjacent cornea become irregularly raised and oedematous (Fig. 5.21). The epithelium of the conjunctiva and cornea breaks down and scleral ulceration ensues.

3. **Surgically induced scleritis** typically starts within 3 weeks of the surgical procedure, but much longer intervals have been reported. Scleritis may be induced by any type of surgery, including strabismus repair, phacoemulsification, trabeculectomy and retinal detachment (Fig. 5.22). The necrotising process starts at the site of surgery and then extends outwards, but, unlike other forms of necrotising disease, it tends to remain localised to one segment.

Investigations

1. **Laboratory.** The commonest association of scleral inflammation is a connective tissue disease. Unfortunately, there are few specific and reliable tests, so the results should be employed as adjuncts to clinical signs. Specific tests include rheumatoid factor, antinuclear antibodies, antineutrophil cytoplasmic antibodies (cANCA –

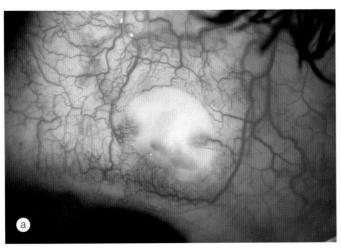

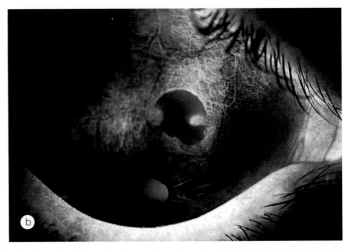

Fig. 5.20 (a) Vaso-occlusive necrotising scleritis with a necrotic patch near the limbus, involving episclera and conjunctiva; (b) fluorescein angiography shows complete lack of perfusion of the necrotic area (Courtesy of Watson, Hazleman, Pavésio and Green, from *The Sclera in Systemic Disorders*, 2nd edition, Butterworth-Heinemann, 2004)

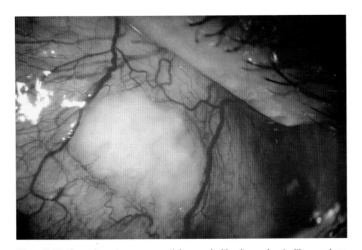

Fig. 5.21 Granulomatous necrotising scleritis in polyarteritis nodosa (Courtesy of P Watson)

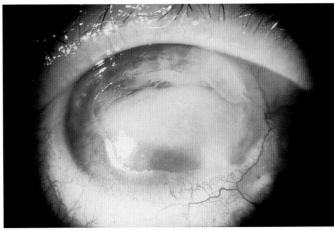

Fig. 5.23 Acute diffuse stromal keratitis with central ulceration (Courtesy of Watson, Hazleman, Pavésio and Green, from *The Sclera and Systemic Disorders*, 2nd edition, Butterworth-Heinemann, 2004)

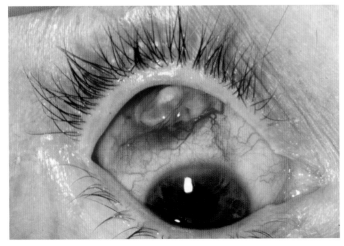

Fig. 5.22 Surgically induced scleritis following scleral buckling for retinal detachment

anti-PR3; pANCA – anti-MPO) and antiphospholipid antibodies.

2. **FA** can aid in deciding if necrotising scleritis is present or is likely to occur. In most patients with necrotising scleritis, there is vascular non-perfusion (see Fig. 5.20b). However, in patients with a systemic vasculitis such as Wegener granulomatosis, the pattern is primarily of transudation, localised areas of vasculitis and new vessel formation.

Complications

1. **Corneal involvement** may take the following forms:

a. *Infiltrative keratitis* may manifest as localised or diffuse acute stromal infiltration (Fig. 5.23) or sclerosing keratitis characterised by chronic thinning and opacification in which the peripheral cornea adjacent to the site of scleritis resembles sclera (Fig. 5.24).

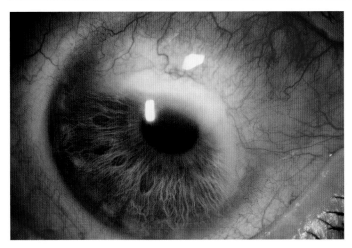

Fig. 5.24 Sclerosing keratitis (Courtesy of Watson, Hazleman, Pavésio, Green. From: *The Sclera and Systemic Disorders*, 2nd edition. Edinburgh: Butterworth-Heinemann, 2004)

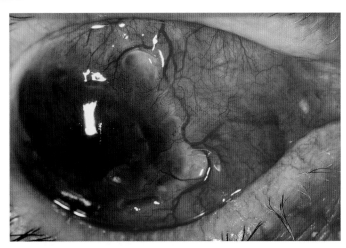

Fig. 5.25 Granulomatous necrotising sclerokeratitis (Courtesy of Watson, Hazleman, Pavésio and Green, from *The Sclera and Systemic Disorders*, 2nd edition, Butterworth-Heinemann, 2004)

b. ***Peripheral ulcerative keratitis*** is characterised by progressive melting and ulceration which may eventually be more serious than the scleritis. In granulomatous scleritis, the destruction extends directly from the sclera into the limbus and cornea (Fig. 5.25). This characteristic pattern is seen in Wegener granulomatosis, PAN and relapsing polychondritis.

> **NB:** Peripheral corneal ulceration can occur at any stage of a necrotising scleritis and, in rare cases, precede its onset.

2. **Uveitis**, if severe, usually denotes aggressive scleritis.

> **NB:** Severe uveitis usually indicates severe scleritis, often necrotising.

3. **Uveal effusion** characterised by exudative retinal and choroidal detachments (see Fig. 5.28) may occur in equatorial scleritis.

4. **Glaucoma** is the most common cause of eventual loss of vision. The intraocular pressure is very difficult to control in the presence of active scleritis.

5. **Hypotony** may be the result of ciliary body detachment, inflammatory damage or ischaemia.

6. **Cataract** is rarely induced by scleritis but may occur in view of the age of the patients affected. Surgery should be performed via a clear corneal incision and always under systemic steroid cover. Surgically induced necrotising scleritis is a potential complication in patients with scleral disease or those with a systemic vasculitis or autoimmune disease associated with scleritis.

7. **Perforation** of the globe as a result of the inflammatory process alone is extremely rare.

Scleromalacia perforans

Scleromalacia perforans is a specific type of necrotising scleritis occurring in elderly women with longstanding rheumatoid arthritis. The use of the word 'perforans' is unfortunate because perforation of the globe is extremely rare, as the integrity of the globe is maintained by a thin, but complete, layer of fibrous tissue.

Diagnosis

1. **Presentation** is with slight non-specific irritation, and keratoconjunctivitis sicca may be suspected; pain is absent and vision unaffected.

2. **Signs**

* Yellow scleral necrotic plaques near the limbus, without vascular congestion (Fig. 5.26a).

* Coalescence and enlargement of necrotic areas (Fig. 5.26b).

* Very slow progression of scleral thinning and exposure of underlying uvea (Figs 5.26c and 5.26d).

Treatment

Treatment may be effective in patients with very early disease, but by the time most patients present, no treatment is either needed or effective. Repair of scleral perforation is very difficult but must be attempted, otherwise phthisis bulbi ensues.

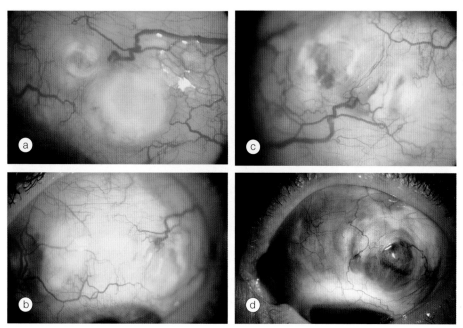

Fig. 5.26 Progression of scleromalacia perforans. (a) Scleral necrotic patches; (b) extension of scleral necrosis; (c and d) progressive scleral thinning and exposure of underlying sclera (Courtesy of Watson, Hazleman, Pavésio and Green, from *The Sclera and Systemic Diseases*, 2nd edition, Butterworth-Heinemann, 2004)

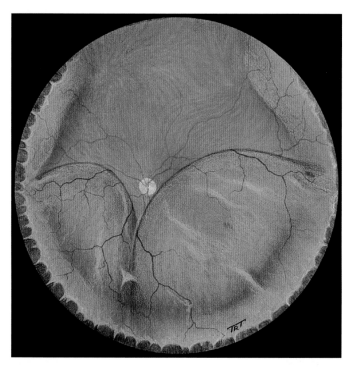

Fig. 5.27 Bullous exudative retinal detachment in posterior scleritis (Courtesy of Watson, Hazleman, Pavésio and Green, from *The Sclera and Systemic Disorders*, 2nd edition, Butterworth-Heinemann, 2004)

Posterior scleritis

Posterior scleritis is a serious, potentially blinding condition, which is often misdiagnosed and treated very late. The age at onset is often under 40 years. The disease is bilateral in 35% of cases. It is important to remember that the inflammatory changes seen in posterior and anterior scleral disease are identical and can arise in both segments simultaneously or separately. The presence of anterior scleritis is a great help if posterior scleritis is suspected, but it only occurs in a minority of cases. Patients with posterior scleritis can go blind extremely rapidly, so correct early diagnosis is crucial. Young patients are usually healthy but about a third of those over the age of 55 years have associated systemic disease.

Diagnosis

1. **Presentation** may be with discomfort or pain. Surprisingly, pain does not correlate with the severity of inflammation but tends to be more severe in those with accompanying myositis. Tenderness to palpation is very common, but photophobia is not a dominant feature.

2. **Signs**

a. **Exudative retinal detachment** occurs in almost 25% of cases (Fig. 5.27).

b. **Uveal effusion** characterised by exudative retinal detachment and choroidal detachment (Fig. 5.28).

c. **Subretinal mass** characterised by a yellowish-brown elevation, the surface of which may manifest lighter-coloured spots (Fig. 5.29); subretinal exudate may also be seen (Fig. 5.30).

d. **Choroidal folds** represent an anterior displacement of the choroid and are usually confined to the posterior pole and run horizontally (Fig. 5.31).

e. **Disc oedema** with an accompanying slight reduction of vision is common. It is caused by spread of the granulomatous process into the orbital tissue and sheaths of the optic nerve. Treatment must not be delayed, as vision can be lost rapidly due to ischaemia.

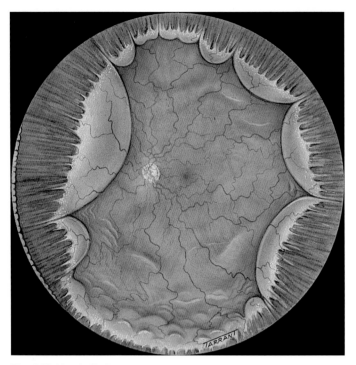

Fig. 5.28 Uveal effusion

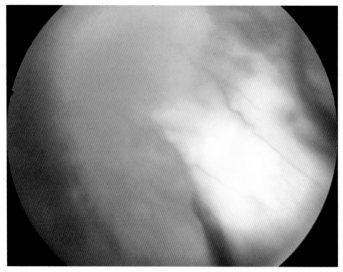

Fig. 5.30 Subretinal exudate in posterior scleritis (Courtesy of P Watson)

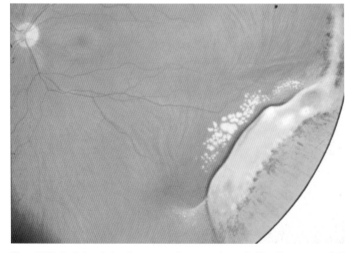

Fig. 5.29 Peripheral fundus mass in posterior scleritis (Courtesy of P Watson)

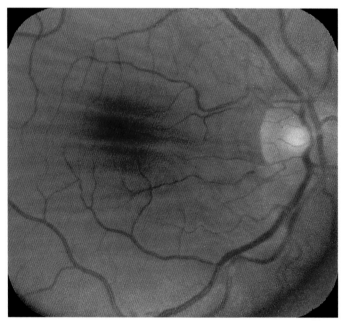

Fig. 5.31 Choroidal folds

NB: About 20% of patients with definite ultrasonic evidence of posterior scleral disease have absolutely no clinical evidence of any abnormality in the posterior segment of the eye.

f. ***Macular oedema*** is not caused by underlying scleritis and is always secondary to some other process, usually disc oedema.

g. ***Myositis*** is common and gives rise to diplopia, pain on eye movement, tenderness to touch, and redness around a muscle insertion.

h. ***Proptosis*** is usually mild and frequently associated with ptosis.

3. Investigations

a. ***Ultrasonography*** is extremely useful in showing increased scleral thickness, scleral nodules, and separation of Tenon capsule from the sclera. Fluid in Tenon space gives rise to the characteristic 'T' sign in which the stem of the T is formed by the optic nerve on its side and the crossbar by the gap containing fluid (Fig. 5.32). Ultrasonography

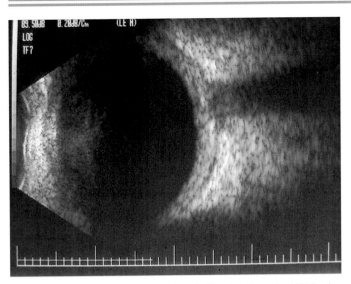

Fig. 5.32 Ultrasonography in posterior scleritis, showing scleral thickening and fluid in sub-Tenon space

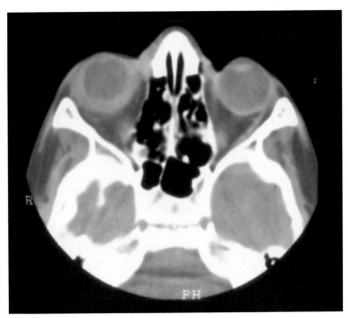

Fig. 5.33 Axial computed tomography in right posterior scleritis, showing scleral thickening and mild proptosis

will also show disc oedema, choroidal folds and retinal detachment.

b. **FA** may be helpful in the differential diagnosis of disc swelling, retinal and choroidal folds, and maculopathy. Serous detachment shows multifocal retinal pigment epithelial leaks, similar to those seen in Vogt–Koyanagi–Harada (VKH) syndrome.

c. **CT and MRI** may show scleral thickening and proptosis (Fig. 5.33).

Differential diagnosis

1. **Subretinal mass** must be differentiated from a granuloma associated with some other pathology, amelanotic choroidal melanoma, choroidal metastasis and choroidal haemangioma.

2. **Choroidal folds**, retinal striae and disc oedema may also occur in orbital tumours, orbital inflammatory disease, thyroid eye disease, papilloedema and hypotony

3. **Exudative retinal detachment** also occurs in VKH syndrome and central serous retinopathy.

Systemic associations of scleritis

Rheumatoid Arthritis

Rheumatoid arthritis (see Ch. 8) is by far the most common systemic association of scleritis. Patients with non-necrotising scleritis usually have mild joint disease, whereas necrotising disease tends to affect patients with severe long-standing rheumatoid disease with extra-articular manifestations, most notably rheumatoid nodules.

Wegener granulomatosis

Wegener granulomatosis is an idiopathic, multisystem, granulomatous disorder characterised by generalised small vessel vasculitis affecting predominantly the respiratory tract and kidneys (see Ch. 8). The disease may be associated with rapidly progressive, necrotising granulomatous scleritis. Because Wegener granulomatosis can be localised to the eye and the orbit, without any systemic involvement, orbital biopsy may be required for diagnosis.

Relapsing polychondritis

Relapsing polychondritis is a rare idiopathic condition characterised by small vessel vasculitis involving cartilage, resulting in recurrent, often progressive, inflammatory episodes involving multiple organ systems (see Ch. 8). It is a common cause of intractable scleritis, which may be non-necrotising or necrotising.

Polyarteritis nodosa

PAN is an idiopathic, potentially lethal, collagen vascular disease affecting medium-sized and small arteries, with frequent aneurysm formation (see Ch. 8). PAN may be associated with aggressive necrotising disease, although other types of scleritis may also occur. Ocular involvement may precede the systemic manifestations by several years.

Systemic lupus erythematosus

Systemic lupus erythematosus (SLE) is an autoimmune, non-organ-specific, connective tissue disease (see Ch. 8). SLE may be associated with anterior diffuse or nodular scleritis. Necrotising scleritis is less common, but is difficult to control if treatment is delayed.

Uncommon associations

1. **Spondyloarthropathies** are occasionally associated with mild diffuse scleritis that may antedate joint involvement.

2. **Behçet syndrome** may rarely be associated with diffuse anterior scleritis, which may occur in the absence of other ocular manifestations.

3. **Sarcoidosis** may rarely manifest scleral nodules.

4. **Gout** may be associated with diffuse episcleritis or scleritis.

Treatment of scleritis

1. **Topical steroids** do not affect the natural history of the scleral inflammation, but may relieve symptoms and oedema in non-necrotising disease.

2. **Systemic NSAIDs** should be used only in non-necrotising disease. There is little to choose between various agents in terms of relief of pain or regression of physical signs. It is unlikely that using them in combination will provide any more relief than using them singly. Because there is a large variation in individual responses to NSAIDs, it is often necessary to try a number of different drugs before finding one that provides adequate relief. Each drug should be given for 2 weeks to assess its efficacy. Guidelines for prescribing an NSAID are as follows:

   - Use a drug with which you are familiar.

   - Prescribe cheaper, established drugs.

   - Prescribe only one drug at a time, in adequate dosage.

   - Choose cyclo-oxygenase 2 (COX-2)-specific drugs for elderly patients or if there is a past history of peptic ulceration, but there are concerns regarding their effects on the cardiovascular system.

   - Prescribe for 2 weeks and review.

3. **Periocular steroid injections** may be used in non-necrotising disease but their effects are usually transient.

4. **Systemic steroids** are used when NSAIDs are inappropriate or ineffective (necrotising disease). The dose of prednisolone is 1.0–1.5 mg/kg/day. If a faster effect is required, the drug should be administered intravenously at a dose of 0.5–1.0 g (1–3 mg/kg) daily.

5. **Cytotoxic agents** are usually necessary whenever disease activity is not completely controlled with steroids alone, or as a steroid-sparing measure in patients requiring very high doses. In patients with an underlying systemic vasculitis such as Wegener granulomatosis or PAN, this form

of therapy may also be life-saving. The most frequently used drugs are cyclophosphamide, which is the drug of choice in Wegener disease, azathioprine, mycophenolate mofetil (CellCept) and methotrexate.

6. **Immune modulators** such as ciclosporin and tacrolimus are less useful as long-term therapy but may be considered as a short-term measure in acute presentations before a cytotoxic agent is able to exert its action.

> **NB:** If pain and headache persist in spite of treatment, there is still active inflammation.

Infective scleritis

1. **Herpes zoster** is the most common infective cause. Necrotising scleritis is extremely resistant to treatment and may result in a punched-out area in the sclera, a very thin atrophic scar or, very occasionally, staphyloma formation or perforation.

2. **Tuberculous** scleritis is rare and difficult to diagnose. The sclera may be infected by direct spread from a local conjunctiva or choroid lesion, or, more commonly, by haematogenous spread. Clinically, involvement may be nodular or necrotising.

3. **Leprosy.** Diffuse scleritis is associated with severe recurrent erythema nodosum leprosum reactions. Nodular scleritis may occur in lepromatous leprosy. Necrotising disease may occur as a result of scleral infection or as part of an immune response.

4. **Syphilis.** Diffuse anterior scleritis may occur in secondary syphilis. Occasionally, scleral nodules may be seen in tertiary syphilis.

5. **Lyme disease.** Scleritis is common but typically occurs long after initial infection.

> **NB:** Once the infective agent has been identified, specific therapy should be initiated. Topical and systemic steroids may also be used to reduce the inflammatory reaction.

FURTHER READING

Akpek EK, Thorne JE, Qazi FA, et al. Evaluation of patients with scleritis for systemic disease. *Ophthalmology* 2004;111:501–506.

Benson WE. Posterior scleritis. *Surv Ophthalmol* 1988;32:297–316.

Biswas J, Mittal S, Ganesh SK, et al. Posterior scleritis: clinical profile and imaging characteristics. *Indian J Ophthalmol* 1998;46:195–202.

Guex-Crosier Y, Durig J. Anterior segment indocyanine green angiography in anterior scleritis and episcleritis. *Ophthalmology* 2003;110:1756–1763.

Isaak BL, Liesegang TJ, Michet CJ Jr. Ocular and systemic findings in relapsing polychondritis. *Ophthalmology* 1986;93:681–689.

Jabs DA, Mudun A, Dunn JP, et al. Episcleritis and scleritis: clinical features and treatment. *Am J Ophthalmol* 2000;130:469–476.

McCluskey PJ, Watson PG, Lightman S, et al. Posterior scleritis: clinical features, systemic associations, and outcome in a large series of patients. *Ophthalmology* 1999;106:2380–2386.

O'Donoghue E, Lightman S, Tuft S, et al. Surgically induced necrotizing scleritis (SINS): precipitating factors and response to treatment. *Br J Ophthalmol* 1992;76:17–21.

Sainz de la Maza M, Jabbur NS, Foster CS. Severity of scleritis and episcleritis. *Ophthalmology* 1994;101:389–396.

Sainz de la Maza M, Foster CS, Jabbur NS. Scleritis associated with systemic vasculitic disease. *Ophthalmology* 1995;102:687–692.

Sen HN, Suhler EB, Al-Khatib SQ. Mycophenolate mofetil in the treatment of scleritis. *Ophthalmology* 2003;110:1750–1755.

Tu EY, Culnertson WW, Pflugfelder SC, et al. Therapy of nonnecrotizing anterior scleritis with subconjunctival corticosteroid injection. *Ophthalmology* 1995;102:718–724.

Tuft S, Watson PG. Progression of scleral disease. *Ophthalmology* 1991;98:467–471.

Watson PG, Hayreh SS. Scleritis and episcleritis. *Br J Ophthalmol* 1976;60:163–191.

Watson PG, Hazleman BL, Pavésio CE, et al, eds. *The Sclera and Systemic Disorders*. 2nd edn. London: Butterworth-Heinemann; 2004.

Uveitis

DEFINITIONS

The uvea is the intermediate vascular coat of the eye which comprises the iris, ciliary body and choroid (Fig. 6.1).

1. **Uveitis**, by strict definition, implies an inflammation of the uveal tract. However, the term is now used to describe many forms of intraocular inflammation involving not only the uveal tract but also the retina and its vessels.

2. **Anterior uveitis** may be subdivided into:

- Iritis, in which the inflammation primarily involves the iris.

- Iridocyclitis, in which both the iris and ciliary body are involved.

3. **Intermediate uveitis** is defined as inflammation predominantly involving the vitreous and peripheral retina.

4. **Posterior uveitis** involves the fundus posterior to the vitreous base.

- Retinitis, with the primary focus in the retina.

- Choroiditis, with the primary focus in the choroid.

- Vasculitis, which may involve veins, arteries, or both.

5. **Panuveitis (diffuse)** implies involvement of the entire uveal tract.

6. **Endophthalmitis** implies inflammation, often purulent, involving all intraocular tissues except the sclera.

7. **Panophthalmitis** involves the entire globe, often with orbital extension.

> **NB:** Anterior uveitis is the most common, followed by posterior, intermediate and panuveitis.

INVESTIGATIONS

Establishing the aetiological diagnosis in uveitis is often challenging. It is based on obtaining an accurate ocular and medical history as well as performing a detailed ocular examination. Laboratory tests may be helpful, but very few conclusively establish the diagnosis. It is not uncommon for an inexperienced clinician to order a battery of investigations in the hope that something will turn up positive and explain the clinical problem. This approach is likely to result in confusing findings which may result in inappropriate treatment that may be harmful to the patient. It is also not a cost-effective way of delivering care. A good example is the common request

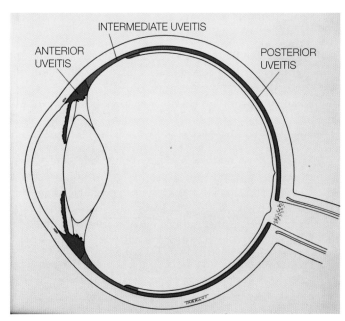

Fig. 6.1 Anatomical classification of uveitis

of toxoplasma serology for patients with any form of uveitis, including anterior.

History

1. **Age** at presentation is very important because certain types of uveitis are confined to patients within a specific age group whilst others may occur at any age. For example:

- Uveitis associated with juvenile idiopathic arthritis (JIA) and ocular toxocariasis typically affects children.

- Birdshot chorioretinopathy and serpiginous choroiditis are more prevalent in the fifth to seventh decades of life.

- HLA-B27-associated uveitis and Behçet syndrome usually affect young adults.

- Acute retinal necrosis and toxoplasmosis may affect individuals of any age group.

> **NB:** It is less common for primary uveitis to first manifest in old age; suspect a masquerade syndrome such as lymphoma.

2. **Gender** is less important than age of onset, although JIA-related uveitis is more common in girls, while HLA-B27 disease typically affects males.

3. **Race** is especially important in conditions such as Behçet syndrome (Mediterranean, Middle Eastern and Asian), sarcoidosis (blacks) and Vogt–Koyanagi–Harada syndrome (Asians and in the USA those with native Indian ancestry).

4. **Geographic location** may be of importance because infectious uveitis – e.g. Lyme disease, presumed ocular histoplasmosis syndrome and diffuse unilateral subacute neuroretinitis – may be endemic in certain locations.

5. **Past ocular history** may occasionally be helpful. For example, recurrent attacks of unilateral acute anterior uveitis would be suggestive of HLA-B27-related disease, whereas a history of previous trauma or surgery would point to the diagnosis of sympathetic ophthalmitis or lens-induced uveitis.

6. **Past medical history** is of paramount importance, particularly in identifying exposure to infectious agents, such as tuberculosis and syphilis, as well as supporting the diagnosis of Behçet syndrome (oral and genital ulcers). Certain medications such as rifabutin and cidofovir may occasionally cause uveitis.

7. **Hygiene and dietary habits** are important when considering infectious diseases such as toxocariasis (history of pica), toxoplasmosis (undercooked meat – ingestion of water in rural areas seems to be a more important factor) and cysticercosis (ingestion of pork in endemic areas).

8. **Sexual practices** are especially important for the diagnosis of syphilis and HIV infection.

9. **Recreational drugs** are a risk factor for HIV infection and fungal endophthalmitis.

10. **Pets.** Cats are linked to the transmission of toxoplasmosis and cat-scratch disease, while exposure to puppies is associated with toxocariasis.

Special investigations

General aspects

1. **Purposes**

- To confirm the diagnosis that is highly suspected from history or examination.

- To exclude a condition which is on the list of differential diagnoses for that presentation.

- Research purposes, which will depend on patient informed consent.

2. **Not indicated**

- Single attack of mild unilateral acute anterior uveitis without suggestion of a possible underlying disease.

- Recognition of a specific uveitis entity such as VKH syndrome, sympathetic ophthalmitis, Fuchs cyclitis and toxoplasma retinitis.

- When a systemic diagnosis compatible with the uveitis is already apparent, as in the case of Behçet syndrome, sarcoidosis, tuberculosis and Reiter syndrome.

3. **Indications**

- Recurrent granulomatous anterior uveitis.

- Intermediate, posterior and diffuse uveitis.

- Bilateral disease.

- Systemic manifestations without a specific diagnosis.

- Confirmation of a suspected ocular picture which depends on the test result as part of the criteria for diagnosis, such as in HLA-A29 testing for birdshot chorioretinopathy.

Non-specific tests

Investigations performed as part of the general evaluation of the patient's health may reveal an active inflammatory process or infection. They are also necessary as baseline when planning systemic immunosuppressive therapy.

1. **Full blood count.** An eosinophil count greater than 5% may indicate a parasitic or allergic process.

2. **Erythrocyte sedimentation rate (ESR) or C-reactive protein (CRP)**, if high, may reflect systemic disease.

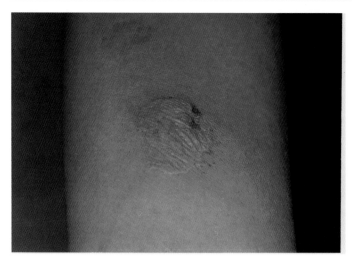

Fig. 6.2 Positive tuberculin skin reaction (Courtesy of U Raina)

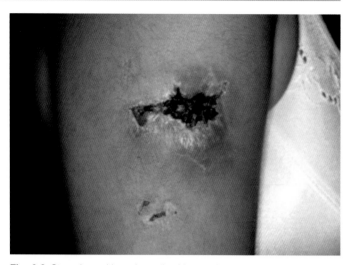

Fig. 6.3 Strongly positive tuberculin skin reaction

3. **Renal function** tests are useful in the diagnosis of tubulo-interstitial nephritis and Wegener granulomatosis.

4. **Liver function** tests are important before and during systemic therapy with immunosuppressive agents.

Skin tests

1. **Tuberculin skin tests (Mantoux and Heaf)** involve the intradermal injection of purified protein derivative of *M. tuberculosis*.

a. **A positive** result is characterised by the development of an induration of 5–14 mm within 48 hours (Fig. 6.2).

b. **A negative** result usually excludes tuberculosis. A false negative may occur in patients with advanced consumptive disease and those on immunosuppressive drugs.

c. **A weakly positive** result does not necessarily distinguish between previous exposure and active disease. This is because most individuals have already received BCG (Bacille Calmette-Guerin) vaccination and will therefore exhibit a hypersensitivity response.

d. **A strongly positive** result (induration >15 mm) is usually indicative of active disease since this level of response is not expected after long exposure to the vaccine (Fig. 6.3).

2. **Pathergy** test (increased dermal sensitivity to needle trauma) is a criterion for the diagnosis of Behçet syndrome, but the results vary and it is only rarely positive in the absence of systemic activity. A positive response is the formation of a pustule following pricking of the skin with a needle (Fig. 6.4).

3. **Leprin test** involves intradermal injection of an extract of leprosy bacilli. It differs from the tuberculin test because it becomes positive after several weeks (Fig. 6.5). It is strongly positive in tuberculoid leprosy but negative in lepromatous disease.

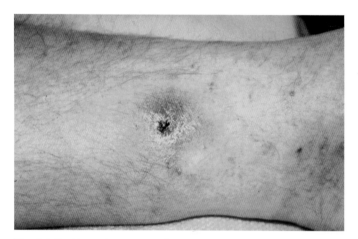

Fig. 6.4 Positive pathergy test in Behçet disease (Courtesy of B Noble)

Serology

SYPHILIS

Because of variable presentation, serology should be performed in all patients with uveitis who require investigation. Serologic tests rely on detection of non-specific antibodies (cardiolipin) or specific treponemal antibodies.

1. **Non-treponemal tests** such as rapid plasma regain (RPR) or Venereal Diseases Research Laboratory (VDRL) are best used to diagnose primary infection, or monitor disease activity or response to therapy based on titre. The patient's serum is mixed with commercially prepared carbon-like cardiolipin antigen (Fig. 6.6). The results may be negative in up to 30% of patients with documented syphilitic uveitis. They also tend to become negative 6–18 months after therapy.

2. **Treponemal antibody tests** are highly sensitive and specific and more useful to prove past infection, or secondary

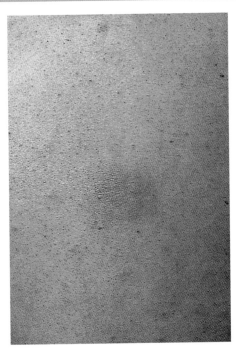

Fig. 6.5 Positive leprin skin test in tuberculoid leprosy (Courtesy of Emond, Welsby and Rowland, from *Colour Atlas of Infectious Diseases*, 4th edition, Mosby, 2003)

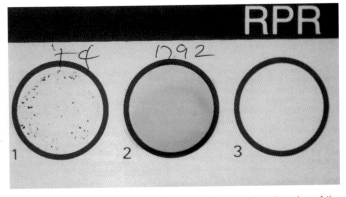

Fig. 6.6 Rapid plasma regain (RPR) for syphilis, showing clumping of the antigenic particles (left) after 4 minutes (Courtesy of Hart and Shears, from *Color Atlas of Medical Microbiology*, 2nd edition, Mosby, 2004)

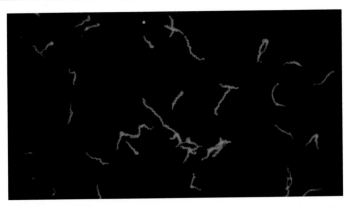

Fig. 6.7 Positive fluorescent treponemal antibody test (FTA-ABS) for syphilis (Courtesy of Mims, Dockrell, Goering, Roitt, Wakelin and Zuckerman, from *Medical Microbiology*, 3rd edition, Mosby, 2004)

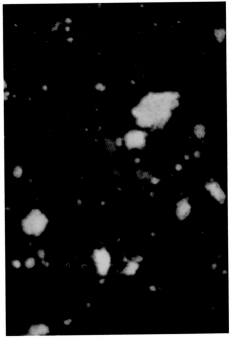

Fig. 6.8 Positive immunofluorescent antibody test (Courtesy of Emond, Welsby and Rowland, from Colour Atlas of Infectious Diseases, 4th edition, Mosby, 2003)

or tertiary forms of clinical infection. The fluorescent treponemal antibody absorption test (FTA-ABS) and the more specific microhaemagglutination treponemal pallidum test (MHA-TP) are most commonly used. The antibody in the patient's serum binds to bacteria and is visualised by a fluorescent dye (Fig. 6.7). The result cannot be titrated and is either positive (reactive) or negative (non-reactive). A positive result always remains positive (serologic scar).

TOXOPLASMOSIS

1. **Dye test (Sabin–Feldman)** utilises live organisms which are exposed to the patient's serum complement. The cell membranes of the organisms are lysed in the presence of the specific anti-toxoplasma IgG, and, as consequence, the organisms fail to stain with methylene-blue dye. This test remains the gold standard for the diagnosis of toxoplasmosis.

2. **Immunofluorescent antibody** tests utilise dead organisms exposed to the patient's serum and anti-human globulin labeled with fluorescein. The results are read using a fluorescent microscope (Fig. 6.8).

3. **Haemagglutination** tests involve coating of lysed organisms onto red blood cells which are then exposed to the patient's serum; positive sera cause the red cells to agglutinate (Fig. 6.9).

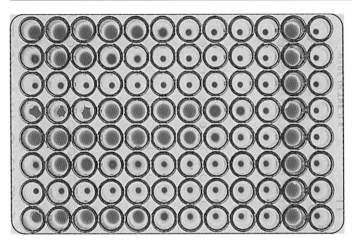

Fig. 6.9 Haemagglutination test (Courtesy of Mims, Dockrell, Goering, Roitt, Wakelin and Zuckerman, from *Medical Microbiology*, 3ʳᵈ edition, Mosby, 2004)

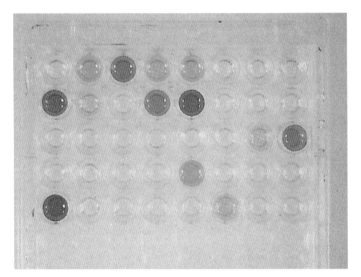

Fig. 6.10 ELISA test showing positive (yellow–brown) and negative wells (Courtesy of Hart and Shears, from *Color Atlas of Medical Microbiology*, 2ⁿᵈ edition, Mosby, 2004)

4. **Enzyme-linked immunosorbent assay (ELISA)** involves binding of the patient's antibodies to an excess of solid-phase antigen (Fig. 6.10). This complex is then incubated with an enzyme-linked second antibody. Assessment of enzyme activity provides measurement of specific antibody concentration. The test can also be used to detect antibodies in the aqueous, which are more specific than those in the serum. The test is also useful in other conditions such as cat-scratch fever and toxocariasis.

Indirect fluorescent antibody tests, haemagglutination and ELISA are comparable to the dye test (gold standard) in sensitivity and specificity. Positive serology only confirms previous exposure to toxoplasmosis and thus will be positive in a high percentage of patients with other types of uveitis. Testing should therefore not be performed routinely and ordered only in patients who have atypical signs in whom a negative result will exclude the diagnosis of toxoplasmosis.

NB: Any positive titre, even in undiluted serum, is significant in the presence of a fundus lesion compatible with toxoplasmic retinitis. Reactivation of ocular disease alone will have no impact on the titre.

ANTINUCLEAR ANTIBODY

Antinuclear antibody (ANA) is mainly used to identify children with JIA who are at high risk of developing anterior uveitis and therefore require closer follow-up.

NB: Rheumatoid factor is relevant only when investigating aetiology of scleritis. It should not be ordered in the work-up of patients with uveitis only.

Enzyme assay

1. **Angiotensin-converting enzyme (ACE)** is a non-specific test which indicates the presence of a granulomatous disease such as sarcoidosis, tuberculosis or leprosy. Elevations occur in up to 80% of patients with sarcoidosis, and it is more likely to be elevated in acute disease. It is normally elevated in children and therefore of less diagnostic value.

2. **Lysozyme** has good sensitivity but less specificity than ACE for the diagnosis of sarcoidosis, but using both tests seems to increase sensitivity and specificity.

HLA tissue typing

1. **HLA-B27** is strongly associated with spondylo-arthropathies, particularly ankylosing spondylitis.

2. **HLA-A29** is strongly associated with birdshot chorioretinopathy.

3. **HLA-B51** is associated with Behçet syndrome.

Fundus angiography

1. **Fluorescein angiography (FA)** is useful in the following conditions:

- Diagnosis and assessment of severity of retinal vasculitis.

- Diagnosis of cystoid macular oedema (CMO) (Fig. 6.11).

- Demonstrating macular ischaemia as the cause of visual loss rather than CMO.

- Differentiation between inflammatory and ischaemic cause of retinal neovascularisation.

- Diagnosis and monitoring of choroidal neovascularisation (CNV) (Fig. 6.12).

NB: FA is less appropriate in choroiditis because deep lesions will be hidden by the choroidal flush. For this reason, more lesions are seen clinically than angiographically in birdshot chorioretinopathy.

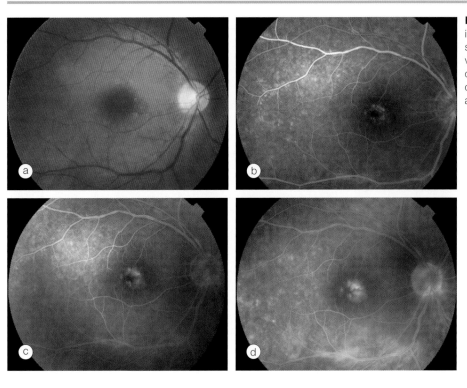

Fig. 6.11 Cystoid macular oedema. (a) Colour image; (b) fluorescein angiography arterial phase shows mild hyperfluorescence due to leakage; (c) venous phase shows increasing hyperfluorescence; (d) late phase shows marked hyperfluorescence that has a 'flower petal' pattern due to accumulation of dye within microcystic spaces

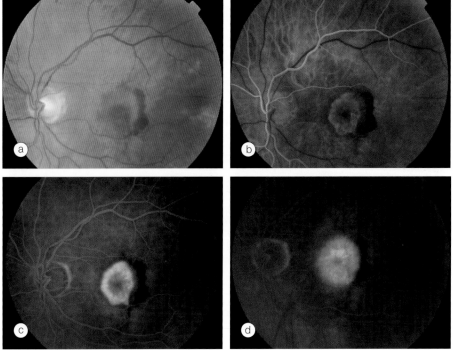

Fig. 6.12 Choroidal neovascularisation (CNV). (a) Colour image shows blood at the macula; (b) fluorescein angiography arterial phase shows 'lacy' hyperfluorescence at the macula due to filling of CNV; (c) venous phase shows marked hyperfluorescence due to leakage from CNV; (d) late phase shows persistent hyperfluorescence due to staining of CNV

2. **Indocyanine green (ICG) angiography** is very suited to choroidal disease because the choroid is visible through the retinal pigment epithelium (RPE). ICG is able to detect non-perfusion of the choriocapillaris and provide information regarding inflammation affecting the stroma (Fig. 6.13).

Ultrasonography

Real-time B-mode scans are of particular value when opaque media hamper adequate fundus examination. In this setting, ultrasonography is of particular value in imaging a retinal detachment or excluding an intraocular mass.

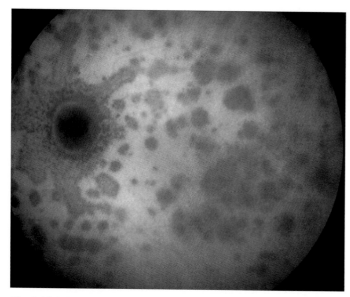

Fig. 6.13 Indocyanine green angiography of multiple evanescent white dot syndrome which shows more numerous lesions than are visible clinically or on fluorescein angiography

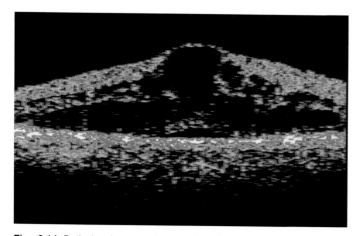

Fig. 6.14 Optical coherence tomography showing very severe cystoid macular oedema

Optical coherence tomography

Optical coherence tomography (OCT) is a non-invasive technique that is as effective as FA in detecting CMO (Fig. 6.14), and is of particular value in eyes with small pupils. It can demonstrate complications of chronic CMO such as lamellar or macular holes and monitor response to treatment.

Biopsy

Histopathology still remains the gold standard for definitive diagnosis of many conditions. Biopsies of the skin or other organs may establish the diagnosis of a systemic disorder associated with the ocular manifestations, such as in sarcoidosis. However, intraocular structures are relatively inac-

cessible to this procedure without running the risk of significant morbidity.

1. **Conjunctiva and lacrimal gland biopsy** may be useful for the diagnosis of sarcoidosis but only in the presence of clinically apparent disease.

2. **Aqueous samples** are not performed routinely. Polymerase chain reaction (PCR) on aqueous may be useful in the diagnosis of viral retinitis. Detection of local production of antibodies is also helpful in establishing an infectious aetiology (Wittmer–Desmonts coefficient).

3. **Vitreous biopsy**, apart from its already well-established role in infectious endophthalmitis, can also be used for the diagnosis of other infectious conditions by obtaining samples for culture and PCR. It is also used for diagnosis of intraocular lymphoma. Obtaining samples with a cutter rather than a needle may be advantageous when a large sample is required. False negative results are due to problems related to the handling of the sample and also depend on the expertise of the pathologist. Complications include cataract, retinal detachment, vitreous haemorrhage and, rarely, endophthalmitis.

4. **Retinal and choroidal biopsies** may be useful in the following conditions:

* Diagnosis not established.

* No response to therapy.

* Further deterioration despite therapy.

* Exclude possibility of malignancy or infection.

The biopsy may be taken by either a transcleral or internal (pars plana) approach, depending on the tissue sample required. Complications include retinal detachment, choroidal haemorrhage and endophthalmitis.

Radiology

1. **Chest X-ray** is frequently requested to exclude tuberculosis and sarcoidosis.

2. **Sacroiliac joint X-ray** is helpful in the diagnosis of a spondyloarthropathy in the presence of symptoms of low back pain and uveitis.

3. **Computed tomography (CT) and magnetic resonance imaging (MRI) scans** of the brain and thorax may be appropriate in the investigation of sarcoidosis, multiple sclerosis and primary intraocular lymphoma. A thorax CT scan may clarify any doubts regarding the presence of hilar adenopathy.

FURTHER READING

Ciardella AP, Prall FR, Borodoker N, et al. Imaging techniques for posterior uveitis. *Curr Opin Ophthalmol* 2004;15:519–530.

Herbort CP, Guex-Crosier Y, LeHoang P. Schematic interpretation of indocyanine green angiography. *Ophthalmology* 1994;2:169–176.

Johnston RL, Tufail A, Lightman S, et al. Retinal and choroidal biopsies are helpful in unclear uveitis of suspected infectious or malignant origin. *Ophthalmology* 2004;111:522–528.

Knox CM, Chandler D, Short GA, et al. Polymerase chain reaction-based assays of vitreous samples for the diagnosis of viral retinitis. Use in diagnostic dilemmas. *Ophthalmology* 1998;105:37–44.

Wade NK. Diagnostic testing in patients with ocular inflammation. *Int Ophthalmol Clin* 2000;40:37–54.

PRINCIPLES OF TREATMENT

The first step in the management of uveitis is the establishment of a correct diagnosis. This depends on the recognition of clinical signs and a good understanding of the natural history of the different entities, supported by adequate laboratory investigations. The distinction between an infectious and autoimmune condition is essential, since therapy will be completely different and the use of immunosuppression will lead to deterioration of an infection, with the potential risk of severe loss of vision. This chapter concentrates on general principles for the management of uveitis. It will deal predominantly with the use of anti-inflammatory and immunosuppressive therapy for the management of immune-mediated uveitis. Antibiotic therapy for infectious diseases will be discussed in the specific sections. It is important to keep in mind that nearly all drugs used to treat uveitis are capable of producing side effects, and this should always be weighted against the decision to treat. Also, it must be emphasised that the use of systemic therapy should be carried out in conjunction with a physician who is competent to deal with complications associated with the underlying disease or therapy.

Mydriatics

Preparations

1. Short-acting

a. **Tropicamide** (0.5% and 1%) has a duration of 6 hours.

b. **Cyclopentolate** (0.5% and 1%) has a duration of 24 hours.

c. **Phenylephrine** (2.5% and 10%) has a duration of 3 hours but no cycloplegic effects.

2. Long-acting

a. **Homatropine** 2% has a duration of up to 2 days.

b. **Atropine** 1% is the most powerful cycloplegic and mydriatic, with a duration of up to 2 weeks.

Indications

1. To promote comfort by relieving spasm of the ciliary muscle and pupillary sphincter, usually with atropine or homatropine, although it is usually unnecessary to use these agents for more than 1–2 weeks. Once the inflammation shows signs of subsiding, they can be replaced by a short-acting preparation.

2. To break down recently formed posterior synechiae with intensive topical mydriatics (atropine, phenylephrine) or subconjunctival injections of Mydricaine (adrenaline, atropine and procaine) in eyes that do not respond to drops. A subconjunctival injection (0.5 ml) of Mydricaine is divided into the four quadrants for maximal effect by pulling from all directions. A good alternative to injections is to insert cotton pledgets soaked in Mydricaine into the superior and inferior fornices for 5 minutes.

NB: Tissue plasminogen activator (12.5 μg in 0.05 ml) injected into the anterior chamber (intracamerally) with a 25-gauge needle will dissolve fibrinous exudate and help break down persistent posterior synechiae.

3. To prevent formation of posterior synechiae following control of acute inflammation by using a short-acting mydriatic that allows some mobility of the pupil and prevents synechiae in the dilated position. In mild chronic anterior uveitis, the mydriatic can be instilled once at bedtime to prevent difficulties with accommodation during the day. Moreover, the pupil should not be kept constantly dilated because posterior synechiae can still form in the dilated position. In young children, constant uniocular atropinisation may induce amblyopia.

NB: Subconjunctival Mydricaine may induce tachycardia and hypertension and should be used with caution in patients with cardiovascular disease.

Steroids

Steroids are the mainstay of treatment. They can be administered (a) *topically*, (b) *by periocular injection*, (c) *intravitreally* or (d) *systemically*. Steroids, by whatever route, generally should be commenced at a high dose and subsequently tapered once the inflammation comes under control.

Topical

Topical steroids are useful only for anterior uveitis, because therapeutic levels are not reached behind the lens. A solution penetrates the cornea better than does a suspension or ointment. Because ointment causes blurring of vision it is usually instilled at bedtime. The frequency of instillation of drops depends on the severity of inflammation.

NB: If a suspension is used (e.g. Pred Forte), the patient must be instructed to shake the bottle vigorously before use since the active component of the preparation will sediment at the bottom of the bottle and exert no effect.

INDICATIONS

1. **Treatment of acute anterior uveitis** is relatively straightforward and depends on the severity of inflammation.

- Initial intensive therapy involves instillation either hourly or every minute for the first 5 minutes of every hour.

- Once the inflammation is well controlled, the frequency should be carefully tapered to 2-hourly, followed by 3-hourly, then q.i.d., and eventually reduced by one drop a week. Treatment can usually be discontinued altogether by 5–6 weeks.

2. **Treatment of chronic anterior uveitis** is more difficult because the inflammation may last for months and even years, so that long-term steroids are often required, with the risk of complications such as cataract and steroid-induced elevation of introcular pressure (IOP).

- Weak steroid preparations, such as rimexolone or loteprednol etabonate, may be attempted, particularly in steroid reactors, as they have much lesser propensity for elevation of IOP, but they are less effective in controlling the inflammation.

- It may be difficult to discontinue therapy since exacerbations are common.

- Exacerbations are initially treated in the same way as acute anterior uveitis. If the inflammation is controlled with no more than +1 aqueous cells, the rate of instillation can be gradually further reduced by one drop per month.

- The classic teaching that only cellular reaction in the anterior chamber represents active inflammation has been challenged. Flare is caused by chronic breakdown of the blood–aqueous barrier, but the intensity of the flare can also indicate an active process, which may respond to therapy. In this regard, the use of the Kowa Flare Meter represents an improvement in the monitoring of these patients. The measurement of the flare gives a direct quantification of the integrity of the blood–aqueous barrier. Unfortunately, this machine is not available in most centres and monitoring then continues to be based on clinical assessment of cells and flare.

NB: Following cessation of treatment, the patient should be re-examined within a short time to ensure that the uveitis has not recurred.

COMPLICATIONS

1. **Elevation of IOP** is common in susceptible individuals (steroid reactors), but long-term exposure to topical steroids may eventually result in ocular hypertension in many patients.

2. **Cataract** can be induced by both systemic and, less frequently, topical steroid administration. The risk increases with dose and duration of therapy.

3. **Corneal** complications, which are uncommon, include secondary infection with bacteria and fungi, recrudescence of herpes simplex keratitis, and corneal melting, which may be enhanced by inhibition of collagen synthesis.

4. **Systemic** side effects are rare but may occasionally occur following prolonged administration, particularly in children.

Periocular injections

GENERAL ASPECTS

1. **Advantages over topical administration**

- Therapeutic concentrations behind the lens may be achieved.

- Water-soluble drugs, incapable of penetrating the cornea when given topically, can enter the eye trans-sclerally when given by periocular injection.

- A prolonged effect can be achieved with long-acting preparations such as triamcinolone acetonide (Kenalog) or depot steroids such as methylprednisolone acetate (Depomedrone).

2. **Indications**

- In unilateral or asymmetric intermediate or posterior uveitis, periocular injections should be considered as first-line therapy to control inflammation and macular oedema.

- In bilateral posterior uveitis, either to supplement systemic therapy or when systemic steroids are contraindicated.

- Poor compliance with topical or systemic medication.

- At the time of surgery in eyes with uveitis.

3. **Complications**

- Globe penetration.

- Elevation of IOP.

- Ptosis.

- Subdermal fat atrophy.

- Extraocular muscle paresis.

- Optic nerve injury.

- Retinal and choroidal vascular occlusion.

TECHNIQUE

1. **Conjunctival anaesthesia**

- A topical anaesthetic such as tetracaine is instilled.

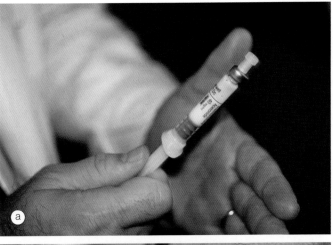

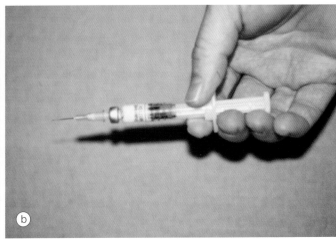

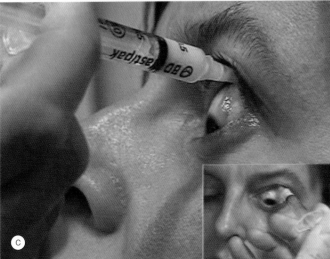

Fig. 6.15 Technique of posterior sub-Tenon injection of steroid (see text)

- A small cotton pledget impregnated with tetracaine (or equivalent) is placed into the superior fornix at the site of injection for 2 minutes.

2. Posterior sub-Tenon injection

- The vial containing the steroid is shaken (Fig. 6.15a).

- 1 ml steroid is drawn up into a 2-ml syringe and the drawing-up needle replaced with a 25-gauge ⅝ inch (16 mm) needle (Fig. 6.15b).

- The patient is asked to look away from the site of injection; most frequently inferiorly when the injection is being given superotemporally.

- The bulbar conjunctiva is penetrated with the tip of the needle, bevel towards the globe, slightly on the bulbar side of the fornix.

- The needle is slowly inserted posteriorly, following the contour of the globe, keeping it as close to the globe as possible. In order not to penetrate the globe accidentally, side-to-side motions are made as the needle is being inserted and the limbus watched; movement of the limbus means that the sclera has been engaged!

- When the needle has been advanced to the hub and cannot be inserted any further (Fig. 6.15c), the plunger is slightly withdrawn and, if no blood has entered the syringe, 1 ml injected. If the needle is too far away from the globe, adequate trans-scleral absorption of steroid will not occur.

3. Orbital floor injection

- The injection is usually performed transcutaneously after skin asepsis.

- A 25-gauge ⅝ inch needle is inserted in the inferior orbital rim and advanced to the hub.

- The plunger is slightly withdrawn to confirm extravascular location and the steroid is injected.

- This is a safer technique than posterior sub-Tenon, but delivers the steroid further away from the globe and is likely, in theory, to result in less intraocular penetration.

Intraocular

1. Injection

- Triamcinolone acetonide (4 mg in 0.1 ml) is an option in the treatment of uveitis and CMO unresponsive to other forms of therapy.

- It produces fast resolution of CMO, lasting about 4 months, and may be used to determine reversibility of visual loss due to CMO.

- Injections may be used following surgery on eyes with uveitis when other forms of prophylaxis are not appropriate.

- Repeated injections should be considered with caution due to significant risk of complications, especially high IOP.

- Other complications include cataract, endophthalmitis (sterile or infectious), hemorrhage and retinal detachment.

2. Slow-release implants are currently undergoing clinical trials.

- The implant (Fig. 6.16), containing an insoluble steroid (fluocinolone acetonide), is implanted via a pars plana incision and sutured to the sclera, similar to a ganciclovir implant used for cytomegalovirus (CMV) retinitis.

- The steroid is continuously released for 3 years and this may obviate the use of long-term systemic steroids.

- Complications are similar to those of intravitreal triamcinolone injection.

Systemic

1. Preparations

a. **Oral** prednisolone 5 mg or 25 mg tablets are the main preparations.

b. **Intravenous injections** of methylprednisolone 1 g/day, repeated for 2 to 3 days, is an option in severe bilateral disease but does not seem to offer any major advantages over high-dose oral therapy.

2. Indications

- Intermediate uveitis unresponsive to posterior sub-Tenon injections.

- Sight-threatening posterior or panuveitis, particularly with bilateral involvement.

- Rarely, anterior uveitis resistant to topical therapy.

3. Contraindications

- Poorly controlled diabetes is a relative contraindication.

- Peptic ulceration.

- Osteoporosis.

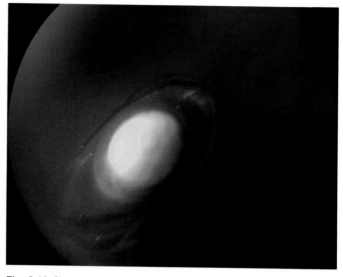

Fig. 6.16 Slow-release steroid implant

- Active systemic infection.

- Psychosis on previous exposure to steroids.

4. General rules of administration

- Start with a large dose and then reduce.

- The starting dose of prednisolone is 1–2 mg/kg/day given in a single morning dose, after breakfast.

- A high level is maintained until a clinical effect is seen, followed by a slow taper over several weeks to avoid reactivation.

- Doses of 40 mg or less for 3 weeks or less do not require gradual reduction.

- Doses of more than 15 mg/day are unacceptable long term, so the use of a steroid-sparing agent has to be considered.

NB: A common cause of failure of treatment is suboptimal dosage.

5. Side effects depend on the dose and duration of administration.

a. **Short-term** therapy may cause dyspepsia, mental changes, electrolyte imbalance, aseptic necrosis of the head of the femur and, very rarely, hyperosmolar hyperglycaemic non-ketotic coma.

b. **Long-term** therapy may cause a cushingoid state (Figs 6.17 and 6.18), osteoporosis, limitation of growth in children, reactivation of infections such as tuberculosis, cataract and exacerbation of pre-existing conditions such as diabetes and myopathy.

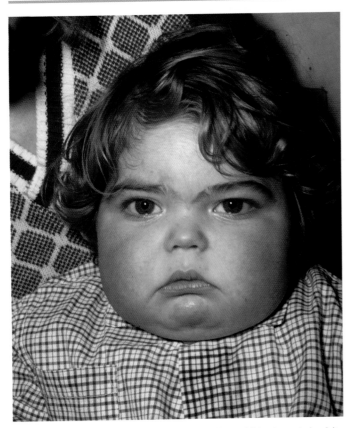

Fig. 6.17 Steroid-induced cushingoid facies in a child, characterised by plethora, swelling and obesity

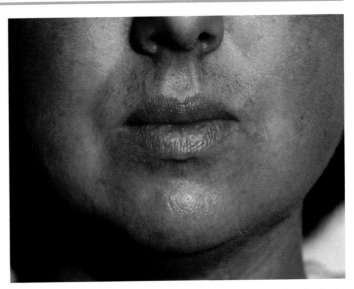

Fig. 6.18 Steroid-induced facial hirsutism and plethora in a female due to systemic steroid administration

Antimetabolites

Indications

1. **Sight-threatening uveitis**, which is usually bilateral, non-infectious, reversible and has failed to respond to adequate steroid therapy.

2. **Steroid-sparing therapy** in patients with intolerable side effects from systemic steroids. Once a patient has been started on an immunosuppressive drug and the appropriate dose ascertained, treatment should continue for 6–24 months, after which gradual tapering and discontinuation of medication should be attempted over the next 3–12 months. However, some patients may require long-term therapy for control of disease activity.

Azathioprine

1. **Indications.** Onset of action takes several weeks but its effects persist after treatment has been discontinued. It is therefore a good option for long-term use in chronic diseases, particularly Behçet syndrome, but not for acute disease.

2. **Regimen**

- Starting dose is 1 mg/kg/day (50-mg tablets) administered once daily or in divided doses.

- After 1–2 weeks, the dose is doubled.

- If appropriate control of inflammation is achieved, the dose of other drugs (e.g. steroids, ciclosporin and tacrolimus) can be tapered.

- Azathioprine is stopped only after the disease has been inactive for over 1 year, ciclosporin or tacrolimus has been withdrawn, and the daily steroid dose is under 7.5 mg.

3. **Side effects.** Bone marrow suppression, gastrointestinal upset and hepatotoxicity are the most important. They can be reversed by dose reduction or temporary withdrawal of the drug.

4. **Monitoring** involves a complete blood count, initially weekly and then every 4–6 weeks, and liver function tests every 12 weeks.

Methotrexate

1. **Indications** are mainly as a steroid-sparing agent in patients with uveitis associated with sarcoidosis and JIA.

2. **Regimen**

- Adult dose is 10–15 mg/week.

- Children require a higher dose (up to 30 mg/week) since the clearance of the drug is increased.

- Folic acid at 2.5–5 mg/day is administered to reduce bone marrow toxicity.

3. **Side effects.** Bone marrow suppression, hepatotoxicity and acute pneumonitis (hypersensitivity reaction) are the most serious but rarely occur with low-dose therapy.

NB: Patients must be warned to abstain from alcohol.

4. **Monitoring** involves a full blood count and liver function tests every 1–2 months. Occasionally, liver biopsies may be required in patients on long-term therapy.

Mycophenolate mofetil

1. **Indications.** A good alternative to azathioprine in unresponsive or intolerant patients. It is not recommended in children.

2. **Dose** is 1 g twice daily (b.d.), which may be increased to 4 g daily.

3. **Side effects** include gastrointestinal disturbance and bone marrow suppression.

4. **Monitoring** involves a full blood count, initially weekly for 4 weeks and then monthly.

Immune modulators

Ciclosporin

1. **Indications.** It is the drug of choice for Behçet syndrome and may also be used in intermediate uveitis, birdshot retinochoroidopathy, VKH syndrome, sympathetic ophthalmitis and idiopathic retinal vasculitis.

2. **Regimen**

- Initial dose is 5 mg/kg/day either as a single daily dose or in two divided doses to avoid serum spikes and renal toxicity.

- Following control of the inflammation, the dose should be tapered to 2–3 mg/kg/day.

- Ciclosporin should not be stopped abruptly, because rebound of inflammation may occur.

3. **Side effects** include nephrotoxicity, hyperlipidaemia, hepatotoxicity, hypertension, hirsutism and gingival hyperplasia. Poorly controlled hypertension and renal disease are relative contraindications. The drug should also be used with caution in patients over 55 years of age, because of less renal reserve.

4. **Monitoring** involves blood pressure measurement and renal and liver function tests every 6 weeks. Serum creatinine level should not be permitted to rise 30% over baseline

Tacrolimus

1. **Indications.** An alternative to ciclosporin in intolerant or unresponsive patients.

2. **Dose.** Maximal is 0.1–0.15 mg/kg, which should be introduced gradually.

3. **Side effects** include hyperglycaemia, neurotoxicity and nephrotoxicity, which are more common than with ciclosporin.

4. **Monitoring** involves blood pressure measurement, renal function tests and blood glucose assessment, initially weekly and then less frequently.

Biological blockers

Biological blockers are used principally for organ transplantation. They have not been licensed for the treatment of ocular inflammatory conditions, but clinical trials are currently in progress.

1. **Interleukin-2 receptor antagonists.** Daclizumab (Zenapax) may be useful to treat uveitis.

2. **Anti-tumour necrosis factor-α antibodies**

a. **Infliximab** (Remicade) shows promise in the treatment of Behçet syndrome. It is given as an intravenous infusion every 8 weeks in a maintenance phase.

b. **Adalimumab** is similar to infliximab but is administered subcutaneously weekly or every other week.

c. **Etanercept** (Embrel) is administered subcutaneously once or twice weekly and seems to be less effective than infliximab in the management of uveitis.

d. **Other** monoclonal antibodies include anakinra and rituximab.

NB: The clinical experience with these agents is very limited and there is concern regarding aggravating tuberculosis and induction of demyelinating disease. The cost is still very high and the long-term effects on the immune system unknown.

FURTHER READING

Degenring RF, Jonas JB. Intravitreal injection of triamcinolone acetonide as treatment for chronic uveitis. Br J Ophthalmol 2003;87:361.

Dick AD, Azim M, Forrester JV. Immunosuppressive therapy for chronic uveitis: optimizing therapy with steroids and cyclosporin A. Br J Ophthalmol 1997;81:1107–1112.

Feldman-Billard S, Lissak B, Benrabah R, et al. Intravenous pulsed methylprednisolone therapy in eye disease. Ophthalmology 2003;110:2369–2371.

Helm CJ, Holland GN. The effects of posterior subtenon injection of triamcinolone acetonide in patients with intermediate uveitis. Am J Ophthalmol 1995;120:55–64.

Jabs DA, Rosenbaum JT. Guidelines for the use of immunosuppressive drugs in patients with ocular inflammatory disorders: recommendations of an expert panel. Am J Ophthalmol 2001;131:679.

Jaffe GJ, Ben-Nun J, Guo H, et al. Fluocinolone acetonide sustained drug device to treat severe uveitis. Ophthalmology 2000;107:2024–2033.

Leslie T, Lois N, Christopoulou D, et al. Photodynamic therapy for inflammatory choroidal neovascularisation unresponsive to immunosuppression. Br J Ophthalmol 2005;89:147–150.

Murphy CC, Ayliffe WH, Booth A, et al. Tumor necrosis factor alpha blockade with infliximab for refractory uveitis and scleritis. Ophthalmology 2004;111:352–356.

Okada AA, Wakabayashi T, Morimura Y, et al. Trans-Tenon's retrobulbar triamcinolone infusion for the treatment of uveitis. Br J Ophthalmol 2003;87:968–971.

Sfikakis PP, Theodossiadis PG, Katsiari CG, et al. Effect of infliximab on sight-threatening panuveitis in Behçet's disease. Lancet 2001;358:295–296.

Tanner V, Kanski JJ, Frith PA. Posterior sub-Tenon's triamcinolone injections in the treatment of uveitis. *Eye* 1998;12:679–685.

ACUTE ANTERIOR UVEITIS

Anterior uveitis is the most common form of uveitis. Acute anterior uveitis (AAU) is the most common form of anterior uveitis, accounting for three-quarters of cases. It is easily recognised due to the severity of symptoms, which will force the patient to seek medical attention.

Clinical features

Symptoms

Presentation is typically with sudden onset of unilateral pain, photophobia and redness, which may be associated with lacrimation.

> **NB:** Patients may notice mild ocular discomfort a few days before the acute attack, when clinical signs are absent.

Signs

1. **Visual acuity** is usually good at presentation, except in very severe cases with hypopyon.

2. **Ciliary (circumcorneal) injection** has a violaceous hue (Fig. 6.19).

3. **Miosis** due to sphincter spasm may predispose to the formation of posterior synechiae unless the pupil is dilated (Fig. 6.20).

4. **Aqueous cells** indicate disease activity and their number reflects disease severity. Grading of cells is performed with a 2 mm long and 1 mm wide slit beam with maximal light intensity and magnification. The findings are recorded in the notes as follows:

   0–5 = 0
   6–10 = +
   11–20 = ++
   21–50 = +++
   >50 = ++++

5. **Anterior vitreous cells** indicate iridocyclitis.

6. **Aqueous flare** reflects the presence of protein due to a breakdown of the blood–aqueous barrier (Fig. 6.21). Flare may be graded by laser inferometry using a flare meter or clinically by observing the degree of interference in the visualisation of the iris using the same settings as for cells:

   just detectable = +
   iris details clear = ++

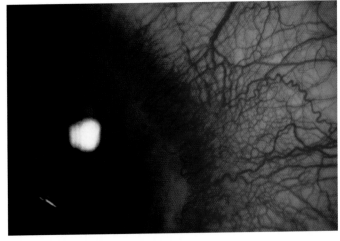

Fig. 6.19 Ciliary injection in acute anterior uveitis

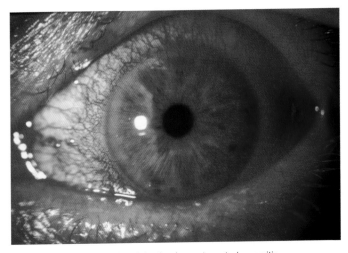

Fig. 6.20 Miosis and ciliary injection in acute anterior uveitis

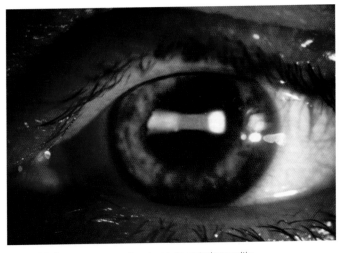

Fig. 6.21 Severe aqueous flare in acute anterior uveitis

ment. In a few patients with many recurrent attacks, the inflammation may eventually become chronic.

2. **Other** uncommon manifestations include scleritis and conjunctivitis.

REITER SYNDROME

Reiter syndrome, also referred to as reactive arthritis, is characterised by the triad of non-specific (non-gonococcal) urethritis, conjunctivitis and arthritis. About 85% of patients with RS are positive for HLA-B27 but the diagnosis is clinical and is based on the presence of arthritis and other characteristic manifestations (see Ch. 8).

1. **AAU** occurs in up to 12% of patients. The prevalence is, however, higher in carriers of HLA-B27.

2. **Conjunctivitis** is very common and usually follows the urethritis by about 2 weeks and precedes the arthritis. The inflammation is usually mild, bilateral and mucopurulent, with a papillary or follicular reaction. Spontaneous resolution occurs within 7–10 days and treatment is not required. Cultures for bacteria are usually negative.

3. **Other** uncommon manifestations include nummular keratitis, scleritis, episcleritis, intermediate uveitis, papillitis, retinal oedema and retinal vasculitis.

PSORIATIC ARTHRITIS

About 7% of patients with psoriasis develop arthritis. Psoriatic arthritis affects both sexes equally and is associated with an increased prevalence of HLA-B27 and HLA-B17 (see Ch. 8).

1. **AAU** is uncommon except in patients with AS.

2. **Other** manifestations include conjunctivitis keratitis in the form of raised, marginal, corneal infiltrates and secondary Sjögren syndrome.

Inflammatory bowel disease

ULCERATIVE COLITIS

Ulcerative colitis is an idiopathic, chronic, relapsing inflammatory disease involving the rectum and extending proximally to involve part or all of the large intestine (see Ch. 8).

1. **AAU** occurs in about 5% of patients and may synchronise with exacerbation of colitis. As expected, uveitis is commoner in patients with associated AS.

2. **Other** manifestations include peripheral corneal infiltrates, conjunctivitis, episcleritis, scleritis and, rarely, posterior segment involvement in the form of papillitis, multifocal choroiditis and retinal vasculitis.

CROHN DISEASE

Crohn disease (regional ileitis) is an idiopathic, chronic, relapsing disease characterised by multifocal, full-thickness, non-caseating granulomatous inflammation of the intestinal wall (see Ch. 8).

1. **AAU** occurs in about 3% of patients.

2. **Other** manifestations include conjunctivitis, episcleritis, peripheral corneal infiltrates and retinal periphlebitis.

Nephritis

TUBULOINTERSTITIAL NEPHRITIS

Tubulointerstitial nephritis and uveitis (TINU) is an uncommon condition usually affecting young women or children. Nephritis is frequently associated with the use of non-steroidal anti-inflammatory drugs (NSAIDs) or antibiotics. Renal disease usually precedes the uveitis.

1. **Presentation** is with constitutional symptoms, proteinuria, anaemia, hypertension and renal failure. The response to systemic steroid therapy is good and the condition resolves within a few months.

2. **Uveitis** is usually anterior, bilateral, non-granulomatous and responds well to steroids. Some cases become chronic and relapsing and may require immunosuppressive therapy. Intermediate and posterior uveitis may also occur.

IGA GLOMERULONEPHRITIS

IgA glomerulonephritis is a common disease in which IgA is found in the glomerular mesangium.

1. **Presentation** is usually in the third to fifth decades with recurrent macroscopic haematuria which may be associated with upper respiratory tract infection.

2. **Ocular manifestations**, which are uncommon, include anterior uveitis, keratoconjunctivitis and scleritis.

Miscellaneous systemic associations

1. **Acute-onset sarcoidosis** may be associated with AAU.

2. **Behçet disease** is characterised by recurrent AAU which may be simultaneously bilateral and associated with a transient mobile hypopyon. It is usually a mild manifestation when compared with posterior segment involvement and usually responds readily to topical therapy.

3. **Syphilis.** AAU occurs in about 4% of patients with secondary syphilis and is bilateral in 50%. The inflammation is usually acute and unless appropriately treated becomes chronic. In some cases, iritis is first associated with dilated iris capillaries (roseolae) which may develop into more localised papules and subsequently into larger yellowish nodules. Various types of postinflammatory iris atrophy may ensue.

4. **Leprosy.** AAU is thought to be caused by immune complex deposition in the uvea. It may be associated with systemic symptoms such as fever and swelling of skin lesions. Intraocular inflammation may be precipitated by initiation or withdrawal of systemic therapy.

5. Relapsing polychondritis may be associated with severe AAU with hypopyon.

FURTHER READING

Amor B. Reiter's syndrome. Diagnosis and clinical features. *Rheum Dis Clin North Am* 1998;24:677–695.

BenEzra D. Bilateral anterior uveitis in interstitial nephritis. *Am J Ophthamol* 1988;106:766–767.

Derzko-Dzulynsky L, Rabinovitch T. Tubulointerstitial nephritis and uveitis with bilateral multifocal choroiditis. *Am J Ophthalmol* 2000;129:805–806.

Kiss S, Letko E, Quamruddin S, et al. Long-term progression, prognosis, and treatment of patients with recurrent ocular manifestations of Reiter's syndrome. *Ophthalmology* 2003;110:1764–1769.

Kotaniemi K, Aho K, Kotaniemi A. Uveitis as a cause of visual loss in arthritides and comparable conditions. *J Rheumatol* 2001;28:309–312.

Mandeville JT, Levinson RD, Holland GN. The tubulointerstitial nephritis and uveitis syndrome. *Surv Ophthalmol* 2001;46:195–208.

Monnet D, Breban M, Hudry C, et al Ophthalmic findings and frequency of extraocular manifestations in patients with HLA-B27 uveitis: a study of 175 cases. *Ophthalmology* 2004;111:802–809.

Paiva ES, Macaluso DC, Edwards A, et al. Characterization of uveitis in patients with psoriatic arthritis. *Ann Rheum Dis* 2000;59:67–70.

Smith JR. HLA-B27-associated uveitis. *Ophthalmol Clin North Am* 2002;15:297–307.

Tay-Kearney ML, Schwam BL, Lowder C, et al. Clinical features and associated systemic diseases of HLA-B27 uveitis. *Am J Ophthalmol* 1996;121:47–56.

Wakefield D, Montanaro A, McCluskey P. Acute anterior uveitis and HLA B-27. *Surv Ophthalmol* 1991;36:223–232.

Specific syndromes

Posner–Schlossman syndrome

Posner–Schlossman syndrome (glaucomatocyclitic crisis) is a rare condition that predominantly affects males from the third to the sixth decades. It is characterised by unilateral, often recurrent, attacks of sudden, sharp elevation in IOP associated with mild anterior uveitis.

The attacks last a few hours to several days and initially the IOP returns to normal following treatment. After many episodes, the IOP may become persistently elevated and some patients develop open-angle glaucoma. The cause of the raised IOP is presumed to be acute trabeculitis; herpes simplex virus (HSV) may play a pathogenetic role.

1. Presentation is with mild discomfort, haloes around lights and slight blurring of vision.

2. Signs

* Corneal epithelial oedema due to a high IOP (40–60 mmHg).

* Mild anterior uveitis with fine white central keratic precipitates (Fig. 6.29).

* The pupil may be slightly dilated.

* Iris heterochromia may occur.

* Gonioscopy shows an open angle.

> **NB:** Unless gonioscopy is performed, the condition may be confused with acute primary angle-closure glaucoma. The absence of peripheral anterior synechiae helps in the differentiation from other inflammatory glaucomas.

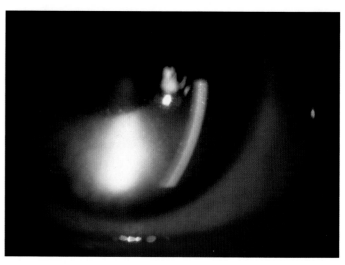

Fig. 6.29 Fine white keratic precipitates and corneal epithelial oedema in Posner–Schlossman syndrome

3. Treatment. Topical steroids are used to control the inflammation and aqueous suppressants are used for the raised IOP. Patients with frequent recurrences may benefit from prophylactic topical steroids.

Schwartz syndrome

Schwartz syndrome is a rare condition characterised by raised IOP in an eye with very mild anterior uveitis and a long-standing shallow retinal detachment associated with a small retinal dialysis. Management involves medical control of IOP followed by repair of the retinal detachment.

FURTHER READING

Jap A, Sivakumar M, Chee SP. Is Posner Schlossman syndrome benign? *Ophthalmology* 2001;108:913–918.

Matsuo N, Takabatake M, Ueno H, et al. Photoreceptor outer segments in the aqueous humor in rhegmatogenous retinal detachment. *Am J Ophthalmol* 1986;101:673–679.

Schwartz A. Chronic open-angle glaucoma secondary to rhegmatogenous retinal detachment. *Am J Ophthalmol* 1973;75:205–211.

Yamamoto S, Pavan-Langston D, Tada R, et al. Possible role of herpes simplex virus in the origin of Posner-Schlossman syndrome. *Am J Ophthalmol* 1995;119:796–798.

Drug-induced uveitis

Rifabutin

Rifabutin is used mainly in the management and prophylaxis of *Mycobacterium avium* complex infections in AIDS patients with low CD4 counts. It is also used with other drugs to treat tuberculosis in immunocompetent patients.

1. **AAU** is typically unilateral and frequently associated with hypopyon; associated vitritis may be mistaken for endophthalmitis.

2. **Treatment** involves withdrawal of the drug or reduction of dose.

> **NB:** Drugs that inhibit metabolism of rifabutin through the cytochrome P450 pathway, such as clarithromycin and fluconazole, will increase the risk of uveitis.

Cidofovir

Cidofovir is used in the management of CMV retinitis in AIDS patients.

1. **AAU** with few cells but a marked fibrinous exudate may develop following several intravenous infusions. Vitritis is common and hypotony may occur with long-term administration.

2. **Treatment** with topical steroids and mydriatics is usually successful, avoiding the need to discontinue therapy.

> **NB:** Intravitreal injection of cidofovir should be used with caution because it carries a high risk of hypotony.

FURTHER READING

Bainbridge JW, Raina J, Shah SM, et al. Ocular complications of intravenous cidofovir for cytomegalovirus retinitis in patients with AIDS. *Eye* 1999;13:353–356.

Bhagat N, Read RW, Rao NA, et al. Rifabutin-associated hypopyon uveitis in human immunodeficiency virus-negative immunocompetent individuals. *Ophthalmology* 2001;108:750–752.

Cunningham ET Jr. Uveitis in HIV positive patients. *Br J Ophthalmol* 2000;84:233–235.

Saran BR, Maguire AM, Nichols C, et al. Hypopyon uveitis in patients with acquired immunodeficiency syndrome treated for systemic *Mycobacterium avium* complex infection with rifabutin. Arch Ophthalmol 1994;112:1159–1165.

Lens-induced uveitis

Lens-induced uveitis is triggered by an immune response to lens proteins.

Phacoanaphylactic endophthalmitis

Phacoanaphylactic endophthalmitis develops days to weeks after traumatic rupture of the lens capsule.

1. **Presentation** is with abrupt reduction in visual acuity and pain which is less severe than in bacterial endophthalmitis.

2. **Signs**

- Anterior uveitis is granulomatous and of variable severity.

- The IOP is frequently high.

- The posterior segment is not involved.

3. **Differential diagnosis** is bacterial endophthalmitis; in doubtful cases, vitreous taps may be required.

4. **Treatment** involves removal of all lens material in conjunction with intensive steroid therapy.

Phacogenic non-granulomatous uveitis

Phacogenic non-granulomatous uveitis develops within 2–3 weeks following lens capsule rupture.

1. **Signs.** Anterior uveitis is less severe and is more chronic than in phacoanaphylactic endophthalmitis.

2. **Differential diagnosis** includes low-grade bacterial and fungal endophthalmitis, sympathetic ophthalmitis and introcular lens-induced inflammation.

3. **Treatment** of mild cases is with topical steroids, but periocular and systemic therapy will be necessary for more intense inflammation. Removal of remaining lens material may also be necessary.

FURTHER READING

Allen JC. Sympathetic uveitis and phacoanaphylaxis. *Am J Ophthalmol* 1987;103:63–83.

Thach AB, Marak GE Jr, McLean IW, et al. Phacoanaphylactic endophthalmitis: a clinicopathologic review. *Int Ophthalmol* 1991;15:271–279.

CHRONIC ANTERIOR UVEITIS

Chronic anterior uveitis (CAU) is less common than the acute type but more unpredictable. It persists for longer than 6 weeks, sometimes even years, and may be associated with remissions and exacerbations. The inflammation may be granulomatous or non-granulomatous. Bilateral involvement is more common than in AAU.

Symptoms

Presentation is insidious and many patients are asymptomatic until the development of complications such as cataract and band keratopathy.

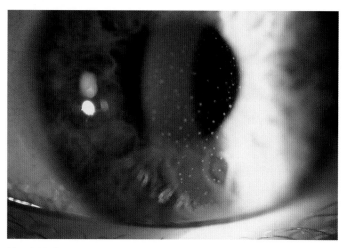

Fig. 6.30 Small keratic precipitates in Fuchs uveitis syndrome

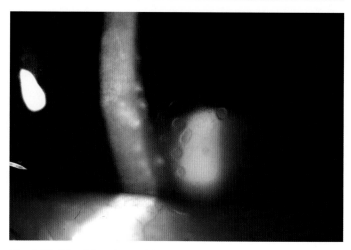

Fig. 6.32 'Ghost' keratic precipitates

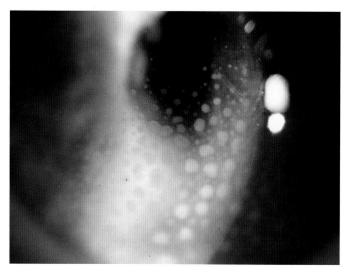

Fig. 6.31 Large 'mutton-fat' keratic precipitates

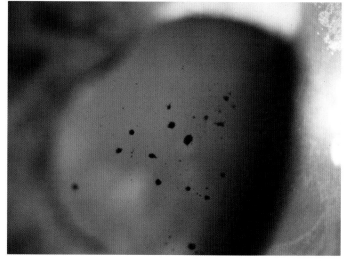

Fig. 6.33 Old pigmented keratic precipitates

> **NB:** Because of the lack of symptoms, patients at risk of developing CAU should be routinely screened; this applies particularly in patients with JIA.

Signs

1. **External.** The eye is usually white or occasionally pink during periods of exacerbation of inflammatory activity.

2. **Aqueous cells** vary in number according to disease activity, but even patients with numerous cells may have no symptoms.

3. **Aqueous flare** may be more marked than cells in eyes with prolonged activity and its severity may act as an indicator of disease activity (contrary to previous teaching).

4. **Keratic precipitates** (KPs) are clusters of cellular deposits on the corneal endothelium, composed of epithelioid cells, lymphocytes and polymorphs. Their characteristics and distribution may indicate the probable type of uveitis.

   - Small stellate KPs, distributed over the entire endothelium, occur in Fuchs uveitis syndrome (Fig. 6.30).

   - Large KPs in granulomatous disease are roundish and have a greasy ('mutton-fat') appearance. They are often more numerous inferiorly and may form in a triangular pattern with the apex pointing up (Fig. 6.31). This is the result of gravity and normal convection flow of aqueous.

   - Resolved 'mutton-fat' KPs leave behind a ground-glass appearance ('ghost' KPs) which is evidence of previous granulomatous inflammation (Fig. 6.32).

   - Longstanding non-granulomatous KPs may become pigmented (Fig. 6.33).

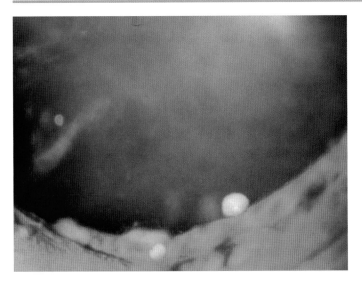

Fig. 6.34 Koeppe nodules

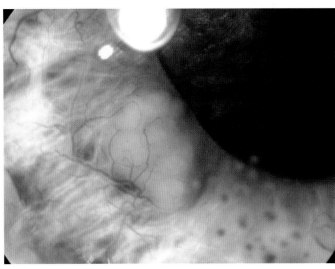

Fig. 6.36 Very large nodule in sarcoid uveitis

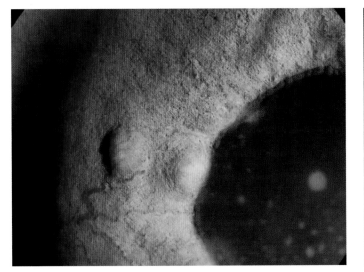

Fig. 6.35 Busacca and Koeppe nodule

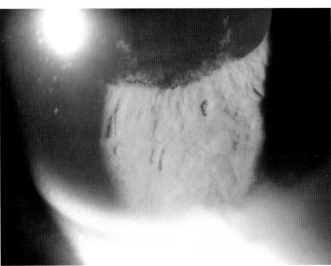

Fig. 6.37 Stromal iris thickening

5. Iris nodules

- Koeppe nodules are small and situated at the pupillary border (Fig. 6.34).

- Busacca nodules are stromal, usually not very large, and are typical of granulomatous inflammation (Fig. 6.35).

- Large pink nodules are characteristic of granulomatous sarcoid uveitis (Fig. 6.36).

6. Iris stromal infiltration giving rise to blunting of the iris crypts and diffuse thickening with a velvety appearance is also typical of sarcoidosis (Fig. 6.37).

7. Posterior synechiae are more common than in AAU and may be extensive and permanent (Fig. 6.38).

8. Gonioscopy may show granulomatous deposits on the trabecular meshwork and peripheral anterior synechiae (Fig. 6.39).

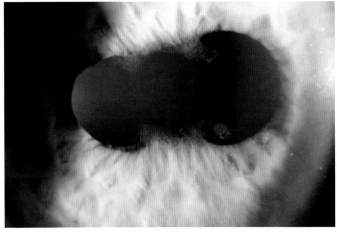

Fig. 6.38 Strong posterior synechiae which cannot be broken by mydriasis

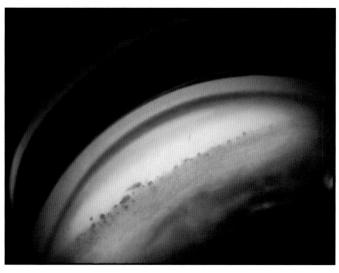

Fig. 6.39 Gonioscopy showing precipitates and small peripheral anterior synechiae in granulomatous inflammation (Courtesy of R Curtis)

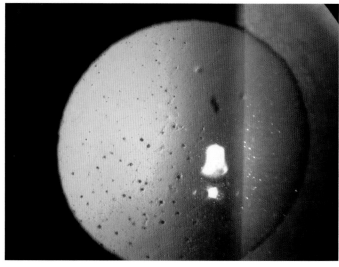

Fig. 6.40 Keratic precipitates in Fuchs uveitis syndrome seen on retro-illumination

Course and prognosis

- The inflammation persists for longer than 6 weeks and in some cases many months or even years.

- Remissions and exacerbations of inflammatory activity are common and it is difficult to determine when the natural course of the disease has come to an end.

- Treatment is more difficult than for AAU and may involve topical and systemic administration.

- As a consequence of the chronicity of the disease, delay in presentation and prolonged therapy, the prognosis is guarded and complications such as cataract and glaucoma are common.

FURTHER READING

Bloch-Michel E, Nussenblatt RB. International Uveitis Study Group recommendations for the evaluation of intraocular inflammatory disease. *Am J Ophthalmol* 1987;103:234–235.

Nussenblatt RB, Palestine AG, Chan CC, et al. Standardisation of vitreal inflammatory activity in intermediate and posterior uveitis. *Ophthalmology* 1985;92:467–471.

Pavesio CE. Clinical features of uveitis. In: Easty DL, Sparrow JM, eds. *Oxford Textbook of Ophthalmology*. Oxford: Oxford University Press; 1999.

Pavesio CE, Nozik RA. Anterior and intermediate uveitis. *Int Ophthalmol Clin* 1990;30:244–251.

Fuchs uveitis syndrome

Fuchs uveitis syndrome (FUS), or Fuchs heterochromic cyclitis, is a chronic anterior uveitis of insidious onset. It typically affects one eye of a young adult, although it can also occur during childhood. Bilateral simultaneous involvement occurs in about 5% of cases. Although FUS accounts for about 4% of all cases of uveitis, it is frequently misdiagnosed and overtreated. The heterochromia (difference in iris colour) may be absent or difficult to detect, particularly in brown-eyed individuals.

Diagnosis

The diagnosis is based mainly on ocular signs, which in early cases may be subtle and easily overlooked.

1. Presentation

- Chronic, annoying vitreous floaters is often the presenting symptom.

- Gradual blurring of vision secondary to cataract formation is common.

- Colour difference between the two eyes.

- Incidental detection.

2. General signs

- Absence of posterior synechiae, except following cataract surgery.

- The KPs are characteristically small, round or stellate, grey–white in colour, and scattered throughout the corneal endothelium and frequently associated with feathery fibrin filaments (Fig. 6.40); they may come and go, but never become confluent or pigmented.

- Iris nodules are common and occur on the pupillary side of the collarette (Fig. 6.41).

- Aqueous humour shows a faint flare and mild cellular reaction.

- Vitritis and stringy opacities may be dense enough to reduce vision (Fig. 6.42).

- Iris crystals may be seen in a minority of cases.

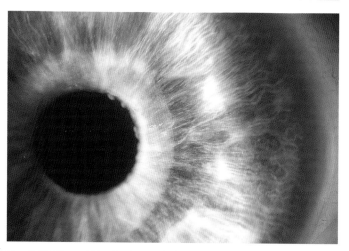

Fig. 6.43 Stromal iris atrophy rendering the sphincter pupillae prominent; also note small pupillary nodules

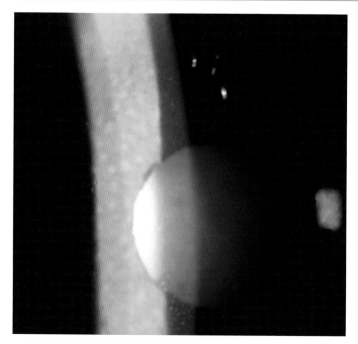

Fig. 6.41 Iris nodule in Fuchs uveitis syndrome; also note cataract

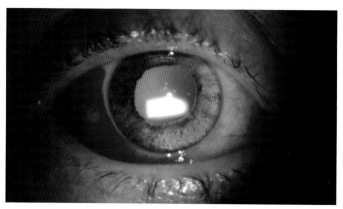

Fig. 6.44 Posterior pigment layer atrophy seen on retroillumination in Fuchs uveitis syndrome; the subconjunctival haemorrhage is due to recent cataract surgery

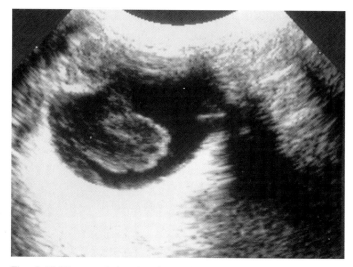

Fig. 6.42 Ultrasound showing dense vitreous opacities in Fuchs uveitis syndrome

3. Diffuse iris atrophy

- The earliest finding is loss of iris crypts.

- Advanced stromal atrophy makes the affected iris appear dull with loss of detail giving rise to a washed-out appearance, particularly in the pupillary zone (Fig. 6.43). The normal radial iris blood vessels appear prominent due to lack of stromal support.

- Posterior pigment layer iris atrophy is best detected by retroillumination (Fig. 6.44).

- Mydriasis resulting from atrophy of the pupillary sphincter may be present.

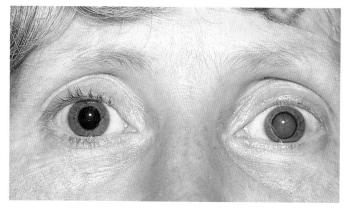

Fig. 6.45 Heterochromia iridis in left Fuchs uveitis syndrome; also note mature cataract

4. Heterochromia iridis is an important and common sign.

- Most frequently, the affected eye is hypochromic (Fig. 6.45).

- It is easily seen in green eyes, but if the iris is blue or deep brown, heterochromia will be difficult to detect.

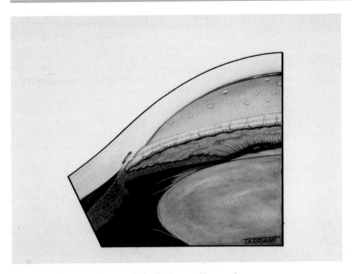

Fig. 6.46 Fine-angle vessels in Fuchs uveitis syndrome

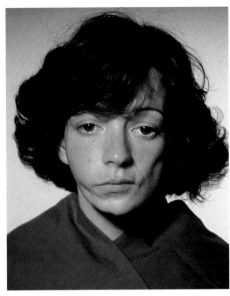

Fig. 6.47 Facial hemiatrophy in Parry–Romberg syndrome (Courtesy of M A Mir, from *Atlas of Clinical Diagnosis*, 2nd edition, Saunders, 2003)

- The nature of heterochromia is determined by the relative degrees of atrophy of the stroma and posterior pigment epithelium, as well as the patient's natural iris colour.

- In blue eyes, predominant stromal atrophy allows the posterior pigmented layer to show through and become the dominant pigmentation, so that the eye may become hyperchromic (reverse heterochromia).

5. **Gonioscopy** may be normal or may show one of the following:

- Fine radial twig-like vessels in the angle (Fig. 6.46), which are probably responsible for the filiform haemorrhages that develop on anterior chamber paracentesis (Amsler sign).

- A membrane obscuring angle details.

- Small, non-confluent, irregular, peripheral anterior synechiae.

6. **Systemic association.** Parry–Romberg syndrome (hemifacial atrophy) is found in a small minority of cases (Fig. 6.47).

Complications

FUS runs a chronic course lasting many years with periods of increased activity. The two main complications are cataract and glaucoma, both of which may be enhanced by the inadvertent use of topical steroids.

1. **Cataract** is extremely common and may be the presenting feature. It does not differ from that associated with other types of anterior uveitis. The results of surgery with posterior chamber intraocular lens implantation are good.

2. **Glaucoma** is a late manifestation which typically develops only after several years of follow-up. It is usually well controlled on topical therapy, but some patients may require trabeculectomy.

Treatment

1. **Topical steroids** are ineffective.

2. **Mydriatics** are unnecessary because posterior synechiae do not occur.

3. **Vitrectomy** may be considered for severe vitreous opacification that is reducing vision or is very disturbing.

Other causes of heterochromia iridis

1. **Hypochromic**

- Congenital.

- Horner syndrome, particularly if congenital.

2. **Hyperchromic**

- Oculodermal melanocytosis (naevus of Ota).

- Ocular siderosis.

- Diffuse iris naevus or melanoma.

- Unilateral use of a topical prostaglandin analogue for glaucoma.

- Sturge–Weber syndrome (rare).

FURTHER READING

Jones NP. Fuchs' heterochromic uveitis: a reappraisal of the clinical spectrum. *Eye* 1991;5:649–661.

Jones NP. Fuchs' heterochromic uveitis: an update. *Surv Ophthalmol* 1993;37:253–272.

La Hey E, Rothova A, Baarsma GS, et al. Fuchs' heterochromic iridocyclitis is not associated with ocular toxoplasmosis. *Arch Ophthalmol* 1992;110:806–811.

O' Neill D, Murray PI, Patel BC, et al. Extracapsular cataract surgery with and without intraocular lens implantation in Fuchs heterochromic cyclitis. *Ophthalmology* 1995;102:1362–1368.

Rothova A, La Hey E, Baarsma GS, et al. Iris nodules in Fuchs' heterochromic uveitis. *Am J Ophthalmol* 1994;118:338–342.

Sherwood DR, Rosenthal RA. Cataract surgery in Fuchs heterochromic iridocyclitis. *Br J Ophthalmol* 1992;76:238–240.

Waters FM, Goodall K, Jones NP, et al. Vitrectomy for vitreous opacification in Fuchs heterochromic uveitis. *Eye* 2000;14:216–218.

Systemic associations

Juvenile idiopathic arthritis

JIA is an inflammatory arthritis of at least 6 weeks duration occurring before the age of 16 years (see Ch. 8). It is by far the most common disease associated with childhood anterior uveitis.

CLASSIFICATION

Classification of JIA is based on the onset and the extent of joint involvement during the first 6 months as follows:

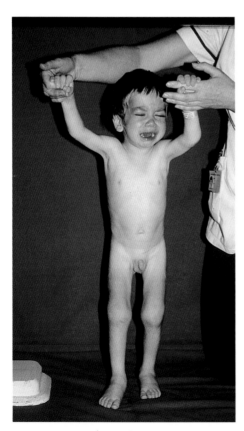

Fig. 6.48 Severe involvement of the knees in pauciarticular-onset juvenile idiopathic arthritis

1. **Pauciarticular-onset** JIA affects four or fewer joints, commonly the knees (Fig. 6.48), and accounts for about 60% of cases. Uveitis affects about 20% of children. Risk factors for uveitis are early onset of JIA, and positive findings for ANA and HLA-DR5.

2. **Polyarticular-onset** JIA affects five or more joints and accounts for a further 20% of cases. Uveitis occurs in about 5% of cases.

3. **Systemic-onset** JIA accounts for about 20% of cases but is not associated with uveitis.

NB: The term 'Still disease' is reserved for patients in this subgroup.

ANTERIOR UVEITIS

In the vast majority of patients, arthritis antedates the diagnosis of uveitis, although, rarely, ocular involvement may precede joint disease by several years.

The intraocular inflammation is chronic, non-granulomatous and bilateral in 70% of cases. It is unusual for unilateral uveitis to become bilateral after more than a year. When bilateral, the severity of inflammation is usually symmetric.

NB: There is no correlation between the activity of joint and eye inflammation.

1. **Presentation** is invariably asymptomatic; the uveitis is frequently detected on routine slit-lamp examination. Even during acute exacerbations with +4 aqueous cells, it is rare for patients to complain, although a few report an increase in vitreous floaters.

NB: Often uveitis may not be suspected until the parents recognise complications such as strabismus, or an abnormal appearance of the eye due to band keratopathy or cataract.

2. **Signs**

- Uninjected eye, even in the presence of severe uveitis.

- Small to medium-sized KPs.

- During acute exacerbations, the entire endothelium shows 'dusting' by many hundreds of cells, but hypopyon is absent.

- Posterior synechiae are common in longstanding undetected uveitis.

NB: Not all children with CAU have or will develop JIA.

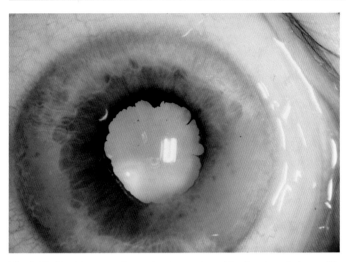

Fig. 6.49 Band keratopathy and mature cataract in chronic anterior uveitis associated with juvenile idiopathic arthritis

3. Prognosis

- In about 10% of cases, the uveitis is mild, with never more than +1 aqueous cells, and persists for less than 12 months.

- About 15% of patients have one attack, which lasts less than 4 months, the severity of inflammation varying from +2 to +4 aqueous cells.

- In 50% of cases, the uveitis is moderate to severe and persists for more than 4 months.

- In 25% of cases, the uveitis is very severe, lasts for several years and responds poorly to treatment. In this subgroup, band keratopathy occurs in 40% of eyes, cataract in 30% and secondary inflammatory glaucoma in 15% (Fig. 6.49).

- Other serious complications include phthisis and amblyopia.

NB: The presence of complications at initial examination appears to be an important risk factor for the development of subsequent complications, regardless of therapy.

4. Treatment with topical steroids is usually effective; acute exacerbations require very frequent instillations. Poor responders to topical administration may benefit from periocular injections. Low-dose methotrexate is useful for steroid resistance.

5. Screening. Because the onset of intraocular inflammation is invariably asymptomatic, it is extremely important to regularly screen children at risk for at least 7 years from the onset of arthritis or until the age of 12 years. The frequency of slit-lamp examination is governed by the various risk factors as follows:

- Systemic onset = not required.
- Polyarticular onset = every 9 months.
- Polyarticular onset + ANA = every 6 months.
- Pauciarticular onset = every 3 months.
- Pauciarticular onset + ANA = every 2 months.

DIFFERENTIAL DIAGNOSIS

1. **Idiopathic juvenile chronic iridocyclitis.** Whilst JIA is the most common systemic association of CAU in children, many patients with juvenile CAU are otherwise healthy. The majority of patients are also girls. As the onset of intraocular inflammation is frequently insidious and asymptomatic, most cases are not diagnosed until visual acuity is reduced from complicated cataract or the parents notice a white patch on the cornea caused by band keratopathy. In a small number of cases, the uveitis is detected by chance.

2. **Other types of juvenile arthritis and uveitis**

a. *Juvenile ankylosing spondylitis* is uncommon and typically affects boys around the age of 10 years. Early diagnosis may be difficult because in children the disease frequently presents with peripheral lower limb arthritis and radiological evaluation of the sacroiliac joints is usually not helpful during the early stages. Just like adults, some children develop AAU.

b. *Juvenile Reiter syndrome* is very rare and is invariably post-dysenteric. A few cases of AAU have been reported.

c. *Juvenile psoriatic arthritis* is relatively uncommon and is characterised by asymmetric involvement of both large and small joints in association with skin lesions and nail pitting. CAU is uncommon.

d. *Juvenile bowel-associated arthritis* is rare. Joint involvement is usually mild and affects large joints in association with either ulcerative colitis or Crohn disease. Anterior uveitis, which may be acute or chronic, has been reported in a few patients.

3. **Juvenile sarcoidosis** is rare and less frequently associated with pulmonary involvement than in adults, and typically manifests with skin, joint and eye disease. Chest radiographs are therefore of less diagnostic value in children with sarcoidosis. Serum ACE may also be misleading, because children have higher normal values than do adults. When uveitis is confined to the anterior segment, it can be confused with JIA-associated uveitis. Unlike JIA-associated uveitis, however, it may be granulomatous and also involve the posterior segment.

4. **Lyme disease** usually presents with intermediate uveitis with significant anterior uveitis, in contrast with pars planitis, where anterior uveitis is insignificant.

5. **Neonatal-onset multisystem inflammatory disease** is a rare, idiopathic, chronic relapsing disease that predomi-

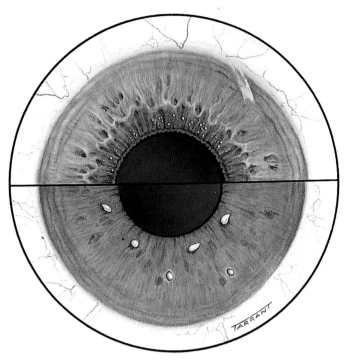

Fig. 6.50 Lepromatous chronic anterior uveitis. (a) Small iris 'pearls' formed from the remains of dead bacteria are pathognomonic; (b) large iris 'pearls' have dropped into the anterior chamber

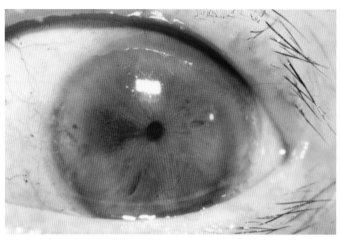

Fig. 6.51 Miosis and iris atrophy in late lepromatous chronic anterior uveitis (Courtesy of T ffytche)

nantly involves the skin, joints and central nervous system (CNS). About 50% of children develop recurrent anterior uveitis. The absence of posterior synechiae and no tendency to glaucoma and cataract formation are characteristic.

Miscellaneous systemic associations

1. **Lepromatous leprosy** (see Ch. 8) may result in CAU as the result of direct invasion of the iris by bacilli. It is characterised by the following:

- Low-grade inflammation associated with the formation of synechiae.

- A pathognomonic sign of lepromatous leprosy is the presence of iris 'pearls' (Fig. 6.50a).

- The 'pearls' slowly enlarge and coalesce, become pedunculated and drop into the anterior chamber, from which they eventually disappear (Fig. 6.50b).

- Eventually, the iris becomes atrophic and the pupil miosed as a result of damage to the sympathetic innervation to the dilator pupillae (Fig. 6.51).

- Treatment involves systemic antibiotics and topical steroids.

2. **Chronic sarcoidosis** in patients with pulmonary disease is associated with granulomatous CAU.

3. **Vogt–Koyanagi syndrome** is associated with granulomatous CAU when recurrent disease occurs.

4. **Other** systemic associations include brucellosis and Lyme disease.

FURTHER READING

Chia A, Lee V, Graham EM, et al. Factors related to severe uveitis at diagnosis in children with juvenile idiopathic arthritis in a screening program. *Am J Ophthalmol* 2003;135:757–762.

Dana MR, Merayo-Lloves J, Schaumberg DA, et al. Visual outcomes prognosticators in juvenile rheumatoid arthritis-associated uveitis. *Ophthalmology* 1997;104:236–244.

Dollfus H, Hafner R, Hofmann HM, et al. Chronic infantile neurological cutaneous and articular/neonatal onset multisystem inflammatory disease syndrome: ocular manifestations in a recently recognized chronic inflammatory disease of childhood. *Arch Ophthalmol* 2000;118:1386–1392.

Edelsten C, Lee V, Bentley CR, et al. An evaluation of baseline risk factors predicting severity in juvenile idiopathic arthritis associated uveitis and other chronic anterior uveitis in early childhood. *Br J Ophthalmol* 2002;86:51–56.

Edelsten C, Reddy MA, Stanford MR, et al. Visual loss associated with pediatric uveitis in English primary and referred centres. *Am J Ophthalmol* 2003;135:676–680.

Espiritu CG. Gelber R. Ostler HB. Chronic anterior uveitis in leprosy: an insidious cause of blindness. *Br J Ophthalmol* 1991;75:273–275.

Foster CS. Diagnosis and treatment of juvenile idiopathic arthritis-associated uveitis. *Curr Opin Ophthalmol* 2003;14:395–398.

Foster CS, Barrett F. Cataract development and cataract surgery in patients with juvenile rheumatoid arthritis-associated iridocyclitis. *Ophthalmology* 1993;100:809–817.

Holland GN. Intraocular lens implantation in patients with juvenile rheumatoid arthritis-associated uveitis: an unresolved management issue. *Am J Ophthalmol* 1996;122:255–257.

Holland GN, Stiehm ER. Special considerations in the evaluation and management of uveitis in children. *Am J Ophthalmol* 2003;135:867–878.

Hoover DL, Khan JA, Giangiacomo J. Pediatric ocular sarcoidosis. *Surv Ophthalmol* 1986;30:215–228.

Kanski JJ. Uveitis in juvenile chronic arthritis: incidence, clinical features and prognosis. *Eye* 1988;2:641–645.

Kanski JJ. Screening for uveitis in juvenile chronic arthritis. *Br J Ophthalmol* 1989;92:225–228.

Kanski JJ. Juvenile arthritis and uveitis. *Surv Ophthalmol* 1990;34:253–267.

Kanski JJ, Shun-Shin A. Systemic uveitis syndromes in childhood; an analysis of 340 cases. *Ophthalmology* 1984;91:1247–1252.

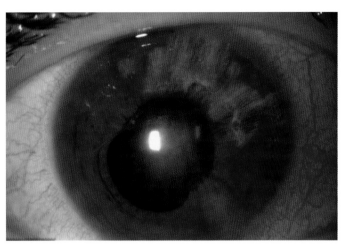

Fig. 6.52 Sectoral iris atrophy and posterior synechiae in herpes zoster chronic anterior uveitis

Kotaniemi K, Kautiainen H, Karma A, et al. Occurrence of uveitis in recently diagnosed juvenile chronic arthritis; a prospective study. *Ophthalmology* 2001;108:2071–2075.

Kuo IC, Fan J, Cunningham ET Jr. Ophthalmic manifestations of neonatal onset multisystem inflammatory disease. *Am J Ophthalmol* 2000;130:856–858.

Petty RE, Smith JR, Rosenbaum JT. Arthritis and uveitis in children: a pediatric rheumatology perspective. *Am J Ophthalmol* 2003;135:879–884.

Prieur A. Chronic infantile neurological cutaneous and articular/neonatal onset multisystem inflammatory disease syndrome. *Arch Ophthalmol* 2000;118:1386–1392.

Rauz S, Murray PI, Southwood TR. Juvenile idiopathic arthritis and uveitis: the classification conundrum. *Eye* 2000;14:817–820.

Tugal-Tutkun I, Harvlikova K, Power WJ, et al. Changing patterns of uveitis in childhood. *Ophthalmology* 1996;103:375–383.

Viral anterior uveitis

Herpes simplex virus

1. **Granulomatous CAU**, which may be associated with trabeculitis and high IOP (hypertensive uveitis), may occur with or without active corneal disease. Iris atrophy, which is often patchy and occasionally sectoral, is common. Spontaneous hyphema is uncommon.

2. **Treatment** involves topical steroids (in the absence of active epithelial disease), mydriatics and oral aciclovir (400 mg five times a day).

Varicella-zoster virus

1. **Granulomatous CAU** affects nearly 50% of the patients with herpes zoster ophthalmicus (HZO), particularly when the rash involves the side of the nose (Hutchinson sign). The inflammation is often mild and asymptomatic, although rarely it may be severe with fibrinous exudation and hypopyon or hyphaema. Residual sectoral iris atrophy is seen in 25% of cases and is thought to be due to occlusive vasculitis (Fig. 6.52).

2. **Treatment** is with topical steroids and mydriatics, although, rarely, systemic steroids may be required.

NB: All patients with HZO must be examined regularly for 6 weeks from the onset of the rash to detect anterior uveitis because it is often asymptomatic.

FURTHER READING

Aylward GW, Claoue CM, Marsh RJ, et al. Influence of oral acyclovir on ocular complications of herpes zoster ophthalmicus. *Eye* 1994;8:70–74.

Cunningham ET Jr. Diagnosing and treating herpetic anterior uveitis. *Ophthalmology* 2000;107:2129–2130.

Sudesh S, Laibson PR. The impact of the herpetic eye disease studies on the management of herpes simplex virus ocular infections. *Curr Opin Ophthalmol* 1999;10:230–233.

Van der Lelij A, Ooijman FM,. Kijlstra A, Rothova A. Anterior uveitis with sectoral iris atrophy in the absence of keratitis: a distinct clinical entity among herpetic eye diseases. *Ophthalmology* 2000;107:1164–1170.

INTERMEDIATE UVEITIS

Intermediate uveitis (IU) is an insidious, chronic disease affecting the extreme retinal periphery and pars plana with cellular inflammation of the vitreous base. The condition may be idiopathic or associated with a systemic disease (see below). Idiopathic IU probably represents an autoimmune reaction to elements in the peripheral retina and is also referred to as pars planitis (PP), especially in the presence of snowbanking. It must be stressed that the presence of snow-banking is not necessary for the diagnosis of PP, although its presence usually indicates a more prolonged and severe process. In tertiary referral centres, IU accounts for up to 15% of all uveitis cases and about 20% of paediatric uveitis. There is no clear evidence of hereditary, racial or geographic factors. PP occurs more commonly in children, while other forms of IU occur in an older age group (25–35 years), reflecting an increase in systemic associations. The diagnosis is essentially clinical, and investigations are carried out to exclude a systemic association, especially in the presence of suggestive findings and in older individuals.

NB: The exact age of onset of IU may be difficult to determine, since a long time may go by before patients become symptomatic.

Symptoms

Presentation is with an insidious onset of blurred vision, often accompanied by vitreous floaters. The initial symptoms are usually unilateral, but the condition is typically bilateral and often asymmetric, and only careful examination of the apparently normal eye may reveal minor abnormalities of the peripheral retina, such as vascular sheathing or localised vitreous condensations.

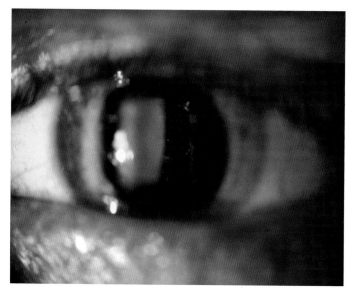

Fig. 6.53 Anterior vitreous cell in mild intermediate uveitis

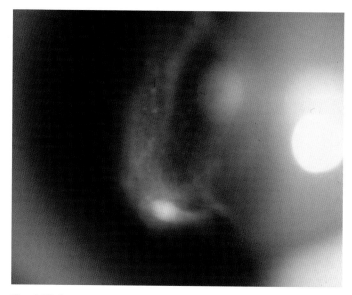

Fig. 6.55 Severe vitritis and one small 'snowball' in intermediate uveitis

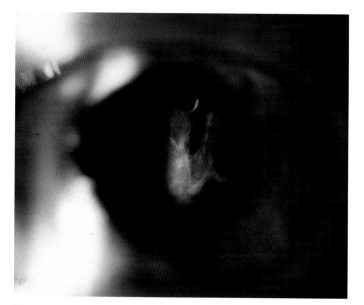

Fig. 6.54 Vitreous condensation in intermediate uveitis

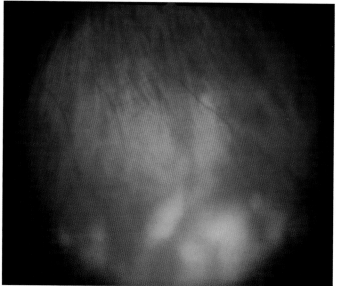

Fig. 6.56 Several large 'snowballs' in severe intermediate uveitis

Signs

1. Anterior uveitis

- In PP, anterior uveitis is mild with small scattered KPs. Occasionally, the KPs have a linear distribution in the inferior cornea and are associated with epithelial oedema (endotheliopathy).

- In the other forms of IU, anterior uveitis can be severe and symptomatic, especially in patients with multiple sclerosis (MS), sarcoidosis and Lyme disease.

2. Vitreous

- Vitreous cells with anterior predominance are universal (Fig. 6.53).

- Vitreous condensation (Fig. 6.54) often results in the formation of 'snowballs' (Fig. 6.55), often most numerous inferiorly (Fig. 6.56). Occasionally, they may be located on the posterior aspect of a posterior vitreous detachment.

- Rarely, the entire vitreous cavity may become opaque (Fig. 6.57).

3. Posterior segment

- Snowbanking is characterised by a grey–white fibrovascular plaque which may occur in all quadrants but is most frequently found inferiorly (Fig. 6.58).

- Peripheral periphlebitis and perivascular sheathing are common, particularly in patients with MS.

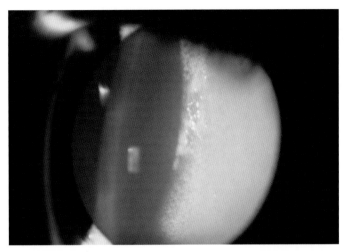

Fig. 6.57 Extensive vitreous opacification in intermediate uveitis

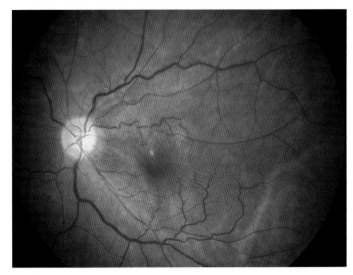

Fig. 6.59 Macular epiretinal membrane in resolved intermediate uveitis (Courtesy of C Barry)

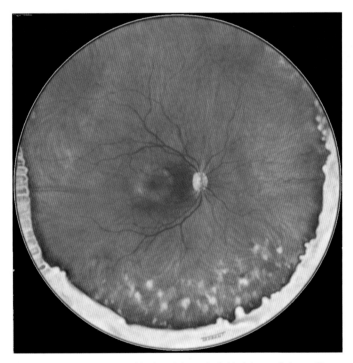

Fig. 6.58 Inferior 'snowbanking' and 'snowballs' in intermediate uveitis

- Neovascularisation may occur on the snowbank or the optic nerve head; the latter usually resolves when inflammatory activity is controlled.

- Subtle disc oedema may be seen in young patients.

Course

- A minority of patients have a benign course with minimal inflammation, which may not require treatment, with spontaneous resolution within several years.

- In other patients, the disease is more severe and prolonged, with episodes of exacerbations that tend to become progressively worse. Snowbanking is a common finding which is associated with CMO and visual loss.

- Disease starting before the age of 10 years tends to be more aggressive, whilst that starting later in life tends to be less severe.

- IU associated with systemic diseases has a variable course depending on the disease and its severity.

- The disease may last as long as 15 years and preservation of vision will depend on control of macular disease. In short-term follow-up of up to 4 years, up to 74% of patients have a visual acuity of 6/12 or better.

Complications

- CMO occurs in 30% of cases and is the major cause of impaired visual acuity.

- Macular epiretinal formation is common (Fig. 6.59).

- Cataract and glaucoma may occur in eyes with prolonged inflammation, particularly if requiring long-term steroid therapy.

- Peripheral retinal vasoproliferative tumours are uncommon.

- Retinal detachment is uncommon, but may occur in advanced cases. The detachment may be tractional, rhegmatogenous and, occasionally, exudative; retinoschisis has also been described.

- Vitreous haemorrhage may occur from the snowbank or disc new vessels, particularly in children with PP.

Management

1. **Medical therapy.** The most common reason to initiate therapy is reduction of vision due to CMO. Initial treat-

ment involves posterior sub-Tenon injections of triamcinolone. Further options in unresponsive cases include systemic steroids and immunosuppressive agents.

2. **Vitrectomy** may be beneficial for CMO as well as the inflammatory process itself. It may therefore be considered following failure of systemic steroids to control CMO but prior to the use of immunosuppressive agents. Other indications for vitrectomy include tractional retinal detachment, severe vitreous opacification, non-resolving vitreous haemorrhage and epiretinal membranes.

3. **Cryotherapy** is currently seldom used but may be considered for peripheral exudative retinal detachments associated with telangiectatic vessels and vasoproliferative tumours.

4. **Laser photocoagulation** of the peripheral retina is useful in eyes with neovascularisation of the vitreous base.

Systemic associations

1. **Multiple sclerosis**-associated IU may precede or antedate the diagnosis of demyelination. MS should be suspected in females in the third to fifth decades, especially if they are carriers of HLA-DR15 (a suballele of HLA-DR2).

> **NB:** Other causes of neurological concomitants of uveitis include VKH syndrome, sarcoidosis, Behçet disease, AIDS, primary CNS lymphoma, herpes virus infections, syphilis, acute posterior multifocal placoid pigment epitheliopathy, Whipple disease and HTLV-1 infection.

2. **Sarcoidosis**-associated IU is relatively uncommon and may antedate the onset of systemic disease. The presence of associated granulomatous anterior uveitis should arouse suspicion.

3. **Lyme disease**-associated IU is often associated with severe anterior uveitis. Information regarding visits to endemic areas and a history of a tick bite should be elicited, and confirmation achieved by serologic testing.

4. **HTLV-1 infection**-associated IU may be associated with extensive periphlebitis but CMO is rare.

Differential diagnosis

Chronic conditions that produce vitritis or peripheral retinal changes mimicking IU include the following:

1. **Fuchs uveitis syndrome** may be associated with severe vitreous inflammation but it is usually unilateral, not associated with CMO and manifests characteristic anterior segment findings.

2. **Primary intraocular lymphoma** may also present with vitritis but the infiltrate is more homogenous and snowballs are absent.

3. **A peripheral toxocara granuloma** may resemble snowbanking and be associated with mild vitritis but it is invariably unilateral.

4. **Other conditions**

- Coats disease is typically unilateral.

- Amyloidosis may produce vitritis without vasculitis or CMO.

- Whipple disease may be associated with vitritis without snowballs.

FURTHER READING

Biousse V, Trichet C, Bloch-Michel E, et al. Multiple sclerosis associated with uveitis in two large clinic-based series. *Neurology* 1999;52:179–181.

Guest S, Funkhouser E, Lightman S. Pars planitis: a comparison of childhood onset and adult onset disease. *Clin Experiment Ophthalmol* 2001;29:81–84.

Henderley DE, Haymond RS, Rao NA, et al. The significance of the pars plana exudate in pars planitis. *Am J Ophthalmol* 1987;103:669–671.

Kaufman AH, Foster CS. Cataract extraction in patients with pars planitis. *Ophthalmology* 1993;100:1210–1217.

Lai WW, Pulido JS. Intermediate uveitis. *Ophthalmol Clin North Am* 2002;15:309–317.

Lauer AK, Smith JR, Robertson JE, et al. Vitreous hemorrhage is a common complication of pediatric pars planitis. *Ophthalmology* 2002;109:95–98.

Malinowski SM, Pulido JS, Folk JC. Long-term visual outcome and complications associated with pars planitis. *Ophthalmology* 1993;100:818–824.

Malinowski SM, Pulido JS, Goeken NE, et al. The association of HLA-B8, B15, DR2, and multiple sclerosis in pars planitis. *Ophthalmology* 1993;100:1199–1205.

Michaelson JB, Friedlaender MH, Nozik L. Lens implant surgery in pars planitis. *Ophthalmology* 1990;97:1023–1026.

Pollack AL, McDonald HR, Johnson RN, et al. Peripheral retinoschisis and exudative retinal detachment in pars planitis. *Retina* 2002;22:719–724.

Raja SC, Jabs DA, Dunn JP, et al. Pars planitis: clinical features and class II HLA associations. *Ophthalmology* 1999;106:594–599.

Schmidt S, Wessels L, Augustin A, et al. Patients with multiple sclerosis and concomitant uveitis/periphlebitis retinae are not distinct from those without intraocular inflammation. *J Neurol Sci* 2001;187:49–53.

Smith JR, Rosenbaum JT. Neurological concomitants of uveitis. *Br J Ophthalmol* 2004;88:1498–1499.

Stavrou P, Baltatzis S, Letko E, et al. Pars plana vitrectomy in patients with intermediate uveitis. *Ocul Immunol Inflamm* 2001;9:141–151.

Tang WM, Pulido JS, Eckels DD, et al. The association of HLA-DR15 and intermediate uveitis. *Am J Ophthalmol* 1997;123:70–75.

Towler HM, Lightman S. Symptomatic intraocular inflammation in multiple sclerosis. *Clin Experiment Ophthalmol* 2000;2:97–102.

Zein G, Berta A, Foster CS. Multiple sclerosis-associated uveitis. *Ocul Immunol Inflamm* 2004;12:137–142.

POSTERIOR UVEITIS

Posterior uveitis (PU) encompasses retinitis, choroiditis and retinal vasculitis. Some lesions may originate primarily in the retina or choroid but often there is involvement of both (retinochoroiditis and chorioretinitis).

Symptoms

Presenting symptoms vary according to the location of the inflammatory focus and the presence of vitritis. For example, a patient with a peripheral lesion may complain of floaters,

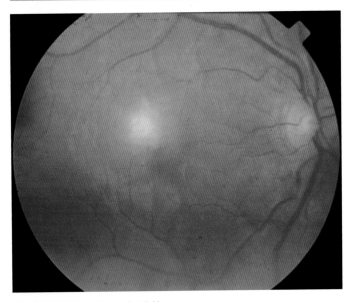

Fig. 6.60 Solitary focus of retinitis

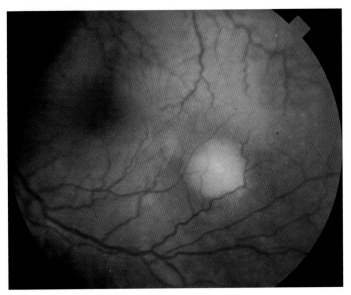

Fig. 6.61 Solitary focus of choroiditis involving the stroma

whereas a patient with a lesion involving the macula will complain of impaired central vision.

Signs

1. **Retinitis** may be focal (solitary) or multifocal. Vitreous involvement reflects inflammatory activity, which can be graded based on the view of the optic disc and posterior retina obtained with an indirect ophthalmoscope and a 20-dioptre lens.

   • Active lesions are characterised by whitish retinal opacities with indistinct borders due to surrounding oedema (Fig. 6.60).

   • As the lesion resolves, the borders become better defined.

   • The retinitis may resolve with minimal sequelae or result in scarring, frequently associated with pigmentary changes.

2. **Choroiditis** may also be focal, multifocal or geographic, but does not usually induce vitritis in the absence of concomitant retinal involvement. The clinical appearance depends on which level the lesions are located.

   • Lesions involving the stroma appear as round, yellow nodules (Fig. 6.61).

   • Lesions primarily involving the choriocapillaris have a more placoid appearance (Fig. 6.62).

   • Inner choroidal lesions may induce RPE dysfunction, which may lead to serous retinal detachment and disruption of photoreceptor function.

   • Resolved choroidal lesions may produce pigmentary changes involving the choroid and RPE.

3. **Retinal** vasculitis may occur as a primary condition or as a secondary phenomenon adjacent to a focus of retinitis.

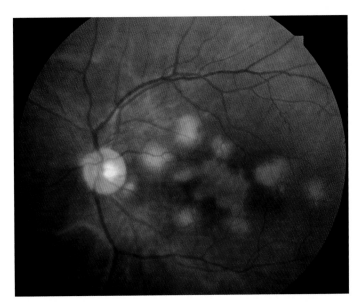

Fig. 6.62 Multifocal placoid choroiditis involving the choriocapillaris

   • Active vasculitis is characterised by yellowish or grey–white, patchy, perivascular cuffing (Fig. 6.63).

   • Quiescent vasculitis may leave perivascular scarring, which should not be mistaken for active disease (Fig. 6.64).

   • Both arteries (periarteritis) and veins (periphlebitis) may be affected, although venous involvement is more common.

A. PARASITIC

Toxoplasma retinitis

Toxoplasma gondii, an obligate intracellular protozoan (see Ch. 8), is the most frequent cause of infectious retinitis in

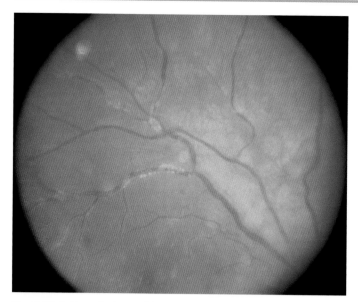

Fig. 6.63 Active retinal vasculitis

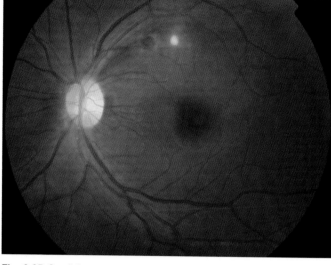

Fig. 6.65 Small focus of toxoplasma retinitis

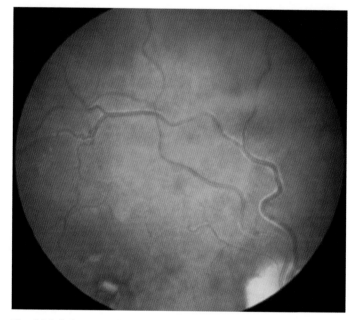

Fig. 6.64 Quiescent retinal vasculitis

immunocompetent individuals. Although some cases may occur as a result of reactivation of prenatal infestation, the vast majority are acquired postnatally. Recurrent episodes of inflammation are common and occur when the cysts rupture and release hundreds of tachyzoites into normal retinal cells. Recurrences usually take place between the ages of 10 and 35 years (average age 25 years) and are uncommon after the age of 50 years. The scars from which recurrences arise may be the residua of previous congenital infestation or, more frequently, remote acquired involvement.

The diagnosis of retinitis caused by toxoplasmosis is based on a compatible fundus lesion and positive serology for toxoplasma antibodies. Any antibody titre is significant because in recurrent ocular toxoplasmosis no correlation exists between the titre and the activity of retinitis.

Diagnostic tests

* Indirect fluorescent antibody test, haemagglutination and ELISA are comparable to the dye test (gold standard) in sensitivity and specificity.

* Positive serology only confirms previous exposure to toxoplasmosis and will therefore be positive in a high percentage of patients with other types of uveitis.

* Testing should therefore not be performed routinely and ordered only in patients who have atypical signs in whom a negative result will exclude the diagnosis of toxoplasmosis.

* Any positive titre, even in undiluted serum, is significant in the presence of a fundus lesion compatible with toxoplasmic retinitis. Reactivation of ocular disease alone will have no impact on the titre.

Clinical features

1. **Presentation** is often with unilateral, sudden onset of floaters, visual loss and photophobia.

2. **Focal retinitis** characterised by a solitary inflammatory focus near an old pigmented scar ('satellite lesion') is typical (Figs 6.65 and 6.66). Very severe vitritis may greatly impair visualisation of the fundus, although the inflammatory focus may still be discernible ('headlight in the fog' appearance) (Figs 6.67 and 6.68).

3. **Associated signs**

* 'Spill-over' anterior uveitis which may be granulomatous (Fig. 6.69).

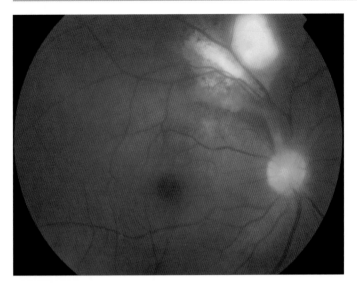

Fig. 6.66 Large focus of toxoplasma retinitis

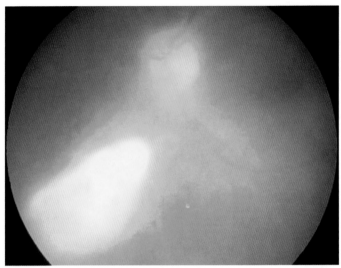

Fig. 6.68 Extremely large focus of toxoplasma retinitis and severe vitreous haze

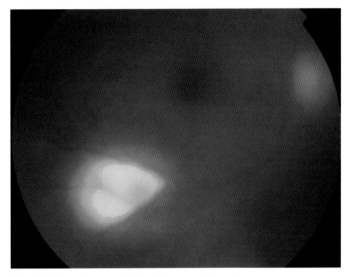

Fig. 6.67 Toxoplasma retinitis with severe vitreous haze

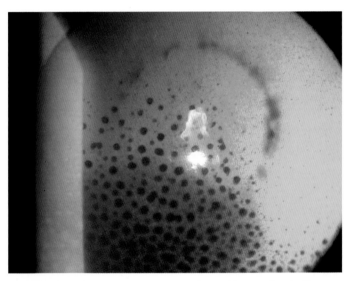

Fig. 6.69 Granulomatous 'spill-over' anterior uveitis associated with toxoplasma retinitis

- Detached posterior hyaloid face covered by inflammatory precipitates.

- Vasculitis which may involve vessels far away from the inflammatory focus (Fig. 6.70).

- Vascular occlusion may occur when a vessel crosses an area of retinitis (Fig. 6.71).

- Small plaques on the surface of retinal arteries, usually in the vicinity of the active area (Kyrieleis plaques).

- Serous retinal detachment adjacent to the focus of activity may rarely be seen (Fig. 6.72).

- Papillitis (inflammation of the optic nerve head) may be secondary to juxtapapillary retinitis (Fig. 6.73).

- Rarely, the optic nerve head itself is the primary site of involvement and the disc swelling may resemble anterior ischaemic optic neuropathy (Fig. 6.74).

Atypical features

Atypical features that may occur in immunocompromised individuals are:

- Absence of pre-existing scars, implying that the infestation has been newly acquired and disseminated to the eye from extraocular sites (Fig. 6.75).

- Extensive confluent areas of retinitis, which may be difficult to distinguish from a viral retinitis (Fig. 6.76).

Course

The rate of healing is dependent on the virulence of the organism, the competence of the host's immune system and especially the size of the lesion.

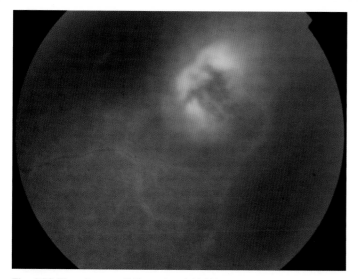

Fig. 6.70 Toxoplasma retinitis and periphlebitis

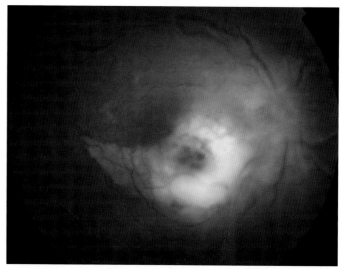

Fig. 6.71 Toxoplasma retinitis associated with periarteritis resulting in branch retinal artery occlusion

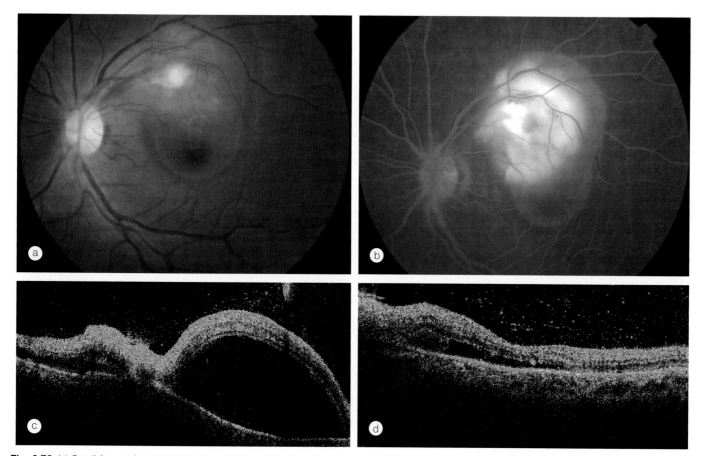

Fig. 6.72 (a) Small focus of toxoplasma retinitis associated with serous detachment at the macula; (b) late-stage FA shows corresponding hyperfluorescence due to pooling of dye; (c) optical coherence tomography (OCT) showing retinal elevation; (d) OCT several weeks later showing nearly complete retinal flattening

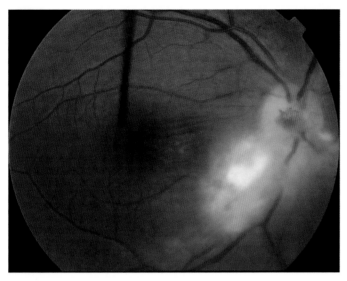

Fig. 6.73 Juxtapapillary toxoplasmosis with small hard exudates at the macula

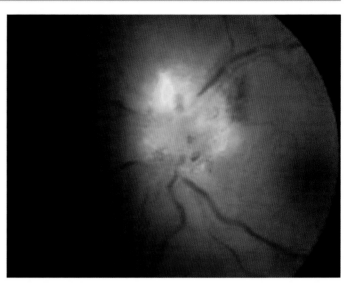

Fig. 6.74 Toxoplasmosis involving the optic nerve head (Courtesy of C de A Garcia)

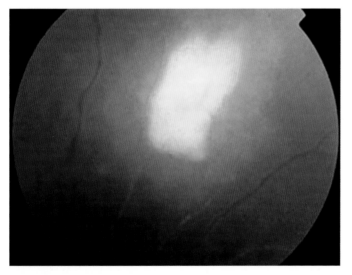

Fig. 6.75 Atypical toxoplasma retinitis not associated with a pre-existing scar (Courtesy of A Garcia)

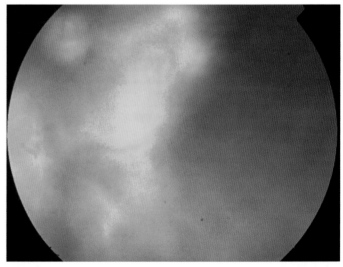

Fig. 6.76 Confluent toxoplasma retinitis in AIDS

In uncompromised hosts, the retinitis heals within 6 to 8 weeks (Fig. 6.77), although symptoms arising from vitreous inflammation take longer to resolve and some vitreous condensation may remain. The inflammatory focus is replaced by a sharply demarcated atrophic scar which becomes progressively pigmented starting at the edges, producing a hyperpigmented border. Resolution of anterior uveitis is a reliable sign of posterior segment healing. After the first attack, the mean recurrence rate within 3 years is about 50% and the average number of recurrent attacks per patient is 2.7.

NB: In elderly patients, the course may be progressive and should be differentiated from viral retinitis and lymphoma.

Complications

Nearly one-quarter of eyes develop serious visual loss as a result of the following complications:

1. **Direct involvement** by the inflammatory focus of the fovea or papillomacular bundle (Fig. 6.78), optic nerve head (see Fig. 6.74) or a major blood vessel (see Fig. 6.71).

2. **Indirect involvement** by epiretinal or vitreoretinal traction may result in macular pucker or tractional retinal detachment.

3. **CNV** at the macula adjacent to chorioretinal scarring is uncommon (Fig. 6.79).

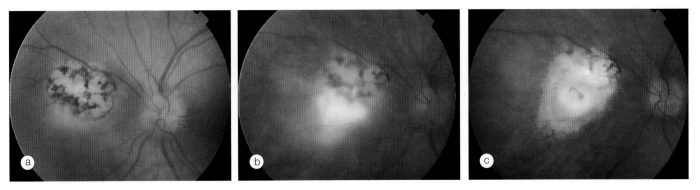

Fig. 6.77 Progression of toxoplasma retinitis. (a) Mild fluffy haze adjacent to an old scar at presentation; (b) after 2 weeks, the area of retinitis is larger and denser; (c) after 7 weeks, the retinitis has nearly resolved

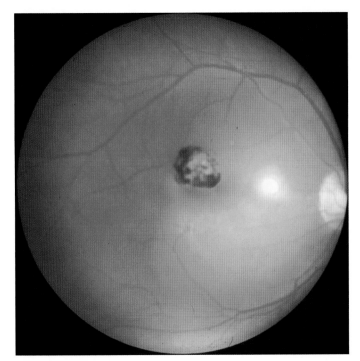

Fig. 6.78 Old toxoplasma scar at the fovea and a fresh focus involving the papillomacular bundle

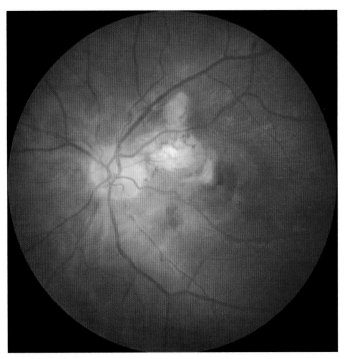

Fig. 6.79 Macular haemorrhage and scarring resulting from secondary choroidal neovascularisation associated with toxoplasma retinitis

Treatment

1. Aims

* To reduce the duration and severity of acute inflammation.

* To reduce the risk of permanent visual loss by reducing the size of the eventual retinochoroidal scar.

* To reduce the risk of recurrences. The intermittent use of antibiotics can reduce recurrences not only during therapy but also over a more prolonged period. The reason for this effect is not clear.

2. Indications.
Unfortunately, there is lack of evidence that treatment with antibiotics achieves any of the above aims, although adjunctive corticosteroids may diminish the duration and severity of inflammatory symptoms. Despite these reservations, however, treatment may be considered for the following vision-threatening lesions:

* A lesion threatening or involving the macula, papillomacular bundle, optic nerve head or a major blood vessel.

* Very severe vitritis, because it may subsequently lead to vitreous fibrosis and tractional retinal detachment.

* In immunocompromised patients, all lesions should be treated irrespective of location or severity. Systemic steroids should be avoided in these patients, but this may need to be reconsidered with immune recovery following highly active antiretroviral therapy (HAART).

3. Regimen.
There is no universally agreed therapeutic regimen and no evidence to support the use of any spe-

cific therapeutic regimen. The use of systemic steroids is important since it is the intense inflammatory activity that causes most damage in the immunocompetent individual. Prednisolone at a dose of 1 mg/kg is given initially and tapered according to clinical response, but steroids should always be used in conjunction with a specific anti-toxoplasma agent.

a. **Clindamycin** 300 mg q.i.d. orally for 3–4 weeks. However, if used alone, it may rarely cause a pseudomembranous colitis secondary to clostridial overgrowth. Treatment of colitis is with oral vancomycin 500 mg 6-hourly for 10 days. The risk of colitis is reduced when clindamycin is used together with a sulphonamide that inhibits clostridial overgrowth.

b. **Sulfadiazine** 1 g q.i.d. for 3–4 weeks. Side effects of sulphonamides include renal stones, allergic reactions and Stevens–Johnson syndrome. Sulfadiazine is usually given in combination with pyrimethamine.

c. **Pyrimethamine** (Daraprim) is a strong anti-toxoplasma agent which may cause thrombocytopenia, leucopenia, and folate deficiency. For this reason, weekly blood counts should be done and the drug used only in combination with oral folinic acid 5 mg three times a week (mixed with orange juice) because this counteracts the side effects. The loading dose is 50 mg, followed by 25–50 mg daily for 4 weeks. In AIDS, pyrimethamine is avoided because of possible pre-existing bone marrow suppression and the antagonistic effect of zidovudine when the drugs are combined.

d. **Co-trimoxazole** (Septrin) is a combination of trimethoprim (160 mg) and sulfamethoxazole (800 mg). When used in oral doses of 960 mg b.d. for 4–6 weeks, it may be effective alone or in combination with clindamycin. Side effects are similar to those of the sulphonamides.

e. **Atovaquone** 750 mg t.i.d. has been used mainly in the treatment of pneumocystosis and toxoplasmosis in AIDS but it is also effective in the treatment of toxoplasma retinitis in immunocompetent individuals. The drug is relatively free of serious side effects but is expensive.

f. **Azithromycin** 500 mg daily is a good alternative to sulfadiazine, being as effective but less toxic.

Vitreoretinal surgery may be necessary in patients with severe vitreous condensations or tractional retinal detachment. Currently it is uncertain whether prophylactic treatment should be undertaken to prevent reactivation of retinal lesions at the time of surgery.

Toxocariasis

Toxocariasis is caused by an infestation with a common intestinal ascarid (roundworm) of dogs called *Toxocara canis* (see Ch. 8).

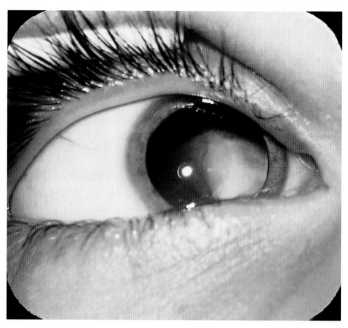
Fig. 6.80 Leucocoria in chronic toxocara endophthalmitis

Diagnostic tests

1. **ELISA** can be used to determine the level of serum antibodies to *Toxocara canis*. When ocular toxocariasis is suspected, exact ELISA titres should be requested, including testing of undiluted serum. Any positive titre is consistent with, but not necessarily diagnostic of, toxocariasis. Thus, it must be interpreted in conjunction with the clinical findings. A positive titre does not therefore exclude the possibility of retinoblastoma.

2. **Ultrasonography** may be useful both in establishing the diagnosis in eyes with hazy media and in excluding other causes of leucocoria.

Chronic endophthalmitis

1. **Presentation** is between the ages of 2 and 9 years with leucocoria (Fig. 6.80), strabismus or unilateral visual loss.

2. **Signs**

- Anterior uveitis and vitritis.

- In some cases, there may be a peripheral granuloma.

- The peripheral retina and pars plana may be covered by a dense greyish-white exudate, similar to the snowbanking seen in pars planitis (Fig. 6.81).

3. **Treatment** with steroids, either periocular or systemic, may be used to reduce the inflammatory activity.

4. **Prognosis** in most cases is very poor and some eyes eventually require enucleation. The main causes of visual loss are:

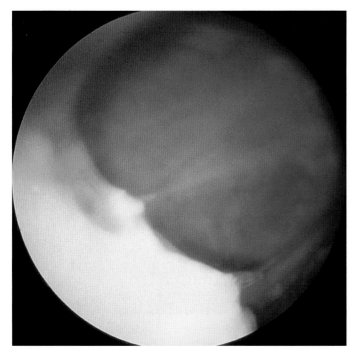

Fig. 6.81 Peripheral exudation and vitreoretinal traction bands in chronic toxocara endophthalmitis (Courtesy of S Lightman)

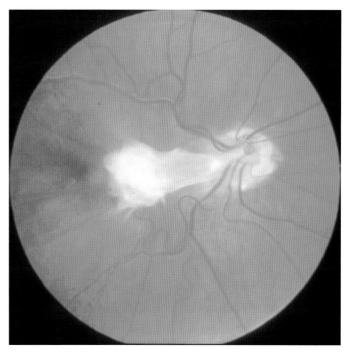

Fig. 6.83 Posterior pole granuloma extending to the disc, associated with vascular tortuosity (Courtesy of C Cunningham)

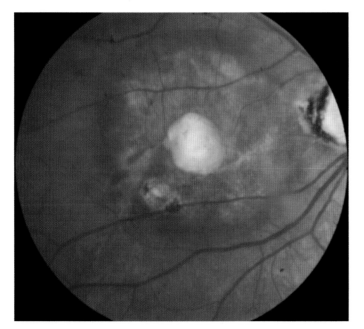

Fig. 6.82 Small posterior pole toxocara granuloma

* Tractional retinal detachment secondary to contraction of vitreoretinal membranes.

* Ocular hypotony and phthisis bulbi caused by separation of the ciliary body from the sclera brought about by contraction of a cyclitic membrane.

* Cataract.

Posterior pole granuloma

1. **Presentation** is typically with unilateral visual impairment between the ages of 6 and 14 years.

2. **Signs**

* Absence of intraocular inflammation.

* Round, yellow–white, solid granuloma which varies between one and two disc diameters in diameter, usually located at the macula (Fig. 6.82) or between the macula and the optic disc.

* Associated findings include vascular distortion (Fig. 6.83) and retinal stress lines (Fig. 6.84); occasionally, the lesion is surrounded by yellow hard exudates (Fig. 6.85).

* A granuloma confined to the optic nerve head is uncommon (Fig. 6.86).

3. **Complications**, which are rare, include tractional retinal detachment (Fig. 6.87) and subretinal haemorrhage.

Peripheral granuloma

1. **Presentation** is usually during adolescence or adult life as a result of visual impairment from distortion of the macula or retinal detachment. In uncomplicated cases, the lesion may remain undetected throughout life.

179

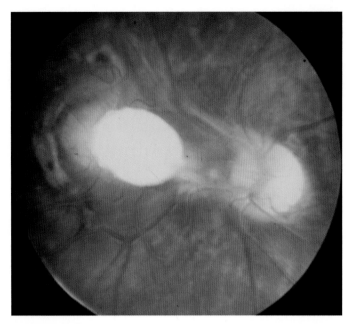

Fig. 6.84 Posterior pole toxocara granuloma with retinal stress lines

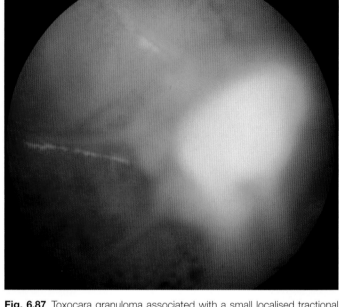

Fig. 6.87 Toxocara granuloma associated with a small localised tractional retinal detachment

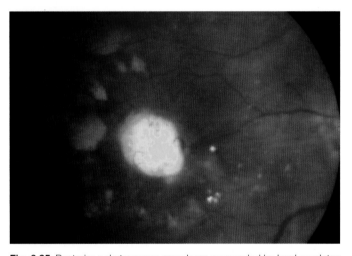

Fig. 6.85 Posterior pole toxocara granuloma surrounded by hard exudates

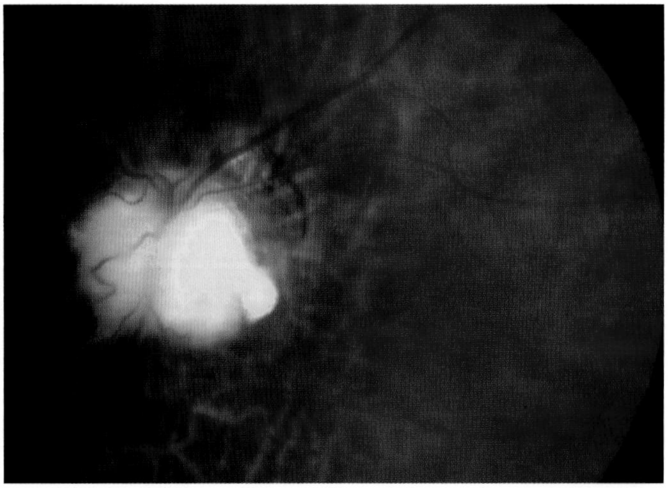

Fig. 6.86 Toxocara granuloma of the optic nerve head (Courtesy of C de A Garcia)

2. **Signs**

- Absence of intraocular inflammation.

- A white hemispherical granuloma located at or anterior to the equator in any quadrant of the fundus (Fig. 6.88).

- Vitreous bands may extend from the lesion to the posterior fundus (Fig. 6.89).

3. **Complications** in severe cases include 'dragging' of the disc and macula (Fig. 6.90) and tractional retinal detachment. The latter may benefit from vitreoretinal surgery.

Onchocerciasis

Onchocerciasis is caused by the filarial parasite *Onchocerca volvulus* which is transmitted by the bite of a blackfly (Simulium) and results in the migration of millions of tiny worms (microfilariae) throughout the body (see Ch. 8).

Signs

1. **The aqueous** may contain live microfilariae, which may be seen floating in the anterior chamber after the patient has bent face down on his knees for a few minutes and then immediately examined on the slit lamp.

2. **Anterior uveitis** may result in pear-shaped pupillary distortion, secondary glaucoma and cataract formation.

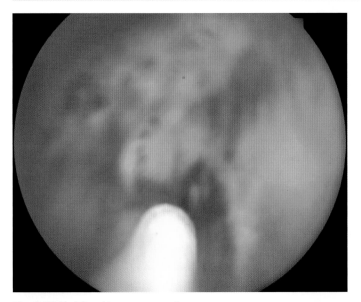

Fig. 6.88 Peripheral toxocara granuloma

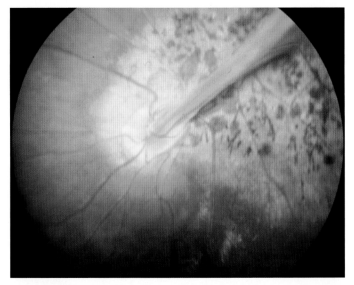

Fig. 6.89 Vitreous band extending between the disc and a peripheral toxocara granuloma

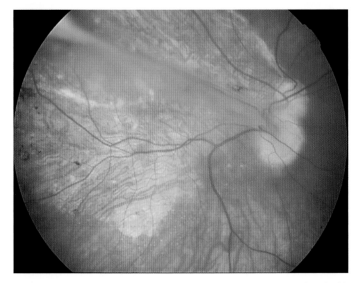

Fig. 6.90 'Dragging' of the disc and macular heterotopia associated with a peripheral toxocara granuloma (Courtesy of C Barry)

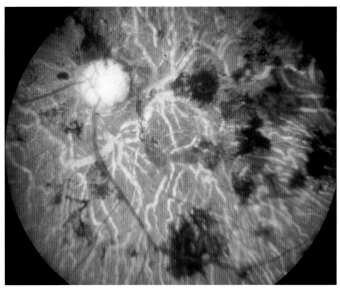

Fig. 6.91 Choroidal 'sclerosis' and pigmentary changes in onchocerciasis

3. **Chorioretinitis** is usually bilateral and predominantly involves the posterior fundus. The severity of involvement varies from atrophy and clumping of the RPE which may resemble choroidal 'sclerosis' (Fig. 6.91) to widespread chorioretinal atrophy (Fig. 6.92); these changes usually take several years to develop.

4. **Other** manifestations include punctate keratitis and sclerosing keratitis (see Ch. 4).

Treatment

Treatment is aimed at eradicating the source of the microfilariae. Ivermectin is currently the drug of choice, but new options are needed. The chorioretinal lesions are irreversible, but anterior uveitis requires topical steroids.

Cysticercosis

Cysticercosis refers to a parasitic infestation by *Cysticercus cellulosae*, the larval form of the pork tapeworm *Taenia solium* (see Ch. 8).

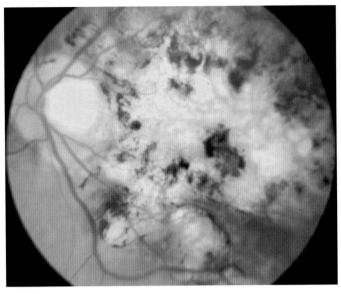

Fig. 6.92 Severe chorioretinal atrophy in onchocerciasis

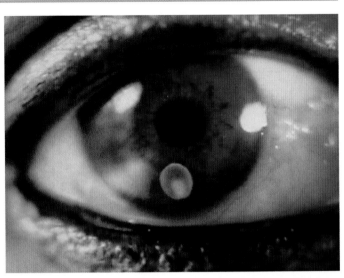

Fig. 6.94 Cysticercus cyst in the anterior chamber (Courtesy of A Pearson)

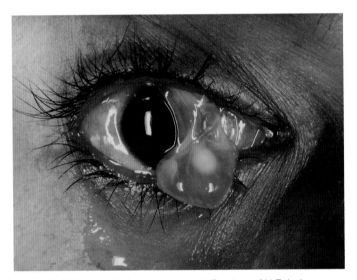

Fig. 6.93 Subconjunctival cysticercus cyst (Courtesy of U Raina)

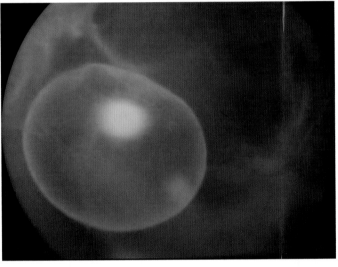

Fig. 6.95 Subretinal cysticercus cyst with overlying retinal detachment (Courtesy of U Raina)

Signs

1. **Subconjunctival** cysts are commonly seen in Asian patients (Fig. 6.93).

2. **Anterior chamber** may show a free-floating cyst (Fig. 6.94).

3. **Subretinal cyst with retinal detachment** (Fig. 6.95). The larvae enter the subretinal space, presumably through the posterior ciliary arteries, and can also pass into the vitreous. The larvae release toxins that incite an intense inflammatory reaction which may ultimately lead to blindness within 3–5 years.

Treatment

Treatment involves surgical removal of the larvae. Subretinal cysts may be removed trans-sclerally and intravitreal cysts transvitreally. Medical therapy with albendazole is not indicated for ocular disease, since it may result in death of the parasite and intense inflammation. Treatment with this drug should be reserved for cases of involvement of the brain parenchyma.

Diffuse unilateral subacute neuroretinitis (DUSN)

DUSN is an inflammatory disease characterised by a motile subretinal nematode that typically causes monocular visual loss in an otherwise healthy individual. *Baylisascaris procyo-*

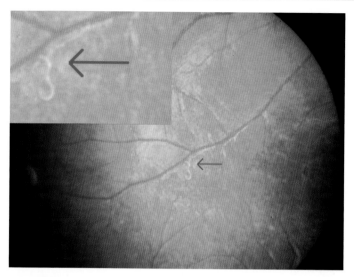

Fig. 6.96 Asymptomatic subretinal nematode (arrows) in early diffuse unilateral subacute neuroretinitis (Courtesy of C de A Garcia)

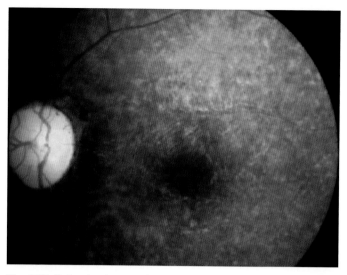

Fig. 6.98 Optic atrophy, vascular attenuation and diffuse RPE degeneration in diffuse unilateral subacute neuroretinitis (Courtesy of C de A Garcia)

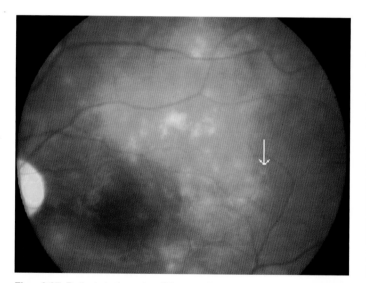

Fig. 6.97 Retinal lesions in diffuse unilateral subacute neuroretinitis (Courtesy of C de A Garcia)

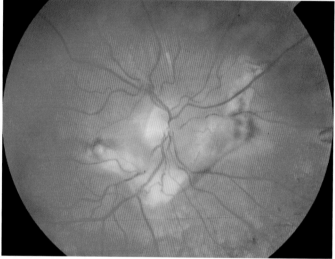

Fig. 6.99 Subretinal scarring in diffuse unilateral subacute neuroretinitis (Courtesy of R Curtis)

nis, an ascarid of the raccoon, has been implicated, but it is possible that different worms are capable of producing the same clinical picture. The nematode may remain viable in the eye for 3 years or longer.

Signs

In choronological order:

- Asymptomatic subretinal nematode (Fig. 6.96).

- Papillitis, retinal vasculitis and recurrent crops of evanescent grey–white outer retinal lesions (Fig. 6.97).

- Optic atrophy, retinal vascular attenuation and diffuse RPE degeneration (Fig. 6.98).

- Subretinal scarring (Fig. 6.99) and tunnels (Fig. 6.100).

Treatment

1. **Laser photocoagulation** of the subretinal nematode. The worm is usually found in areas where fresh outer retinal lesions are seen. It is difficult to hit the worm with single laser burns because it moves quickly. It must therefore be first surrounded by a ring of burns, which restricts its movement, and then the entire area is treated with heavy burns.

2. **Systemic** treatment with albendazole may be beneficial.

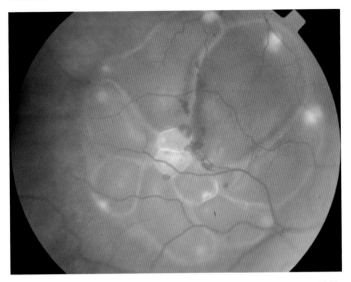

Fig. 6.100 Subretinal tunnels in diffuse unilateral subacute neuroretinitis (Courtesy of R Curtis)

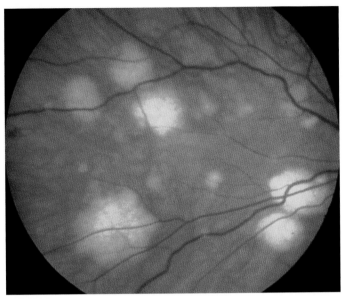

Fig. 6.101 Multifocal choroidal pneumocystosis (Courtesy of S Mitchell)

Choroidal pneumocystosis

Pneumocystis carinii, an opportunistic protozoan parasite, is a major cause of morbidity and mortality in AIDS. The presence of choroidal involvement can be an important sign of extrapulmonary systemic dissemination. Most patients with choroiditis have received inhaled pentamidine as prophylaxis against *P. carinii* pneumonia. In contrast with systemic prophylaxis, this protects only the lungs, allowing the organisms to disseminate throughout the body.

Signs

- Variable number of flat, yellow, round, choroidal lesions, scattered throughout the posterior pole, which are frequently bilateral and not associated with vitritis (Fig. 6.101).

- The lesions may coalesce and produce large geographic patches (Fig. 6.102).

- Alterations of the RPE may occur, overlying some lesions, and serous detachment may rarely occur.

- Even when the fovea is involved, there is little, if any, impairment of visual acuity.

Treatment

Intravenous trimethoprim and sulfamethoxazole or parenteral pentamidine induces resolution within several weeks (Fig. 6.103).

Ophthalmomyiasis interna

Ophthalmomyiasis is invasion of the eye or adnexa by larvae of flies, often by the rodent botfly larva (maggot) of the *Cuterebra* and *Hypoderma* species. The larvae usually gain

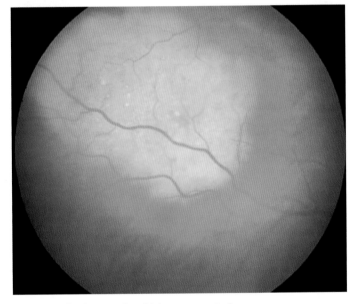

Fig. 6.102 Coalescent choroidal pneumocystosis

access to the posterior segment from the conjunctival fornices through the peripheral sclera and choroid. Ocular involvement occurs in about 5% of all cases of myiasis.

Signs

- The larvae travel in the subretinal space, leaving characteristic grey–white tracks in the RPE (Fig. 6.104), which later become depigmented streaks dotted with focal pigment proliferation that may involve the fovea and cause visual impairment.

- The larvae may also penetrate the vitreous.

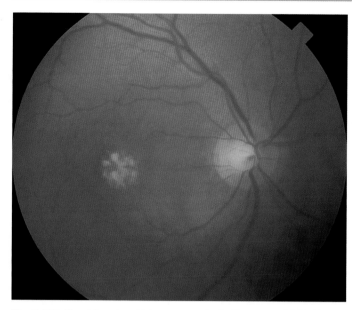

Fig. 6.103 Resolving choroidal pneumocystosis (Courtesy of A Dick)

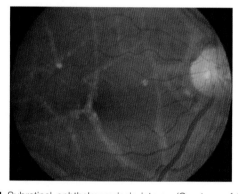

Fig. 6.104 Subretinal ophthalmomyiasis interna (Courtesy of Podos and Yanoff, from *Textbook of Ophthalmology*, Volume 9, Mosby, 1991)

Treatment

Treatment may involve iridectomy, vitrectomy, and retinotomy to remove maggots. Retinal breaks must be sealed by laser photocoagulation or eventually cryotherapy. Destruction of the organism can also be attempted directly with argon laser, and usually results in minimal or no inflammation. It is interesting to note that a dead intraocular larva does not usually produce significant inflammation.

FURTHER READING

Bosch-Driessen EH, Rothova A. Sense and nonsense of corticosteroid administration in the treatment of ocular toxoplasmosis. *Br J Ophthalmol* 1998;82:858–860.

Bosch-Driessen EH, Rothova A. Recurrent ocular disease in postnatally acquired toxoplasmosis. *Am J Ophthalmol* 1999;128:421–425.

Bosch-Driessen LEH, Berendschot TTJM, Ongkosuwito JV, et al. Ocular toxoplasmosis: clinical features and prognosis of 154 patients. *Ophthalmology* 2002;109:869–878.

Bosch-Driessen LH, Verbraak FD, Suttorp-Schulten MSA, et al. A prospective, randomized trial of pyrimethamine and azithromycin vs pyrimethamine and sulfadiazine for the treatment of ocular toxoplasmosis. *Am J Ophthalmol* 2002;134:34–40.

de Souza EC, Abujamra S, Nakashima Y, et al. Diffuse bilateral subacute neuroretinitis: first patient with documented nematodes in both eyes. *Arch Ophthalmol* 1999;117:1349–1351.

Dugel PU, Rao NA, Forster DJ, et al. Pneumocystis carinii choroiditis after long-term aerosolized pentamidine therapy. *Am J Ophthalmol* 1990;110:113–117.

Fardeau C, Romand S, Rao NA, et al. Diagnosis of toxoplasmic retinochoroiditis with atypical clinical features. *Am J Ophthalmol* 2002;134:196–203.

Freeman WR, Gross JG, Labelle J, et al. Pneumocystis carinii choroidopathy. A new clinical entity. *Arch Ophthalmol* 1989;107:863–867.

Gass JD, Braunstein RA. Further observations concerning the diffuse unilateral subacute neuroretinitis syndrome. *Arch Ophthalmol* 1983;101:1689–1697.

Gilbert RE, Stanford MR. Is ocular toxoplasmosis caused by prenatal or postnatal infection? Perspective. *Br J Ophthalmol* 2000;84:224–226.

Goldberg MA, Kazacos KR, Boyce WM, et al. Diffuse unilateral subacute neuroretinitis. Morphometric, serologic, and epidemiologic support for Baylisascaris as a causative agent. *Ophthalmology* 1993;100:1695–1701.

Holland GN. Reconsidering the pathogenesis of ocular toxoplasmosis. *Am J Ophthalmol* 1999;128:502–505.

Holland GN. Ocular toxoplasmosis: a global reassessment. Part I: Epidemiology and course of disease. LX Edward Jackson Memorial Lecture. *Am J Ophthalmol* 2003;136:973–988.

Holland GN. Ocular toxoplasmosis: a global reassessment. Part II: Disease manifestations and management. LX Edward Jackson Memorial Lecture. *Am J Ophthalmol* 2004;137:1–17.

Holland GN, Lewis KG. An update on current practices in the management of ocular toxoplasmosis. *Am J Ophthalmol* 2002;134:102–114.

Holland GN, Lewis KG, O'Connor GR. Ocular toxoplasmosis. A 50th anniversary tribute to the contributions of Helenor Campbell Wilder Foerster. *Arch Ophthalmol* 2002;120:1081–1084.

Johnson MW, Greven GM, Jaffe GJ, et al. Atypical, severe toxoplasmic retinochoroiditis in elderly patients. *Ophthalmology* 1997;104:48–57.

Moshfeghi DM, Dodds EM, Couto CA, et al. Diagnostic approaches to severe, atypical toxoplasmosis mimicking acute retinal necrosis. *Ophthalmology* 2004;111:716–725.

Pavesio CE, Lightman S. Toxoplasma gondii and ocular toxoplasmosis: pathogenesis. *Br J Ophthalmol* 1996;80:1099–1107.

Pearson PA, Piracha AR, Sen HA, et al. Atovaquone for treatment of toxoplasma retinochoroiditis in immunocompetent patients. *Ophthalmology* 1999;106:148–153.

Phelan MJ, Johnson MW. Acute posterior ophthalmomyiasis interna treated with photocoagulation. *Am J Ophthalmol* 1995;119:106–107.

Rao NA, Zimmerman PL, Boyer D, et al. A clinical, histopathologic, and electron microscopic study of Pneumocystis carinii choroiditis. *Am J Ophthalmol* 1989 107:218–228.

Rosenblatt MA, Cunningham C, Teich S, et al. Choroidal lesions in patients with AIDS. *Br J Ophthalmol* 1990 74:610–614.

Rothova A, Bosch-Driessen EH, van Loon NH, et al. Azithromycin for ocular toxoplasmosis. *Br J Ophthalmol* 1998;82:1306–1308.

Sabrosa NA, Zajdenweber M. Nematode infections of the eye: toxocariasis, onchocerciasis, diffuse unilateral subacute neuroretinitis, and cysticercosis. *Ophthalmol Clin North Am* 2002;15:351–356.

Sharma T, Sinha S, Shah N, et al. Intraocular cysticercosis; clinical characteristics and visual outcome after vitreoretinal surgery. *Ophthalmology* 2003;110:996–1004.

Shields JA. Ocular toxocariasis: a review. *Surv Ophthalmol* 1984;28:361–381.

Silvera C, Belfort R Jr, Muccioli C, et al. The effect of long-term intermittent trimethoprim/sulfamethoxazole treatment on recurrences of toxoplasma retinochoroiditis. *Am J Ophthalmol* 2002;134:41–46.

Slusher MM, Holland WD, Weaver RG, et al. Ophthalmomyiasis interna posterior. Subretinal tracks and intraocular larvae. *Arch Ophthalmol* 1979;97:885–887.

Stanford MR, See SE, Jones LV, et al. Antibiotics for toxoplasmic retinochoroiditis. An evidence-based systematic review. *Ophthalmology* 2003;110:926–932.

Wan WL, Cano MR, Pince KJ, et al. Echographic characteristics of ocular toxocariasis. *Ophthalmology* 1991;98:28–32.

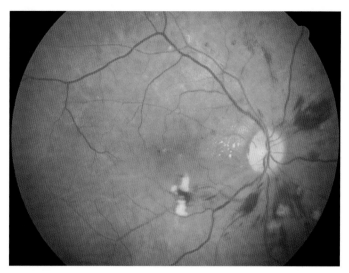

Fig. 6.105 HIV microangiopathy (Courtesy of C Barry)

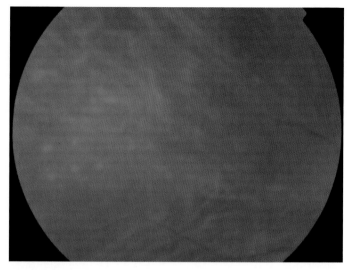

Fig. 6.106 HIV retinitis

B. VIRAL

HIV microangiopathy

Retinal microangiopathy is the most frequent retinopathy in patients with AIDS, developing in up to 70% of patients, and is associated with a declining CD4+ count. Postulated causes of the microangiopathy include immune complex deposition, HIV infection of the retinal vascular endothelium, haemorheological abnormalities and abnormal retinal haemodynamics.

1. **Signs.** Cotton-wool spots, which may be associated with retinal haemorrhages and capillary abnormalities (Fig. 6.105).

2. **Differential diagnosis.** The lesions may be mistaken for early CMV retinitis. However, in contrast to CMV retinitis, the cotton-wool spots are usually asymptomatic and almost invariably disappear spontaneously after several weeks.

HIV retinitis

Signs

* Anterior uveitis and vitritis.

* Small, irregular, grey–white or yellow lesions located in the midperipheral and anterior fundus (Fig. 6.106).

* The lesions may slowly enlarge or remain static.

Treatment

The response to antiretroviral therapy is good, but not to aciclovir or ganciclovir; the visual prognosis is good.

Cytomegalovirus retinitis

CMV retinitis is the most common ocular opportunistic infection among patients with AIDS (see Ch. 8). Since the

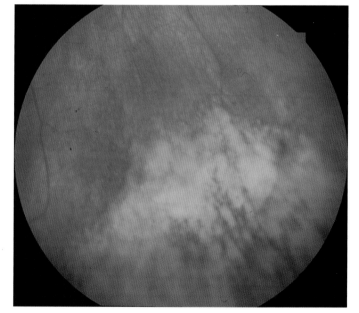

Fig. 6.107 Indolent cytomegalovirus retinitis

advent of HAART, its incidence has declined and its rate of progression reduced, even in patients with low CD4+ T-cell counts. It also appears that the rates of second eye involvement and retinal detachment are less than in the pre-HAART era.

Signs

1. **Indolent** CMV retinitis frequently starts in the periphery and progresses slowly. It is characterised by a mild granular opacification which may be associated with a few punctate haemorrhages but no vasculitis (Figs 6.107 and 6.108).

2. **Fulminating** retinitis is characterised by the following:

* Mild vitritis.

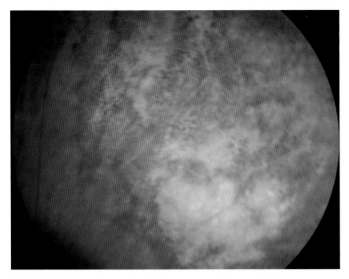

Fig. 6.108 More advanced indolent cytomegalovirus retinitis

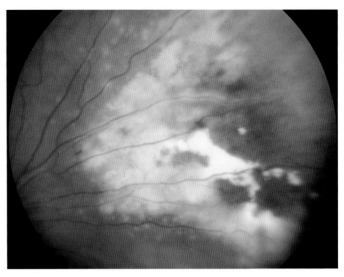

Fig. 6.110 More advanced fulminating cytomegalovirus retinitis

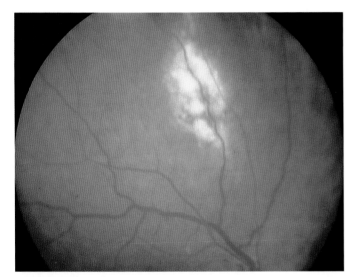

Fig. 6.109 Early vasculitis in fulminating cytomegalovirus retinitis

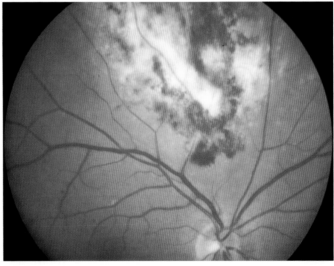

Fig. 6.111 Severe fulminating cytomegalovirus retinitis

- Vasculitis with perivascular sheathing and opacification (Fig. 6.109).

- Dense, white, well-demarcated, geographical area of confluent opacification (Fig. 6.110).

- Retinal haemorrhages may develop either within the area of retinitis or along its leading edge (Fig. 6.111).

- Slow but relentless 'brushfire-like' extension along the course of the retinal vascular arcades and may involve the optic nerve head (Fig. 6.112).

- Without treatment, the entire retina becomes involved within a few months (Fig. 6.113).

- Regression is characterised by fewer haemorrhages and less opacification, followed by diffuse atrophic and mild pigmentary changes (Fig. 6.114).

Complications

1. **Macular** complications include necrosis, epiretinal membranes, cystoid oedema and hard exudates (Fig. 6.115).

2. **Retinal detachment** may occur as a result of large posterior breaks caused by severe retinal necrosis (Fig. 6.116).

Treatment

1. **Ganciclovir** is initially given intravenously (induction) 5 mg/kg every 12 hours for 2–3 weeks, then 5 mg/kg every 24 hours.

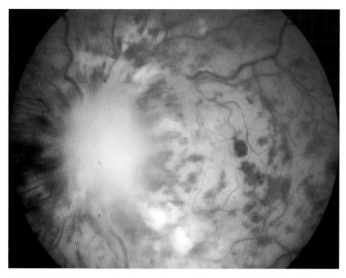

Fig. 6.112 Optic nerve involvement provoking a central retinal vein occlusion in severe cytomegalovirus retinitis

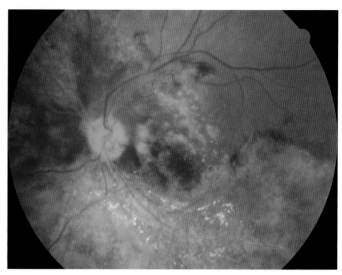

Fig. 6.114 Regressing cytomegalovirus retinitis of the same eye as in the previous figure (Courtesy of L Merin)

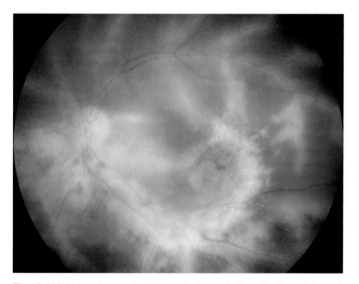

Fig. 6.113 Very advanced cytomegalovirus retinitis with frosted branch angiitis (Courtesy of L Merin)

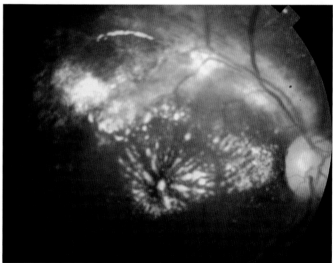

Fig. 6.115 Hard exudates at the macula in cytomegalovirus retinitis

- Patients with stable retinitis may be treated with oral ganciclovir 300–450 mg daily for prophylaxis and maintenance. Ganciclovir is effective in 80% of patients, but 50% subsequently relapse and require reinduction of therapy.

- The drug carries a high risk of bone marrow suppression, which often forces interruption of treatment. Ganciclovir can also be administered as a prodrug (valganciclovir) with improved gastrointestinal absorption and is as effective as intravenous therapy for treatment and prophylaxis (induction dose of 900 mg b.d. and maintenance of 900 mg daily).

2. **Intravenous foscarnet**, unlike ganciclovir, may also improve life expectancy. The initial dose is 60 mg/kg every 8 hours for 2–3 weeks and then 90–120 mg every 24 hours. Its side effects include nephrotoxicity, electrolyte disturbances and seizures. Foscarnet can also be given intravitreally (2.4 mg in 0.1 ml).

3. **Intravitreal ganciclovir**

a. **Slow-release devices** (Vitrasert) appear to be as effective as intravenous therapy (Fig. 6.117). The duration of efficacy is 8 months, which is superior to intravenous therapy with either ganciclovir or foscarnet (average 60 days). However, Vitrasert does not protect the fellow eye from retinitis and has no systemic effect.

b. **Intravitreal injections** (2.0–2.5 mg in 0.1 ml) represent another alternative and should be attempted first whenever a decision to insert an intravitreal implant is made,

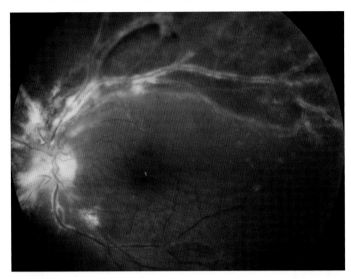

Fig. 6.116 Large posterior retinal break and localised retinal detachment in cytomegalovirus retinitis (Courtesy of C Barry)

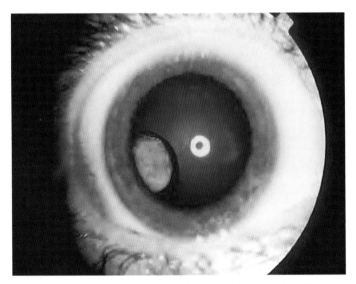

Fig. 6.117 Slow-release intravitreal implant containing ganciclovir (Courtesy of V Tanner)

since it is important to test the response to the drug before proceeding with a more invasive procedure. Both may cause serious complications such as cataract, vitreous haemorrhage, retinal detachment and endophthalmitis.

4. **Intravenous cidofovir**, 5 mg/kg once weekly for 2 weeks and then every 2 weeks, may be used when other agents are unsuitable. It must be administered in combination with probenecid. Side effects include nephrotoxicity and neutropenia. Cidofovir may cause anterior uveitis, usually after several infusions, but this normally responds well to topical steroid therapy. Cidofovir can also be given intravitreally (15–20 μg in 0.1 ml), but, unlike ganciclovir, it is extremely toxic and may cause severe inflammation, which may occasionally result in hypotony and even phthisis bulbi.

5. **Intravitreal fomivirsen** has a different mechanism of action from other agents. Adverse effects include anterior uveitis, vitritis, cataract and, rarely, retinopathy. The experience with this drug is not as good as with the others mentioned above, since its introduction coincided with the use of HAART, which was associated with a reduction in the frequency of CMV retinitis.

6. **Vitreoretinal surgery** for retinal detachment often involves the use of silicone oil tamponade because of the presence of multiple posterior breaks.

Prognosis

* Without treatment, the eye becomes blind within 6 weeks to 6 months.

* With treatment, there is a 95% response, with decrease in size of the lesions. However, there is a 100% relapse rate within 2 weeks when treatment is discontinued and a 50% relapse rate within 6 months in patients on maintenance therapy.

* Since the introduction of HAART therapy, the incidence of CMV retinitis has decreased and many patients have had their treatment of retinitis stopped after immune recovery (CD4 > 100–150).

* Unfortunately, many patients with HAART-induced immune recovery develop intraocular inflammation, which may result in chronic vision-limiting complications, including macular oedema and epiretinal membrane formation. The former may respond, at least transiently, to steroid therapy or valganciclovir. However, the results are not satisfactory and immune-recovery inflammation is now a common cause of new visual loss in patients with AIDS-related CMV retinitis.

Progressive outer retinal necrosis (PORN)

PORN is a rare but devastating necrotising retinitis caused by varicella-zoster virus (VZV), which behaves aggressively, probably because of the profound immunosuppression of the host. The name is actually not appropriate since it is only in the early stages that the infection is limited to the outer retina and there is rapid progression to a full-thickness retinal necrosis. Although it occurs predominantly in AIDS it may also occur in patients with drug-induced immunosuppression.

Diagnosis

1. **Presentation** is with rapidly progressive visual loss which is initially unilateral in 75% of cases.

2. **Signs**, in chronological order:

* Minimal anterior uveitis.

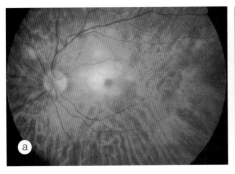
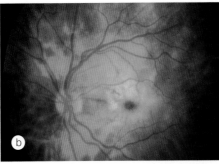
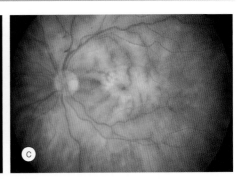

Fig. 6.118 Progression of macular involvement in progressive outer retinal necrosis (Courtesy of T Margolis. From: Varicella-zoster virus retinitis in patients with the acquired immunodeficiency syndrome. *Am J Ophthalmol* 1991;112:119–131.).

- Multifocal, yellow–white, retinal infiltrates with minimal vitritis.

- Early macular involvement (Fig. 6.118).

- Rapid confluence and full-thickness retinal necrosis (Fig. 6.119).

> **NB:** Vitreous inflammation is usually late and reflects extensive retinal necrosis.

3. **Investigations.** Specific PCR-based diagnostic assay for VZV DNA may be performed on vitreous samples.

Treatment

1. **Medical** treatment with intravenous ganciclovir, alone or in combination with foscarnet, or intravitreal foscarnet is often disappointing and most patients become blind in both eyes within a few weeks as a result of macular necrosis or retinal detachment. In addition, 50% of patients are dead 5 months after diagnosis.

2. **Vitreoretinal surgery** for retinal detachment also yields poor results, although silicone oil tamponade and relaxing retinotomies may occasionally salvage ambulatory vision.

Acute retinal necrosis (ARN)

ARN is a rare but devastating necrotising retinitis. It typically affects otherwise healthy individuals of all ages. Males are more frequently affected than females by a 2 : 1 ratio. ARN is a biphasic disease which tends to be caused by herpes simplex (HSV) in younger patients and VZV in older individuals; rarely, CMV or Epstein-Barr virus is implicated. Some patients have a past history of HSV encephalitis, many years before developing ARN, and, occasionally, encephalitis and ARN develop simultaneously.

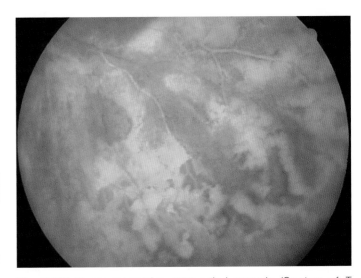

Fig. 6.119 Severe progressive outer retinal necrosis (Courtesy of T Margolis)

Diagnosis

1. **Presentation** is initially unilateral and varies according to severity. Some patients develop severe visual impairment over a few days associated with pain, whereas others have an insidious onset with mild visual symptoms such as floaters.

2. **Signs**, in chronological order:

- Anterior granulomatous uveitis is universal and unless the fundus is examined the diagnosis may be missed.

- Peripheral retinal periarteritis associated with multifocal, deep, yellow–white retinal infiltrates (Fig. 6.120).

- Gradual confluence of lesions (Fig. 6.121).

- Vitritis is universal (Fig. 6.122).

- Progressive full-thickness retinal necrosis (Figs 6.123 and 6.124).

- The posterior pole is usually spared (Fig. 6.125), so visual acuity may remain fairly good despite severe necrosis of

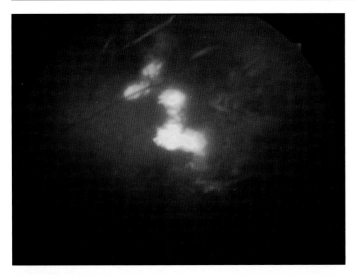

Fig. 6.120 Peripheral periarteritis and retinal infiltrates in early acute retinal necrosis

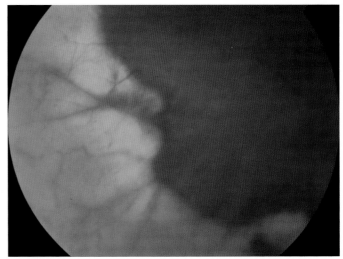

Fig. 6.123 Full-thickness necrosis in acute retinal necrosis

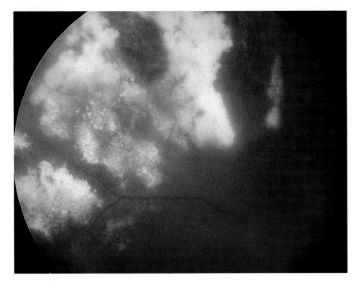

Fig. 6.121 Confluence of infiltrates in acute retinal necrosis

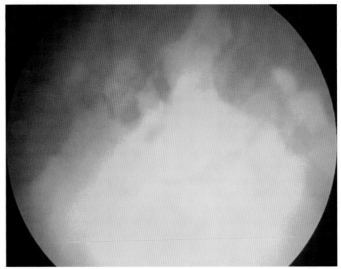

Fig. 6.124 Advanced acute retinal necrosis

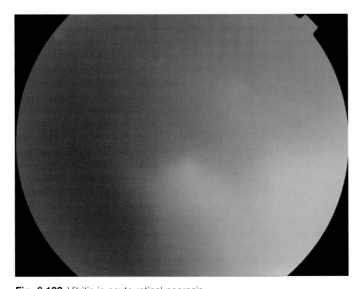

Fig. 6.122 Vitritis in acute retinal necrosis

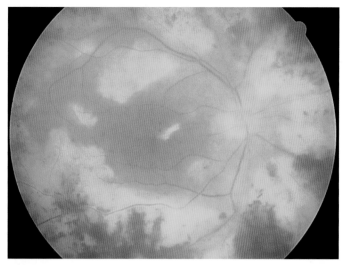

Fig. 6.125 Advanced acute retinal necrosis with relative macular sparing

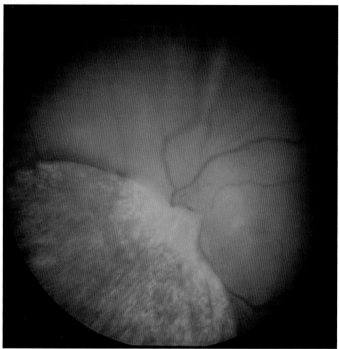

Fig. 6.127 Retinal detachment in acute retinal necrosis

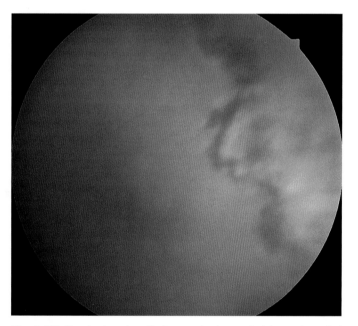

Fig. 6.126 Resolved acute retinal necrosis demarcated by a pigmented border

Treatment

1. **Systemic aciclovir**, initially given intravenously (10 mg/ kg every 8 hours) for 10–14 days and then orally 800 mg five times daily for 6–12 weeks, may hasten resolution of the acute retinal lesions and reduce the risk of second eye involvement, but it does not prevent retinal detachment. Recurrences may occur in some patients and long-term therapy may be required.

2. **Systemic steroids** may be started 24 hours after initiation of antiviral therapy and are usually indicated in severe cases, especially those showing optic nerve involvement.

NB: Prophylactic laser photocoagulation aimed at limiting posterior spread of retinitis has been largely abandoned.

Prognosis

The prognosis is relatively poor, with 60% of patients having a final visual acuity of less than 6/60 as a result of the following:

- Rhegmatogenous retinal detachment associated with retinal holes at the margin of uninvolved and involved zones (Fig. 6.127). The anatomic results of treatment by vitrectomy are excellent.

- Tractional retinal detachment, which is less common and caused by secondary condensation and fibrosis of the vitreous base.

the surrounding retina, but papillitis may occur early and result in visual loss.

- Other signs include choroidal thickening and retinal haemorrhages.

- The acute lesions resolve within 6–12 weeks, leaving behind a transparent necrotic retina with hyperpigmented borders (Fig. 6.126).

NB: Unless the patient receives appropriate treatment, the second eye becomes involved in 30% of patients, usually within 2 months, although in some patients the interval may be much longer.

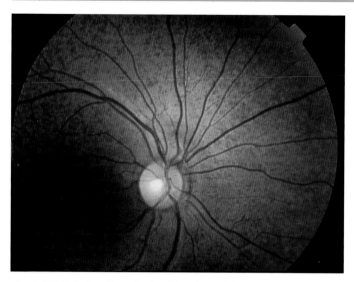

Fig. 6.128 Rubella retinopathy involving the periphery

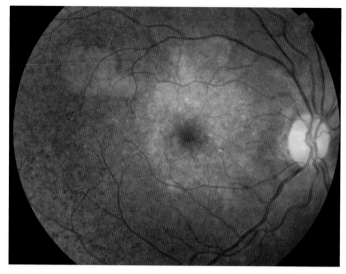

Fig. 6.129 Rubella retinopathy involving the posterior pole

- Ischaemic optic neuropathy caused by thrombotic arteriolar occlusion and infiltration of the optic nerve by inflammatory cells.

- Occlusive periphlebitis.

Differential diagnosis

The diagnosis of ARN may be difficult in certain cases because the clinical presentations range from focal to extensive involvement and the clinical course may be mild or fulminating. The following conditions should be considered in differential diagnosis.

1. **Behçet syndrome** is also characterised by panuveitis, retinitis and necrotising periarteritis. However, the onset and course are more chronic, systemic symptoms are present, and anterior uveitis is non-granulomatous.

2. **CMV retinitis** has a more gradual onset and vitritis is mild or absent.

3. **PORN** occurs predominantly in AIDS, has a more rapid course, and there is minimal intraocular inflammation.

4. **Atypical peripheral toxoplasma retinitis** may simulate ARN when it manifests as a large focus or multiple smaller foci of peripheral necrotising retinitis without adjacent pigmented scars. This may occur in immunosuppressed or elderly patients.

Congenital rubella

Rubella (German measles) is usually a benign febrile exanthema. Congenital rubella results from transplacental transmission of virus to the foetus from an infected mother, usually during the first trimester of pregnancy (see Ch. 8).

1. **Anterior uveitis** may result in iris atrophy.

2. **Retinopathy** is a common manifestation, but the exact incidence is unknown because cataracts frequently impair visualisation of the fundus.

- 'Salt and pepper' pigmentary disturbance involving the periphery (Fig. 6.128) and posterior pole (Fig. 6.129).

- Prognosis is usually good, although a small percentage of eyes may later develop CNV.

3. **Other** manifestations include cataract, microphthalmos, glaucoma, keratitis and extreme refractive errors.

Subacute sclerosing panencephalitis

Subacute sclerosing panencephalitis is a chronic, progressive, neurodegenerative and usually fatal disease of children caused by the measles virus.

1. **Systemic features** include insidious personality change followed by progressive psychomotor deterioration, myoclonus and seizures. Death ensues within years.

2. **Posterior uveitis** is characterised by papillitis, macular oedema, whitish retinal infiltrates and choroiditis (Fig. 6.130).

FURTHER READING

Anninger WV, Lomeo MD, Dingle J, et al. West Nile virus-associated optic neuritis and chorioretinitis. *Am J Ophthalmol* 2003;136:1183–1185.

Balansard B, Bodaghi B, Cassoux N, et al. Necrotizing retinopathies simulating acute retinal necrosis. *Br J Ophthalmol* 2005;89:96–101.

Belfort R Jr. The ophthalmologist and the global impact of the AIDS epidemic. LV Edward Jackson Memorial Lecture. *Am J Ophthalmol* 2000;129:1–8.

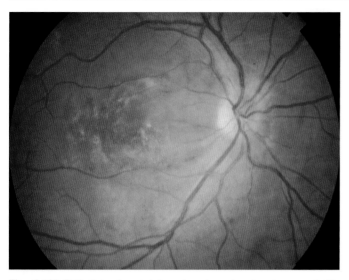

Fig. 6.130 Retinal involvement in subacute sclerosing panencephalitis (Courtesy of Z Bashshur)

Berker N, Batman C, Guven A, et al. Optic atrophy and macular degeneration as initial presentations of subacute sclerosing panencephalitis. *Am J Ophthalmol* 2004;138:879–881.

Cunningham ET Jr, Levinson RD, Jampol LM, et al. Ischemic maculopathy in patients with acquired immunodeficiency syndrome. *Am J Ophthalmol* 2001;132:727–733.

Curi AL, Muralha A, Muralha L, et al. Suspension of anticytomegalovirus maintenance therapy following immune recovery due to highly active antiretroviral therapy. *Br J Ophthalmol* 2001;85:471–473.

Duker JS, Blumenkranz MS. Diagnosis and management of the acute retinal necrosis (ARN) syndrome. *Surv Ophthalmol* 1991;35:327–343.

Engstrom RE, Holland GA, Margolis TP, et al. The progressive outer retinal necrosis syndrome: a variant of necrotizing herpetic retinopathy in patients with AIDS. *Ophthalmology* 1994;101:1488–1502.

Ganatra JB, Chandler D, Santos C, et al. Viral causes of the acute retinal necrosis syndrome. *Am J Ophthalmol* 2000;129:166–172.

Givens KT, Lee DA, Jones T, et al. Congenital rubella syndrome: ophthalmic manifestations and associated systemic disorders. *Br J Ophthalmol* 1993;77:358–363.

Goldberg DE, Wang H, Azen SP, et al. Long term visual outcome of patients with cytomegalovirus retinitis treated with highly active antiretroviral therapy. *Br J Ophthalmol* 2003;87:853–855.

Henderson HWA, Mitchell SM. Treatment of immune recovery vitritis with local steroids. *Br J Ophthalmol* 1999;83:540–545.

Hodge WG, Boivin J-F, Shapiro SH, et al. Clinical risk factors for cytomegalovirus retinitis in patients with AIDS. *Ophthalmology* 2004;111:1326–1333.

Holland GN. Standard diagnostic criteria for the acute retinal necrosis syndrome. Executive Committee of the American Uveitis Society. *Am J Ophthalmol* 1994;117:663–667.

Holland GN. Treatment options for cytomegalovirus retinitis. A time for reassessment. *Arch Ophthalmol* 1999;117:1549–1550.

Holland GN. New issues in the management of patients with AIDS-related cytomegalovirus retinitis. Commentary. *Arch Ophthalmol* 2000;118:704–706.

Jabs DA, Bolton SG, Dunn JP, et al. Discontinuing anticyclomegalovirus therapy in patients with immune reconstitution after combination antiretroviral therapy. *Am J Ophthalmol* 1998;126:817–822.

Jabs DA, Martin BK, Forman MS, et al. Cytomegalovirus resistance to ganciclovir and clinical outcomes of patients with cytomegalovirus retinitis. *Am J Ophthalmol* 2003;135:26–34.

Jabs DA, Van Natta ML, Thorne JE, et al. Course of cytomegalovirus retinitis in the era of highly active antiretroviral therapy. 1. Retinitis progression. *Ophthalmology* 2004;111:2224–2231.

Jabs DA, Van Natta ML, Thorne JE, et al. Course of cytomegalovirus retinitis in the era of highly active antiretroviral therapy. 2. Second eye involvement and retinal detachment. *Ophthalmology* 2004;111:2232–2239.

Kashiwase M, Sata T, Yamauchi Y, et al. Progressive outer retinal necrosis caused by herpes simplex virus type 1 in a patient with acquired immunodeficiency syndrome. *Ophthalmology* 2000;107:790–794.

Kempen JH, Jabs DA, Wilson LA, et al. Risk of visual loss in patients with cytomegalovirus retinitis and the acquired immunodeficiency syndrome. *Arch Ophthalmol* 2003;121:466–476.

Kempen JH, Martin BK, Wu AW, et al. The effect of cytomegalovirus retinitis on the quality of life of patients with AIDS in the era of highly active antiretroviral therapy. *Ophthalmology* 2003;110:987–995.

Kuppermann BD, Holland GN. Immune recovery uveitis. *Am J Ophthalmol* 2000;130:103–106.

Macdonald JC, Karavellas MP, Torriani FJ, et al. High active antiretroviral therapy-related immune recovery in AIDS patients with cytomegalovirus retinitis. *Ophthalmology* 2000;107:877–883.

Mitchell SM, Membrey WL, Youle MS, et al. Cytomegalovirus retinitis after initiation of highly active antiretroviral therapy: a 2 year prospective study. *Br J Ophthalmol* 1999;83:652–655.

Pavesio CE, Mitchell SM, Barton K, et al. Progressive outer retinal necrosis syndrome (PORN) in AIDS patients: a different appearance of varicella-zoster retinitis. *Eye* 1995;9:271–276.

Pavesio CE, Conrad DK, McCluskey PJ, et al. Delayed acute retinal necrosis after herpetic encephalitis. *Br J Ophthalmol* 1997;81:415–416.

Raina J, Bainbridge JWB, Shah SM. Decreased visual acuity in patients with cytomegalovirus retinitis and AIDS. *Eye* 2000;14:8–12.

Sarrafizadeh R, Weinberg DV, Huang C-F. An analysis of lesion size and location in newly diagnosed cytomegalovirus retinitis. *Ophthalmology* 2002;109:119–125.

Tran TH, Stanescu D, Caspers-Velu L, et al. Clinical characteristics of acute HSV-2 retinal necrosis. *Am J Ophthalmol* 2004;137:872–879.

Vitravene Study Group. A randomized controlled clinical trial of intravenous fomivirsen for treatment of newly diagnosed peripheral cytomegalovirus retinitis in patients with AIDS. *Am J Ophthalmol* 2002;133:467–474.

Vitravene Study Group. Randomized dose-comparison studies of intravenous fomivirsen for treatment of cytomegalovirus retinitis that has reactivated or is persistently active despite other therapies in patients with AIDS. *Am J Ophthalmol* 2002;133:475–483.

Vitravene Study Group. Safety of intravenous fomivirsen for treatment of cytomegalovirus retinitis in patients with AIDS. *Am J Ophthalmol* 2002;133:484–498.

Wang LK, Kansal S, Pulido JS. Photodynamic therapy for the treatment of choroidal neovascularization secondary to rubella retinopathy. *Am J Ophthalmol* 2002;134:790–792.

Yoser SL, Forster DJ, Rao NA. Systemic viral infections and their retinal and choroidal manifestations. *Surv Ophthalmol* 1993;37:313–352.

C. FUNGAL

Presumed ocular histoplasmosis syndrome (POHS)

Histoplasmosis is caused by *Histoplasma capsulatum* acquired by inhalation of infective mycelia fragments and/or spores with dust particles. The organisms then pass via the bloodstream to the spleen, liver and, on occasion, the choroid, setting up multiple foci of granulomatous inflammation. Although ocular histoplasmosis has never been reported in patients with active, systemic histoplasmosis, eye disease has an increased prevalence in areas where histoplasmosis is endemic, such as the Mississippi–Missouri river valley. Patients with ocular involvement show an increased prevalence of HLA-B7 and HLA-DR2. A significant association exists between the HLA-DR15/HLA-DQ6 haplotype and development of CNV in POHS.

NB: It must be stressed that organisms have never been isolated from the eyes, hence the name presumed ocular histoplasmosis syndrome, and it is thought that the eye disease represents an immunologic-mediated response in individuals previously exposed to the fungus.

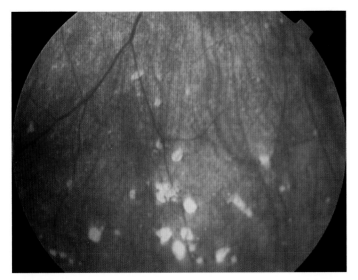

Fig. 6.131 Peripheral 'histo' spots in presumed ocular histoplasmosis syndrome

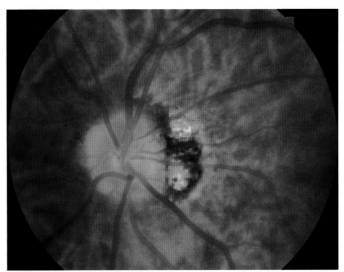

Fig. 6.134 Focal peripapillary atrophy in presumed ocular histoplasmosis syndrome

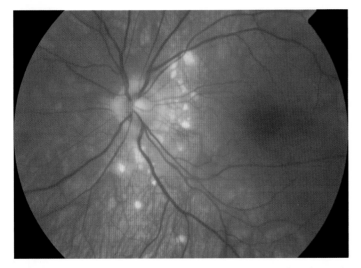

Fig. 6.132 Central 'histo' spots in presumed ocular histoplasmosis syndrome

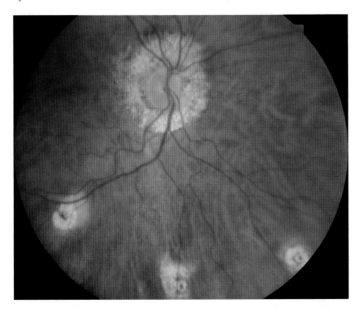

Fig. 6.133 Circumferential peripapillary atrophy and 'histo' spots in presumed ocular histoplasmosis syndrome

General signs

POHS is asymptomatic unless it causes a maculopathy. The earliest symptom of macular involvement is metamorphopsia. The following types of fundus lesion are seen, which are bilateral in 60% of cases.

1. **Absence of intraocular inflammation.**

2. **Acute stage** may manifest localised swelling of the choroid, which may also lead to changes in the overlying RPE.

3. **Atrophic 'histo' spots** consist of roundish, slightly irregular, yellowish-white lesions about 200 µm in diameter. Small pigment clumps may be present within or at the margins of the scars. The lesions are scattered in the mid-retinal periphery (Fig. 6.131) and the posterior pole (Fig. 6.132).

4. **Peripapillary atrophy** may be diffuse or focal or a combination of both.

- Diffuse, circumferential, choroidal atrophy extends up to half a disc diameter beyond the disc margin (Fig. 6.133).

- Focal peripapillary lesions are less common and are irregular and 'punched out', resembling the peripheral spots (Fig. 6.134).

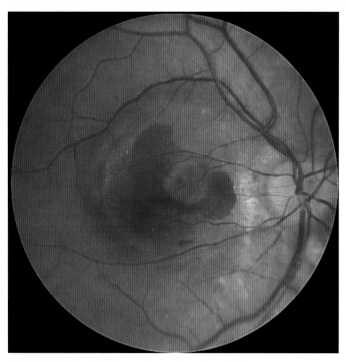

Fig. 6.135 Subretinal haemorrhage from choroidal neovascularisation in presumed ocular histoplasmosis syndrome (Courtesy of C Barry)

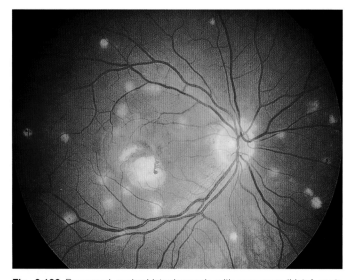

Fig. 6.136 Presumed ocular histoplasmosis with numerous 'histo' spots and a disciform scar at the macula associated with previous choroidal neovascularisation

Exudative maculopathy

1. **Exudative (wet) maculopathy** associated with CNV is a late manifestation that usually develops between the ages of 20 and 45 years in about 5% of eyes. In most cases, CNV is associated with an old macular 'histo' spot, although occasionally it develops within a peripapillary lesion. Very rarely, the CNV occurs in the absence of a pre-existing scar.

2. **The clinical course** of maculopathy is variable and follows one of the following patterns:

- The CNV may initially leak fluid and give rise to metamorphopsia, blurring of central vision and a scotoma. Careful slit-lamp biomicroscopy with a fundus contact lens shows that the macula is elevated by serous fluid and an underlying focal yellow–white or grey lesion. In 12% of eyes, the subretinal fluid absorbs spontaneously and visual symptoms regress.

- A dark green–black ring frequently develops on the surface of the yellow–white lesion and bleeding occurs into the subsensory retinal space, causing a marked drop in visual acuity. In a few eyes, the subretinal haemorrhage resolves and visual acuity improves.

- In some cases, the initial CNV remains active for about 2 years, giving rise to repeated macular haemorrhages (Fig. 6.135). This finally causes a profound and permanent impairment of central vision resulting from the development of a fibrous disciform scar at the fovea (Fig. 6.136). Patients with maculopathy in one eye and an asymptomatic atrophic macular scar in the other are likely to develop a disciform lesion in the second eye. They should therefore test themselves every day with an Amsler grid to detect early metamorphopsia because, without treatment, 60% of eyes with CNV have a final visual acuity of less than 6/60.

3. **Treatment of CNV**

a. *Systemic steroids* may halt progression of the CNV and prevent recurrence after subfoveal surgery.

b. *Argon laser photocoagulation* for extrafoveal CNV.

c. *Photodynamic therapy* for subfoveal CNV.

d. *Surgical removal* of CNV may be indicated in selected cases.

e. *Intravitreal triamcinolone acetonide* is relatively safe and effective for both subfoveal and juxtafoveal CNV.

Cryptococcosis

Cryptococcus neoformans is a yeast that enters the body through inhalation (see Ch. 8). Ocular involvement is present in approximately 6% of patients with cryptococcal meningitis.

1. **Signs**

- Meningitis-associated manifestations are the most common and include papilloedema, ophthalmoplegia, ptosis, optic neuropathy and sixth nerve palsy.

- Multifocal choroiditis (Fig. 6.137).

- Iris infiltration, keratitis and conjunctival granuloma have been reported.

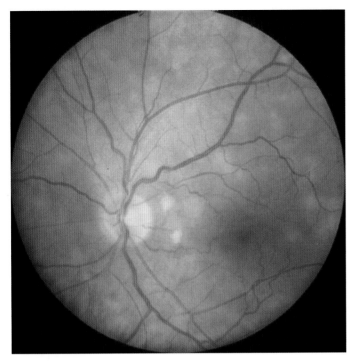

Fig. 6.137 Multifocal cryptococcal choroiditis (Courtesy of A Curi)

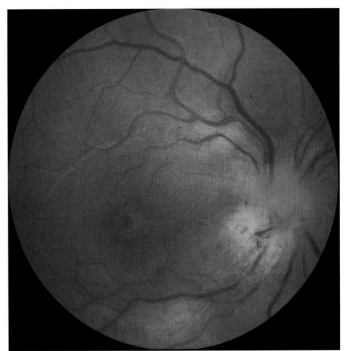

Fig. 6.138 Severe papillitis (Courtesy of P Saine)

2. **Treatment** of sight-threatening lesions is with intravenous amphotericin, oral fluconazole and itraconazole.

FURTHER READING

Carney MD, Combs JL, Waschler W. Cryptococcal choroiditis. *Retina* 1990;10:27–32.

Charles NC, Boxrud CA, Small EA. Cryptococcosis of the anterior segment in acquired immune deficiency syndrome. *Ophthalmology* 1992;99:813–816.

Kestelyn P, Taelman H, Bogaerts J, et al. Ophthalmic manifestations of infections with Cryptococcus neoformans in patients with the acquired immunodeficiency syndrome. *Am J Ophthalmol* 1993;116:721–727.

Macular Photocoagulation Study Group. Five-year follow-up of fellow eyes in individuals with ocular histoplasmosis and unilateral extrafoveal or juxtafoveal choroidal neovascularization. *Arch Ophthalmol* 1996;114:677–688.

Rechtman E, Allen VD, Danis RP, et al. Intravitreal triamcinolone for choroidal neovascularization in ocular histoplasmosis syndrome. *Am J Ophthalmol* 2003;136:739–741.

Rosenfeld PJ, Saperstein DA, Bressler NM, et al. Verteporfin in Ocular Histoplasmosis Study Group. Photodynamic therapy with verteporfin in ocular histoplasmosis: uncontrolled, open-label 2-year study. *Ophthalmology* 2004;111:1725–1733.

Saperstein DA, Rosenfeld PJ, Bressler NM, et al. Verteporfin in Ocular Histoplasmosis (VOH) Study Group. Photodynamic therapy of subfoveal choroidal neovascularization with verteporfin in the ocular histoplasmosis syndrome: one-year results of an uncontrolled, prospective case series. *Ophthalmology* 2002;109:1499–1505.

Sheu SJ, Chen YC, Kuo NW, et al. Endogenous cryptococcal endophthalmitis. *Ophthalmology* 1998;105:377–381.

Spencer WH, Chan C-C, Shen DF, et al. Detection of Histoplasma capsulatum DNA in lesions of chronic ocular histoplasmosis syndrome. *Arch Ophthalmol* 2003;121:1551–1555.

Submacular Surgery Trials Research Group. Surgical vs observation of subfoveal choroidal neovascularization, either associated with ocular histoplasmosis syndrome or idiopathic. *Arch Ophthalmol* 2004;122:1597–1611.

D. BACTERIAL

Cat-scratch disease

Cat-scratch disease (benign lymphoreticulosis) is a subacute infection caused by *Bartonella henselae*, a Gram-negative rod. The infection is transmitted by the scratch or bite of an apparently healthy cat (see Ch. 8). Ocular involvement occurs in about 6% of cases.

Diagnosis

Neuroretinitis is the most common manifestation. It is characterised by the following:

1. **Presentation** is with unilateral, painless visual impairment, which starts gradually and then becomes most marked after about a week.

2. **Signs**, in chronological order:

- Visual acuity is impaired to a variable degree.

- Papillitis associated with peripapillary and macular oedema, which may be associated with venous engorgement and splinter-shaped haemorrhages in severe cases (Fig. 6.138).

- A macular star figure composed of hard exudates subsequently ensues (Fig. 6.139).

- After several months, visual acuity improves, with first resolution of papillitis (Fig. 6.140) and then hard exudates, although initially the exudates may increase as disc swelling is resolving.

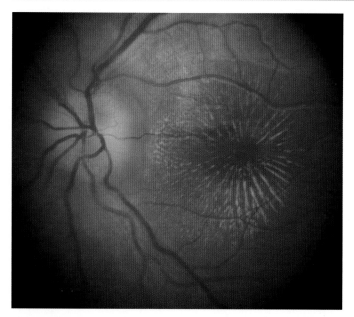

Fig. 6.139 Papillitis and macular star (Courtesy of L Merin)

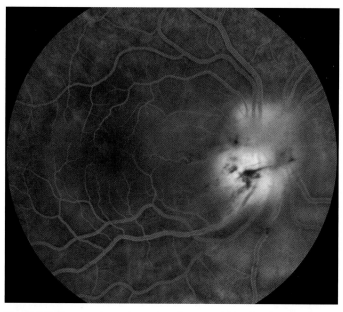

Fig. 6.141 Fluorescein angiography of neuroretinitis showing disc hyperfluorescence due to leakage (Courtesy of P Saine)

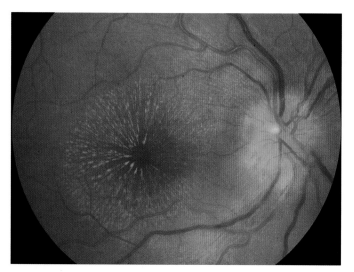

Fig. 6.140 Resolving papillitis

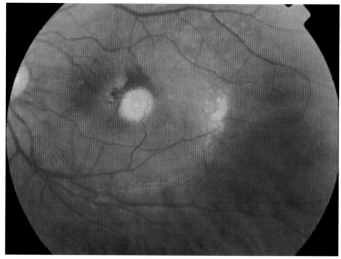

Fig. 6.142 Focal choroiditis in cat-scratch disease (Courtesy of A Curi)

• The fellow eye occasionally becomes involved, but recurrences in the same eye are uncommon.

3. **FA** shows leakage from superficial disc vessels (Fig. 6.141).

4. **Systemic investigations** include serology for *B. henselae* and PCR.

Other ocular manifestations

Other less common ocular manifestations include Parinaud oculoglandular syndrome, focal choroiditis (Fig. 6.142), intermediate uveitis, exudative maculopathy, retinal vascular occlusion and panuveitis.

Treatment

Treatment is with oral doxycycline or erythromycin, with or without rifampicin; the organism is also sensitive to ciprofloxacin and co-trimoxazole.

Whipple disease

Whipple disease (intestinal lipodystrophy) is a rare, chronic, bacterial infection with *Tropheryma whippelii* that primarily involves the gastrointestinal tract and its lymphatic drainage. It occurs mostly in white middle-aged men and is fatal if untreated.

Systemic features

1. **Presentation** is with weight loss, arthralgia, diarrhoea and abdominal pain.

2. **Extraintestinal** involvement includes primarily the CNS, lungs, heart, joints and eyes.

3. **Diagnostic tests**

* Jejunal biopsy shows infiltration of small intestinal mucosa by 'foamy' macrophages that stain with periodic acid–Schiff. Electron microscopy shows small rod-shaped bacilli within the macrophages.

* PCR on vitreous samples in patients with ocular involvement may be used to detect the 16S ribosomal RNA gene sequences which correspond to *T. whippelii*.

4. **Treatment** is primarily with trimethoprim–sulfamethoxazole; the organism is also usually sensitive to tetracycline, erythromycin, penicillin, streptomycin and chloramphenicol.

Ocular features

1. **Secondary to CNS involvement** includes gaze palsy, nystagmus, ophthalmoplegia, papilloedema and optic atrophy

2. **Intraocular inflammation** in the form of vitritis, retinitis, retinal haemorrhages and cotton-wool spots, and multifocal choroiditis may occur with or without concomitant CNS disease.

Nocardia

Nocardia asteroides, a Gram-positive aerobic bacterium, is a cause of opportunistic infections in immunocompromised patients, particularly with lymphomas, long-term pulmonary disease and long-term systemic steroid therapy. Ocular involvement is, however, rare (see Ch. 8).

Diagnosis

1. **Presentation** is with floaters, decreased vision, photophobia and ocular pain.

2. **Signs**

* Anterior uveitis and vitritis.

* Chorioretinitis with subretinal abscess formation is the hallmark (Fig. 6.143).

* Retinal detachment may occur.

3. **Investigations** include vitreous biopsy, pars plana vitrectomy, and fine-needle aspiration of chorioretinal lesions.

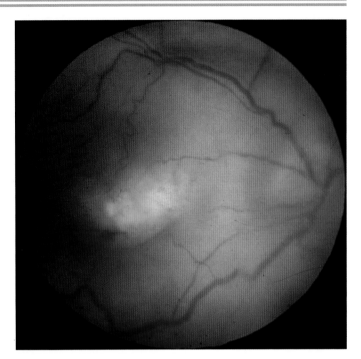

Fig. 6.143 Subretinal abscess in nocardia infection

Treatment

Because of its rarity, the optimal therapeutic regimen has not been established. Intravitreal amikacin and imipenem, and intravenous ceftriaxone may be effective, but the prognosis is often poor.

FURTHER READING

Avila MP, Jalkh AE, Feldman E, et al. Manifestations of Whipple's disease in the posterior segment of the eye. *Arch Ophthalmol* 1984;102:384–390.

Chan RY, Yannuzzi LA, Foster CS. Ocular Whipple's disease. Earlier definitive diagnosis. *Ophthalmology* 2001;108:2225–2231.

Cunningham ET, Koehler JE. Ocular bartonellosis. *Am J Ophthalmol* 2000;130:340–349.

Davitt B, Gehers K, Bowers T. Endogenous Nocardia endophthalmitis. *Retina* 1998;18:71–73.

Fish RH, Hogan RN, Nightingale SD, et al. Peripapillary angiomatosis associated with cat-scratch neuroretinitis. *Arch Ophthalmol* 1992;110:323.

Gray AV, Michels KS, Lauer AK, et al. Bartonella henselae infection associated with neuroretinitis, central retinal artery and vein occlusion, neovascular glaucoma, and severe visual loss. *Am J Ophthalmol* 2004;137:187–189.

Marth T, Raoult D. Whipple's disease. *Lancet* 2003;361:239–246.

Ng EWM, Zimmer-Galler IE, Green WR. Endogenous Nocardia asteroides endophthalmitis. *Arch Ophthalmol* 2002;120:210–212.

Nishimura JK, Cook BE, Pach JM. Whipple disease presenting as posterior uveitis without prominent gastrointestinal symptoms. *Am J Ophthalmol* 1998;126:130–132.

Ormerod LD, Skolnick KA, Menosky MM, et al. Retinal and choroidal manifestations of cat-scratch disease. *Ophthalmology* 1998;105:1024–1031.

Reed JB, Scales DK, Wong MT, et al. Bartonella henselae neuroretinitis in cat scratch disease. Diagnosis, management and sequelae. *Ophthalmology* 1998;105:459–466.

Solley WA, Martin DF, Newman NJ, et al. Cat scratch disease: posterior segment manifestations. *Ophthalmology* 1999;106:1546–1553.

Suhler EB, Lauer AK, Rosenbaum JT. Prevalence of serologic evidence of cat scratch disease in patients with neuroretinitis. *Ophthalmology* 2000;107:871–876.

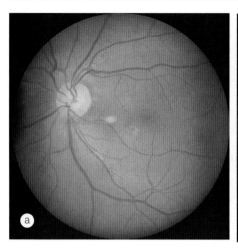

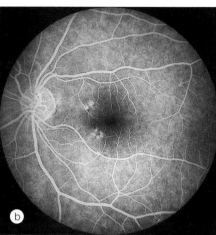

Fig. 6.144 (a) Retinal pigment epitheliitis; (b) fluorescein angiography showing corresponding focal hyperfluorescence (Courtesy of M Prost)

Williams JG, Edward DP, Tessler HH et al. Ocular manifestations of Whipple disease: an atypical presentation. *Arch Ophthalmol* 1998;116:1232–1234.

E. MISCELLANEOUS

Acute retinal pigment epitheliitis

Acute retinal pigment epitheliitis is a rare, idiopathic, self-limiting inflammatory condition of the macular RPE. It typically affects young adults, and although there is no treatment, the visual prognosis is excellent. The condition is unilateral in 75% of cases.

Diagnosis

1. **Presentation** is with sudden-onset impairment of central vision, which may be associated with metamorphopsia.

2. **Signs**

- Absence of intraocular inflammation.

- The fovea shows a blunted reflex with discrete clusters of a few, subtle, small, brown or grey spots at the level of the RPE which may be surrounded by hypopigmented yellow halos (Fig. 6.144a).

- These lesions tend to appear 1 to 2 weeks after the onset of symptoms. The loss of visual function is out of proportion to the changes seen in the macula.

3. **FA** may be normal or show small hyperfluorescent dots with hypofluorescent centres ('honeycomb' appearance) without leakage (Fig. 6.144b).

4. **Electro-oculogram** (EOG) is subnormal.

Prognosis

The condition is self-limiting and does not require treatment. After 6–12 weeks, the acute fundus lesions resolve spontaneously and visual acuity returns to normal, although innocuous residual pigment clumping at the fovea may remain. Recurrences are uncommon.

Acute macular neuroretinopathy

Acute macular neuroretinopathy is a rare, idiopathic, self-limiting condition that typically affects healthy females between the second and fourth decades of life.

The disease may affect one or both eyes and may be preceded by a flu-like illness. Occasionally, it may be associated with multiple evanescent white dot syndrome (MEWDS) and idiopathic blind spot enlargement syndrome, as well as with the use of intravenous iodine contrast agents, oral contraceptives and trauma.

Diagnosis

1. **Presentation** is with sudden decrease of visual acuity and paracentral scotomas.

2. **Signs**

- Absence of intraocular inflammation.

- Darkish, brown–red, wedge-shaped lesions in a 'flower petal' arrangement around the centre of the macula (Fig. 6.145).

- Amsler grid and perimetry reveal remarkable correspondence of the lesions with the shape and location of the scotoma.

- FA and the electroretinogram (ERG) are usually normal.

Prognosis

The condition is self-limiting and does not require treatment. Within several months, visual symptoms gradually improve and the lesions fade but do not completely resolve for many years. Recurrences are uncommon. Visual impairment may be temporary or permanent.

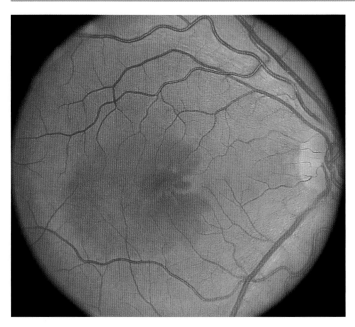

Fig. 6.145 Acute macular neuroretinopathy (Courtesy of J Donald Gass, from *Stereoscopic Atlas of Macular Disease*, Mosby, 1997)

Acute idiopathic maculopathy

Acute idiopathic maculopathy is a very rare condition that typically affects young adults. It is most frequently unilateral and may be preceded by a flu-like illness.

Diagnosis

1. **Presentation** is with a unilateral sudden and severe loss of vision with the presence of a central scotoma.

2. **Signs**

- Wedge-shaped detachment of the sensory retina at the macula with an irregular outline (Fig. 6.146a).

- Smaller, greyish, subretinal thickening at the level of the RPE beneath the sensory detachment is frequently present.

- Iritis, papillitis and mild vitritis may be present.

3. **FA** in the early phase shows minimal subretinal hypo-fluorescence and hyperfluorescence beneath the sensory retinal detachment (Fig. 6.146b). The mid-venous phases show two levels of hyperfluorescence, one from staining of the subretinal thickening at the level of the RPE, and the second from pooling of dye within the subretinal space (Fig. 6.146c). The late phase shows complete staining of the overlying sensory retinal detachment (Fig. 6.146d).

Fig. 6.146 Acute idiopathic maculopathy (see text) (Courtesy of S Milewski)

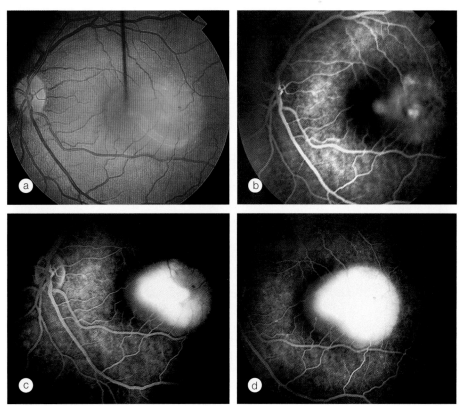

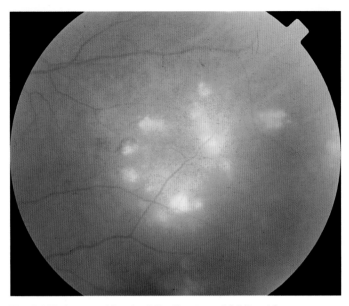

Fig. 6.147 Acute multifocal retinitis (Courtesy of S Milewski)

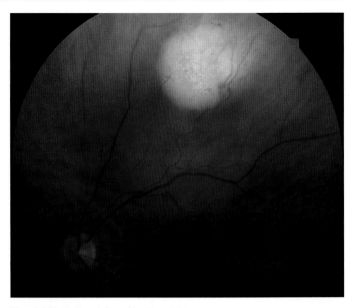

Fig. 6.148 Solitary idiopathic choroiditis

Prognosis

The condition is self-limiting and no treatment is required. Within a few weeks, the exudative changes resolve, with nearly complete recovery of vision. Innocuous residual RPE atrophic changes which may have a 'bull's eye' pattern remain.

Acute multifocal retinitis

Acute multifocal retinitis is a very rare, frequently bilateral condition that typically affects healthy, young to middle-aged adults. It may be preceded by a flu-like illness, usually 1 to 2 weeks before the onset of the visual symptoms. It has been postulated by some that acute multifocal retinitis may be an unusual presentation of cat-scratch disease.

Diagnosis

1. **Presentation** is with sudden onset of mild visual loss.

2. **Signs**

* Bilateral, multiple areas of retinitis posterior to the equator (Fig. 6.147).

* Mild vitritis and disc oedema are frequent.

* A macular star is present in a few cases.

* Small retinal branch artery occlusions occur in a minority of cases.

Prognosis

The condition is self-limiting and treatment is not required. After 2–4 months, the fundus lesions resolve and visual acuity returns to normal.

Solitary idiopathic choroiditis

Solitary idiopathic choroiditis is a distinct clinical entity that may give rise to diagnostic problems as it may simulate other pathology.

Diagnosis

1. **Presentation** is with mild visual loss and floaters.

2. **Signs**

* Vitritis is present during active disease.

* Discrete, post-equatorial, dull-yellow, nummular choroidal elevation with an ill-defined margin (Fig. 6.148).

* Associated findings include adjacent subretinal fluid and a macular star figure away from the main lesion.

* As the inflammation resolves, the lesion develops a better-defined margin with resolution of subretinal fluid and exudation

* Occasional features include retinal vascular dilatation and focal retinal haemorrhages.

NB: The lesions tend to be small, so ultrasonography is of little diagnostic value.

Treatment

Lesions with active inflammation respond well to systemic steroids. Most inactive lesions either remain stable or resolve without treatment.

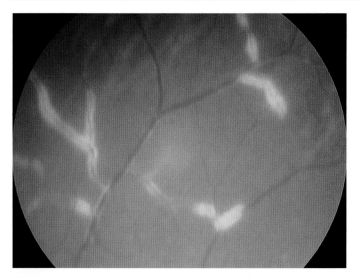

Fig. 6.149 Frosted branch angiitis

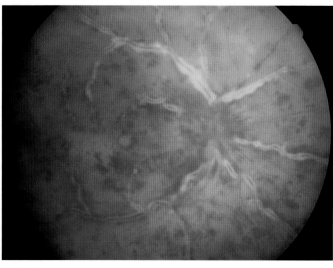

Fig. 6.150 Frosted branch angiitis and venous occlusion (Courtesy of C Barry)

Differential diagnosis

1. **Inflammatory conditions** that may resemble solitary choroidal granuloma, including sarcoidosis, tuberculosis, toxocariasis, nodular posterior scleritis, syphilis and cat-scratch disease.

2. **Amelanotic tumours** such as amelanotic melanoma, metastasis, circumscribed choroidal haemangioma, choroidal osteoma or retinal astrocytoma.

Frosted branch angiitis (FBA)

FBA describes a characteristic fundus picture that may represent a specific syndrome (primary form) or a common immune pathway in response to multiple infective agents.

1. **Secondary** FBA may be associated with infectious retinitis, most notably CMV retinitis, but it may also occur in association with other conditions such as glomerulonephritis and central retinal vein occlusion.

2. **Primary** FBA is extremely rare and typically affects children and young adults.

Diagnosis

1. **Presentation** is with a subacute bilateral visual loss, floaters or photopsia.

2. **Signs**

- Visual acuity is usually very poor.

- Florid translucent retinal perivascular sheathing of both arterioles and venules (Fig. 6.149).

- Variable anterior uveitis and vitritis, and retinal oedema are common.

- Uncommon findings include papillitis, retinal haemorrhages and punctate hard exudates (Fig. 6.150).

Treatment

Treatment is with systemic and topical steroids, but the optimal regimen has not been established. The primary form has a good visual prognosis, but significant visual loss may result in secondary forms.

Acute zonal occult outer retinopathy

The acute zonal outer retinopathies (AZOR) are a group of very rare, idiopathic syndromes characterised by acute onset of loss of one or more zones of visual field caused by damage to the retinal receptor elements. Although AZOR are rare, it is important to be aware of their existence, to save the patient inappropriate and unrewarding medical and neurological investigations.

Acute zonal occult outer retinopathy (AZOOR) is the most common of the AZOR syndromes. It typically affects healthy, young, frequently myopic women, some of whom have an antecedent viral-like illness. Although autoimmunity has been implicated, there are several factors that suggest that AZOOR is probably not primarily an autoimmune disease: asymmetric nature of retinal involvement, lack of improvement with steroids, and difficulty in detecting circulating retinal antibodies.

Diagnosis

1. **Presentation** is with acute loss affecting one or more zones of the visual field, which is frequently associated with photopsia. The temporal field is frequently involved

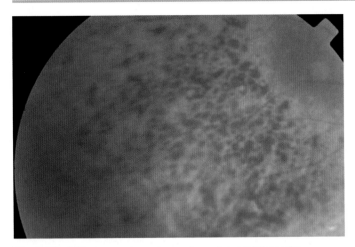

Fig. 6.151 RPE changes in acute zonal occult outer retinopathy

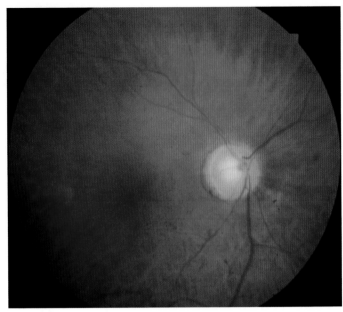

Fig. 6.152 Vascular attenuation, optic atrophy and mild RPE changes in cancer-related retinopathy

but the central field is usually spared; bilateral involvement occurs in 50% of patients.

2. **Signs**, in chronological order:

- Normal fundus.

- Several weeks later, there may be mild vitritis, attenuation of retinal vessels in the affected zone and, occasionally, periphlebitis, particularly in patients with large visual field defects.

- The zones may enlarge, or, less frequently, they remain the same or improve.

- In 50% of cases, visual field loss stabilises within 4–6 months.

- Late findings are characterised by RPE clumping and arteriolar narrowing in the involved area (Fig. 6.151), although if the retinal cells survive, the fundus remains normal.

3. **Perimetry** should include both peripheral and central visual fields because large peripheral zones of visual field loss may go undetected if only central fields are tested. Visual field loss does not correlate with retinal findings.

4. **ERG** characteristically shows a-wave and b-wave amplitude reduction and delayed 30-Hz flicker.

5. **EOG** shows absence or severe reduction of the light rise.

Prognosis

The prognosis is relatively good, with a final visual acuity of 6/12 in at least one eye in 85% of cases. A recurrence rate of 25% to the affected eye and delayed involvement of the fellow eye may occur.

Cancer-associated retinopathy

Paraneoplastic retinopathies are rare diseases with subtle but specific features that may be missed by the unsuspecting observer. Many of the patients present with visual symptoms

before the primary malignancy is diagnosed. It is therefore important for practising clinicians to be familiar with these syndromes to allow early diagnosis of the disease and initiate investigations to unveil the underlying malignancy. The two types are cancer-associated retinopathy (CAR) and melanoma-associated retinopathy (MAR). The most common underlying malignancy in CAR is small cell bronchial carcinoma, followed by gynaecological and breast cancer.

Diagnosis

1. **Symptoms**

- Subacute bilateral visual loss over weeks to months.

- Visual symptoms precede the diagnosis of malignancy in half the cases.

- Positive visual phenomenon of shimmering or flickering lights.

- Progressive reduction of visual acuity, colour impairment, glare, photosensitivity and central scotoma attributed to cone dysfunction.

- Night blindness, impaired dark adaptation, ring scotoma and peripheral field loss due to rod dysfunction.

2. **Signs**

- Fundus often appears normal on presentation.

- Attenuated arterioles, optic disc pallor and mild RPE changes develop as the disease progresses (Fig. 6.152).

- Vitreous cells and vascular inflammation may be seen but are usually mild.

3. Investigations

a. **ERG** is severely attenuated under photopic and scotopic condition; dark adaptation is abnormal.

b. **Lumbar puncture** may show elevated cerebrospinal fluid (CSF) protein and lymphocytosis.

c. **Search for an underlying malignancy.**

Prognosis

The prognosis for both vision and life is poor. Treatment of the primary malignancy does not improve vision. Systemic steroids may be tried but there is no good evidence for their efficacy.

Melanoma-associated retinopathy

MAR differs from CAR because it affects patients with established metastatic cutaneous melanoma prior to the development of the visual symptoms. Male preponderance is 4.5 to 1. The specific antigen responsible has not been identified, but autoantibodies from MAR sera react against bipolar cells in human retina. Clinical and electrophysiological data also implicate the bipolar cells as the primary abnormality in MAR.

Diagnosis

1. Symptoms are shimmering or flickering lights and nyctalopia.

2. Signs

- Visual acuity and colour vision are normal or mildly impaired.

- Visual field shows normal central field, general constriction, peripheral depression and midperipheral scotoma – central scotomas are infrequently seen.

- Fundus appears normal initially.

- RPE irregularity, retina arteriolar attenuation and optic disc pallor are seen in longstanding cases.

- Vitritis and retinal periphlebitis may be present.

3. ERG shows marked reduction of dark-adapted and light-adapted b-wave and preservation of a-wave (normal photoreceptor function). Both the amplitude and implicit time of the b-wave are abnormal. MAR is characterised by a 'negative ERG', similar to the pattern seen in congenital stationary night blindness.

Prognosis

Despite the lack of treatment, the visual prognosis is good and most patients maintain stable vision.

NB: Immunosuppressive therapy should be avoided as this may enhance metastatic disease.

FURTHER READING

Amin P, Cox TA. Acute macular neuroretinopathy. *Arch Ophthalmol* 1998;116:112–113.

Arai M, Nao-I N, Sawada A, et al. Multifocal electroretinogram indicates visual field loss in acute zonal occult outer retinopathy. *Am J Ophthalmol* 1998;126:446–449.

Chan JW. Paraneoplastic retinopathies and optic neuropathies. *Surv Ophthalmol* 2003;48:12–38.

Cunningham ET Jr, Schatz H, McDonald HR, et al. Acute multifocal retinitis. *Am J Ophthalmol* 1997;123:347–357.

Foster RE, Gutman FA, Myers SM, et al. Acute multifocal inner retinitis. *Am J Ophthalmol* 1991;111:673–681.

Francis PJ, Marinescu A, Fitzke FW, et al. Acute zonal occult outer retinopathy: towards a set of diagnostic criteria. *Br J Ophthalmol* 2005;89:70–73.

Freund, KB, Yannuzzi LA, Barile GR, et al. The expanding clinical spectrum of unilateral acute idiopathic maculopathy. *Arch Ophthalmol* 1996;114:555–559.

Gass JDM. The acute zonal outer retinopathies. *Am J Ophthalmol* 2000;130:655–657.

Gass JDM, Agarwal A, Scott IU. Acute zonal occult outer retinopathy: a long-term follow-up study. *Am J Ophthalmol* 2002;134:329–339.

Kleiner RC, Kaplan HJ, Shakin JL, et al. Acute frosted retinal periphlebitis. *Am J Ophthalmol* 1988;106:27–34.

Luttrull JK. Acute retinal pigment epitheliitis. *Am J Ophthalmol* 1997;123:127–129.

Prost M. Long-term observations of patients with acute retinal pigment epitheliitis. *Ophthalmologica* 1989;199:84–89.

Shields JA, Shields CL, Dermici H, et al. Solitary idiopathic choroiditis: the Richard Beaver lecture. *Arch Ophthalmol* 2002;120:311–319.

Sugin SL, Henderley DE, Friedman SM, et al. Unilateral frosted branch angiitis. *Am J Ophthalmol* 1991;111:682–685.

Thirkill CE, Roth AM, Keltner JL. Cancer-associated retinopathy. *Arch Ophthalmol* 1987;105:372–375.

Turbeville SD, Cowan LD, Gass JD. Acute macular neuroretinopathy: a review of the literature. *Surv Ophthalmol* 2003;48:1–11.

Vander JF, Masciulli L. Unilateral frosted branch angiitis. *Am J Ophthalmol* 1991;112:477–478.

Walker S, Iguchi A, Jones NP. Frosted branch angiitis: a review. *Eye* 2004;18:527–533.

Yannuzzi LA, Jampol LM, Rabb MF, et al. Unilateral acute idiopathic maculopathy. *Arch Ophthalmol* 1991;109:1411–1416.

PANUVEITIS

Sarcoidosis

Sarcoidosis is a T-lymphocyte-mediated, non-caseating granulomatous inflammatory disorder of unknown cause. The clinical spectrum of disease varies from mild single-organ involvement to potentially fatal multisystem disease that can affect almost any tissue (see Ch. 8).

Anterior uveitis

1. Acute anterior uveitis typically affects patients with acute-onset sarcoid and usually responds well to topical therapy.

2. Chronic granulomatous anterior uveitis tends to affect older patients with chronic pulmonary disease. It is characterised by 'mutton-fat' keratic precipitates and iris

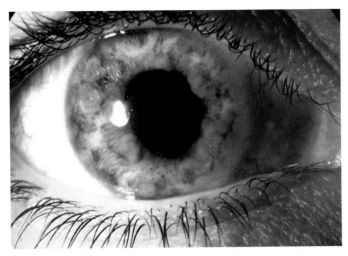

Fig. 6.153 Granulomatous anterior uveitis in sarcoidosis

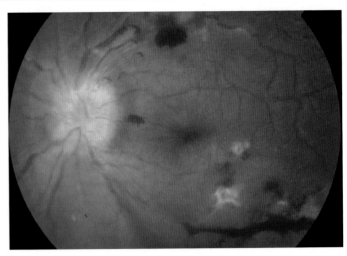

Fig. 6.155 Occlusive periphlebitis and disc oedema in sarcoidosis

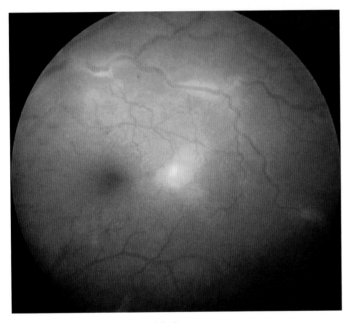

Fig. 6.154 Periphlebitis in sarcoidosis

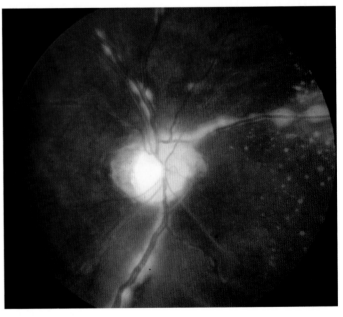

Fig. 6.156 'Candlewax' drippings in severe sarcoid periphlebitis (Courtesy of P Morse)

nodules (Fig. 6.153). Treatment is more difficult than for acute anterior uveitis; periocular and systemic steroids may be required. Longstanding inflammation may lead to cataract, glaucoma, band keratopathy and CMO.

Intermediate uveitis

Intermediate uveitis is uncommon and may antedate the onset of systemic disease. The presence of associated granulomatous anterior uveitis should arouse suspicion.

Posterior uveitis

The posterior segment is involved in about 25% of patients with ocular sarcoid and may take the following forms:

SIGNS

1. **Retinal periphlebitis** varies in severity.

- Periphlebitis is characterised by yellowish or grey–white perivenous sheathing (Fig. 6.154).

- Occlusive periphlebitis is uncommon (Fig. 6.155).

- Perivenous exudates referred to as 'candlewax drippings' (*en taches de bougie*) are typical of severe sarcoid periphlebitis (Fig. 6.156).

2. **Choroidal infiltrates** are uncommon and vary in appearance:

- Multiple, small, pale-yellow infiltrates that may have a 'punched-out' appearance and are often most numerous inferiorly are most common (Fig. 6.157).

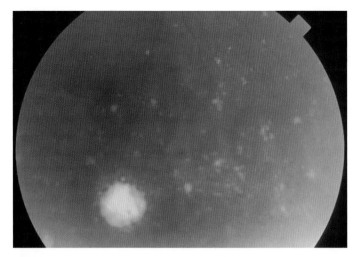

Fig. 6.157 Small peripheral choroidal sarcoid granulomas

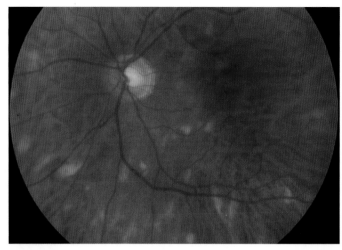

Fig. 6.160 Multifocal sarcoid choroiditis

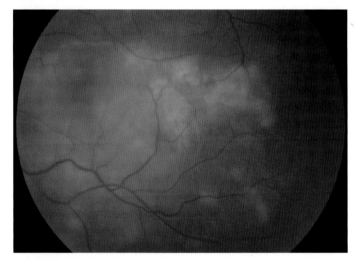

Fig. 6.158 Confluent choroidal infiltrates in sarcoidosis

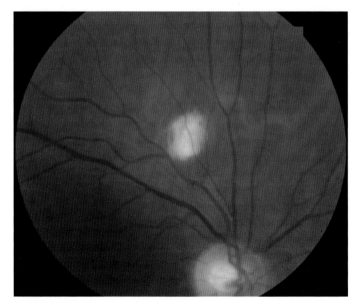

Fig. 6.159 Solitary choroidal sarcoid granuloma

- Multiple, large, confluent infiltrates which may have amoeboid margins are less common (Fig. 6.158).

- Solitary choroidal granulomas are the least common (Fig. 6.159).

3. **Multifocal choroiditis** (Fig. 6.160) carries a guarded visual prognosis because it may cause loss of central vision as a result of secondary CNV which may be peripapillary (Fig. 6.161) or associated with a chorioretinal scar (Fig. 6.162).

4. **Retinal granulomas** are small, discrete, yellow lesions (Fig. 6.163).

5. **Dalen–Fuchs nodules** represent cellular infiltrates between the RPE and Bruch membrane which disappear once the inflammation has resolved but leave corresponding areas of RPE atrophy.

> **NB:** Dalen–Fuchs nodules may also occur in sympathetic ophthalmitis and VKH syndrome.

6. **Peripheral retinal neovascularisation** may develop as a result of retinal capillary dropout (Fig. 6.164). In black patients, it may be mistaken for proliferative sickle-cell retinopathy.

7. **Optic nerve** involvement may take the following forms:

- Focal granulomas, which do not usually affect vision (Fig. 6.165).

- Papilloedema, which is usually secondary to involvement of the CNS, may occur in the absence of other ocular manifestations.

- Persistent disc oedema is a frequent finding in patients with retinal or vitreous involvement.

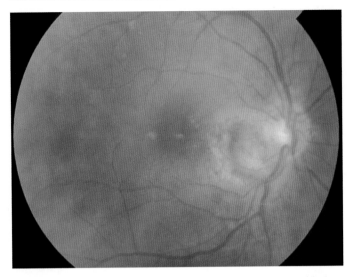

Fig. 6.161 Peripapillary scar choroidal neovascularisation in sarcoidosis

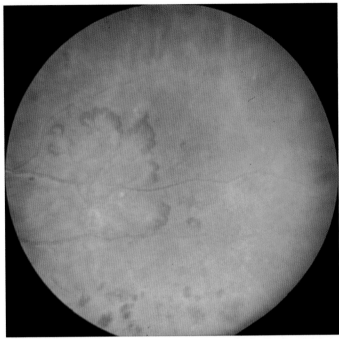

Fig. 6.164 Peripheral retinal neovascularisation in sarcoidosis

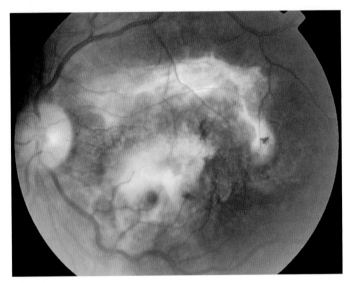

Fig. 6.162 Macular disciform lesion associated with chorioretinal scarring in sarcoidosis

TREATMENT

Treatment of vision-threatening posterior segment disease may be with posterior sub-Tenon steroid injections or systemic steroids. Rarely, ciclosporin or methotrexate is required.

Differential diagnosis of posterior segment sarcoid

1. Small choroidal lesions

- Multifocal choroiditis with panuveitis.
- Birdshot chorioretinopathy.
- Tuberculosis.

2. Large choroidal infiltrates

- Metastatic tumour.
- Large cell lymphoma.
- Harada disease.
- Serpiginous choroidopathy.

3. Periphlebitis

- Tuberculosis.
- Behçet syndrome.
- CMV retinitis.

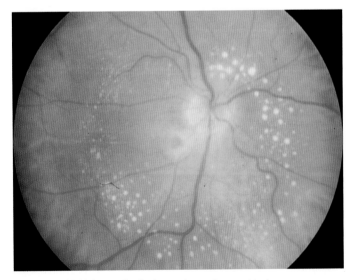

Fig. 6.163 Multiple small retinal granulomas in sarcoidosis

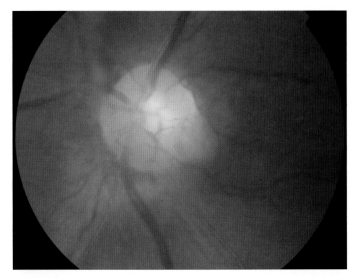

Fig. 6.165 Disc granuloma in sarcoidosis

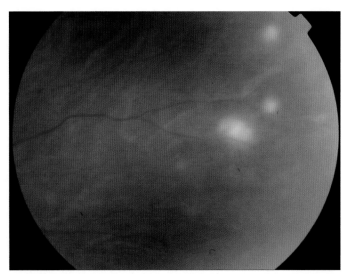

Fig. 6.167 Retinal infiltrates in Behçet disease

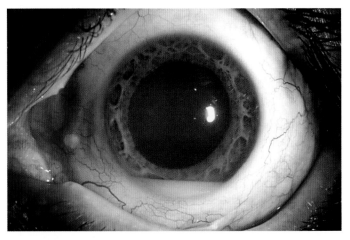

Fig. 6.166 Hypopyon in Behçet disease (Courtesy of B Noble)

FURTHER READING

Brod RD. Presumed sarcoid choroidopathy mimicking birdshot retinochoroidopathy. *Am J Ophthalmol* 1990;109:357–358.

Dana MR, Merayo-Lloves J, Schaumberg DA, et al. Prognosticators for visual outcome in sarcoid uveitis. *Ophthalmology* 1996;103:1846–1853.

Dev S, McCallum RM, Jaffe GJ. Methotrexate treatment for sarcoid-associated panuveitis. *Ophthalmology* 1999;106:111–118.

Edelsten C, Pearson A, Joyles E, et al. The ocular and systemic prognosis of patients presenting with sarcoid uveitis. *Eye* 1999;13:748–753.

Johns CJ, Michele TM. The clinical management of sarcoidosis: a 50-year experience at the Johns Hopkins Hospital. *Medicine* 1999;78:65–111.

Lobo A, Barton K, Minassian D, et al. Visual loss in sarcoid-related uveitis. *Clin Experiment Ophthalmol* 2003;31:310–316.

Power WJ, Neves RA, Rodriguez A, et al. The value of combined serum angiotensin-conversion enzyme and gallium scan in the diagnosis of ocular sarcoidosis. *Ophthalmology* 1995;102:2007–2011.

Rothova A. Ocular involvement in sarcoidosis. Perspectives. *Br J Ophthalmol* 2000;84:110–116.

Smith JA, Foster CS. Sarcoidosis and its ocular manifestations. *Int Ophthalmol Clin* 1996;36:109–125.

Stavrou P, Linton S, Young DW, et al. Clinical diagnosis of ocular sarcoid. *Eye* 1997;11:365–370.

Thorne JE, Brucker AJ. Choroidal white lesions as early manifestations of sarcoidosis. *Retina* 2000;20:8–15.

Behçet syndrome

Behçet syndrome (BS) is an idiopathic, multisystem disease characterised by recurrent episodes of orogenital ulceration and vasculitis which may involve small, medium and large veins and arteries (see Ch. 8). Ocular complications occur in up to 95% of men and 70% of women with BS. Eye disease typically occurs within 2 years of the onset of oral ulceration, but rarely the delay may be as long as 14 years. Conversely, intraocular inflammation is the presenting manifestation in about 10% of cases. It is unusual for the systemic and ocular manifestations to develop simultaneously. Ocular disease is usually bilateral and only in 6% does it remain uniocular.

Signs

1. **Acute recurrent anterior uveitis**, which may be simultaneously bilateral and frequently associated with a transient mobile hypopyon in a relatively white eye (Fig. 6.166). It is often a mild manifestation when compared with posterior segment involvement and usually responds well to topical steroids.

2. **Retinal infiltrates** are white, superficial, necrotic, cellular lesions seen during the acute stage of the systemic disease (Fig. 6.167); they heal without scarring.

3. **Retinal vasculitis** may involve both veins (Fig. 6.168) and arteries and result in ischaemic retinopathy which may involve the macula (Fig. 6.169). Retinal neovascularisation may occur in eyes with significant retinal capillary dropout.

4. **Vascular leakage** may give rise to diffuse retinal oedema, CMO and disc oedema.

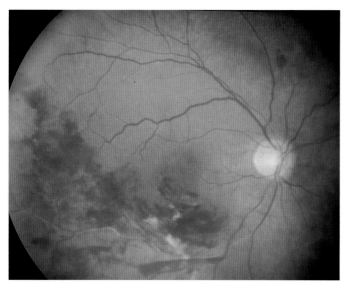

Fig. 6.168 Occlusive retinal periphlebitis in Behçet syndrome resulting in branch vein occlusion (Courtesy of A Dick)

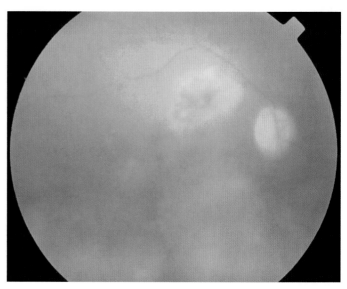

Fig. 6.170 Severe vitritis and retinitis in Behçet syndrome

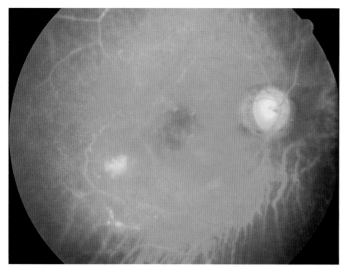

Fig. 6.169 Severe ischaemic retinopathy in Behçet syndrome

5. **Vitritis**, which may be severe and persistent, is universal in eyes with active disease (Fig. 6.170).

6. **Other manifestations**, which are uncommon, include conjunctivitis, conjunctival ulcers, episcleritis, scleritis, and ophthalmoplegia from neurological involvement.

Treatment of posterior uveitis

1. **Systemic steroids** may shorten the duration of an inflammatory episode but are not effective long term, so an additional agent is usually required.

2. **Azathioprine** does not act fast enough in acute disease but is effective for long-term treatment. Patients with low serum levels of thiopurine methyltransferase are at increased risk of developing side effects from azathioprine,

whereas those with high levels are less likely to benefit from therapy.

3. **Alkylating agents**, including chlorambucil and cyclophosphamide, are capable of inducing remission for long periods following discontinuation of therapy, but their toxicity is especially worrying in young patients. They are still useful in resistant aggressive disease involving the posterior segment.

4. **Ciclosporin** is effective and rapidly acting but is associated with nephrotoxicity, particularly at doses higher than 5 mg/kg/day; relapses after cessation often limit its use.

5. **Subcutaneous interferon alfa-2a** (6 million units daily) is very effective for mucocutaneous lesions and may also be used to treat ocular disease resistant to high-dose steroids. Side effects are dose-dependent and include flu-like symptoms, hair loss, itching and depression.

6. **Intravitreal sustained-release steroid implants** are currently under investigation. They are capable of releasing fluocinolone acetonide over a 3-year period and prevent recurrent attacks of uveitis. Their main complications are cataract and glaucoma.

7. **Biological agents** such as infliximab (Remicade) are currently undergoing clinical trials and show promise in treating retinal vasculitis.

Prognosis

The prognosis is guarded and about 20% of eyes become blind despite treatment. The end stage of posterior segment involvement is characterised by optic atrophy, vascular attenuation, chronic sheathing and variable chorioretinal scarring (Fig. 6.171).

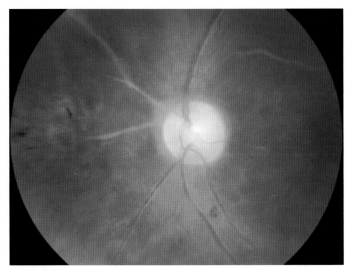

Fig. 6.171 End-stage Behçet syndrome

International Study Group for Behçet's disease. Evaluation of diagnostic ('classification') criteria in Behçet's disease – towards internationally agreed criteria. *Br J Rheumatol* 1992;31:299–308.

Kotter I, Zierhut M, Eckstein AK, et al. Human recombinant interferon alfa-2a for the treatment of Behçet's disease with sight threatening posterior or panuveitis. *Br J Ophthalmol* 2003;87:423–431.

Matsuo T, Itami M, Nakagawa H. The incidence and pathology of conjunctival ulceration in Behçet's syndrome. *Br J Ophthalmol* 2002;86:140–143.

Ohno S, Nakamura S, Hori S, et al. Efficacy, safety, and pharmacokinetics of multiple administration of infliximab in Behçet's disease with refractory uveoretinitis. *J Rheumatol* 2004;31:1362–1368.

Sakamoto M, Akazawa K, Nishioka Y, et al. Prognostic factors of vision in patients with Behçet's disease. *Ophthalmology* 1995;102:317–321.

Sfikakis PP, Theodossiadis PG, Katsiari CG, et al. Effect of infliximab on sight-threatening panuveitis in Behçet's disease. *Lancet* 2001;358:295–296.

Stanford MR. Behçet's syndrome. New treatments for an old disease [Editorial]. *Br J Ophthalmol* 2003;87:381–382.

Toker E, Kozokoglu H, Acar N. High dose intravenous steroid therapy for severe posterior segment uveitis in Behçet disease. *Br J Ophthalmol* 2002;86:521–523.

Tugal-Tutkun I, Urgancioglu M. Childhood-onset uveitis in Behçet disease: a descriptive study of 36 cases. *Am J Ophthalmol* 2003;136:1114–1119.

Tugal-Tutkun I, Onal S, Altan-Yaycioglu R, et al. Uveitis in Behçet disease: an analysis of 880 patients. *Am J Ophthalmol* 2004;138:373–380.

Verity DH, Wallace GR, Vaughan RW, et al. Behçet's disease: from Hippocrates to the third millennium. *Br J Ophthalmol* 2003;87:1175–1183.

Differential diagnosis

In patients with suggestive ocular findings but lack of classical systemic manifestations, the diagnosis becomes uncertain, especially due to the lack of definitive laboratory tests. It is therefore important to consider the following conditions:

1. **Recurrent anterior uveitis with hypopyon** may occur in spondyloarthropathies. However, the uveitis is not usually simultaneously bilateral and the hypopyon is not mobile because it is frequently associated with a fibrinous exudate. In BS, uveitis is frequently simultaneously bilateral and the hypopyon shifts with gravity as the patient changes head position.

2. **Retinal vasculitis** may be associated with sarcoidosis. However, sarcoid vasculitis involves only veins in a segmental manner and is rarely occlusive. In contrast, BS usually affects both arteries and veins, is diffuse, frequently occlusive and is associated with vitritis, which is uncommon in sarcoid-related vasculitis.

3. **Retinal infiltrates** similar to those in BS may be seen in viral retinitis such as the acute retinal necrosis syndrome. However, in viral retinitis, the infiltrates eventually coalesce. Multiple retinal infiltrates also occur in idiopathic acute multifocal retinitis. In contrast to BS, the clinical course is favourable, with return to normal vision within 2–4 months of onset.

FURTHER READING

Demiroglu H, Barista I, Dundar S. Risk factor assessment and prognosis of eye involvement in Behçet disease in Turkey. *Ophthalmology* 1997;104:701–705.

International Behçet's Study Group. Criteria for diagnosis of Behçet's disease. *Lancet* 1990;335:1078–1080.

Vogt–Koyanagi–Harada syndrome (VKH)

VKH syndrome is an idiopathic, multisystem, autoimmune disease against melanocytes, causing inflammation of melanocyte-containing tissues such as the uvea, ear and meninges (see Ch. 8).

Signs

1. **Anterior uveitis** is usually non-granulomatous during the acute phase but shows granulomatous features during recurrences which typically involve only the anterior segment. IOP may become elevated in cases of inflammatory infiltration of the ciliary body and anterior displacement of the lens–iris diaphragm.

2. **Posterior segment involvement** occurs in patients with Harada disease and is frequently bilateral. In chronological order, the findings are as follows:

- Diffuse choroidal infiltration.

- Multifocal detachments of the sensory retina and disc oedema (Fig. 6.172).

- Exudative retinal detachment (Fig. 6.173).

- The chronic phase is characterised by diffuse RPE atrophy (sunset-glow fundus) which may be associated with peripheral, small, discrete atrophic spots, which are usually labelled Dalen–Fuchs nodules (Fig. 6.174).

NB: Although uncommon, VKH may also affect children, who tend to have more aggressive disease and a poorer visual prognosis than adults.

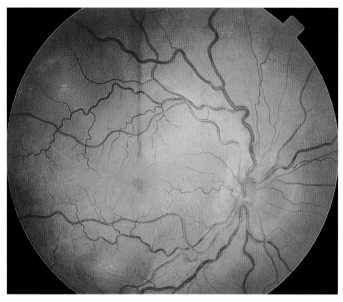

Fig. 6.172 Multifocal serous retinal detachments in Harada disease

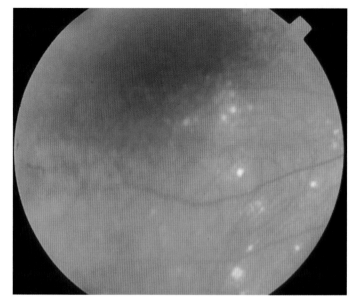

Fig. 6.174 'Sunset-glow' fundus with scattered depigmented spots in Harada disease

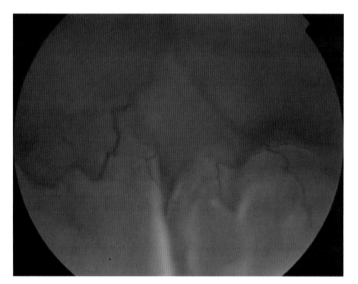

Fig. 6.173 Exudative inferior retinal detachment in Harada disease

Diagnostic tests

1. **CSF analysis** shows pleocytosis with predominant small lymphocytes in about 80% of patients within 1 week and 97% within 3 weeks of disease onset.

2. **FA** shows multifocal hyperfluorescent dots at the level of the RPE and the accumulation of dye in the subretinal space (Fig. 6.175). The chronic phase shows areas of hyperfluorescence due to RPE window defects.

3. **ICG** demonstrates areas of choroidal inflammatory vasculopathy and hypofluorescent dark spots, which probably represent choroidal granulomas. Pinpoint leakage from RPE is also seen. ICG is useful in monitoring the evolu-

tion of the choroidal inflammation and the effect of therapy.

4. **Ultrasonography** may be helpful in cases of poor visualisation of the fundus, and may show diffuse thickening of the posterior choroid, serous retinal detachment and vitreous opacities.

Complications

1. **Cataract** develops in 10% to 35% of patients with VKH, as a consequence of longstanding inflammation and use of steroids.

2. **Glaucoma** is less common.

3. **CNV and subretinal fibrosis** are responsible for significant visual loss. Subretinal fibrosis (Fig. 6.176) has been associated with long duration of the disease and may occur in as many as 40% of the cases.

Treatment

Posterior segment involvement is treated with intravenous or high-dose oral steroids. Steroid-resistant patients may require ciclosporin. Eyes with subfoveal CNV may benefit from surgical excision or photodynamic therapy.

NB: The prognosis depends on early recognition and aggressive control of the early stages of the disease. Late diagnosis or incorrect initial therapy is more likely to be associated with a guarded prognosis, with only 50% of patients having a final visual acuity better than 6/12.

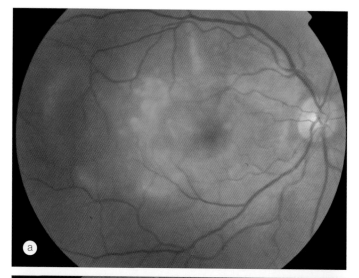

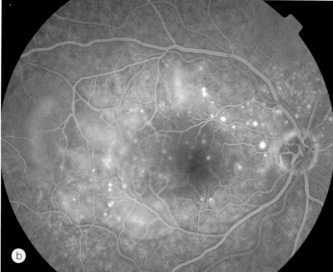

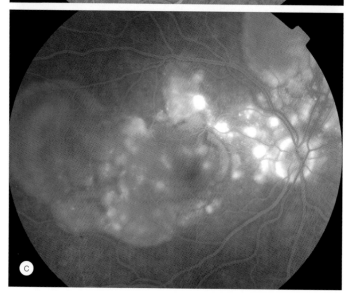

Fig. 6.175 (a) Multifocal serous retinal detachments in Harada disease; (b) fluorescein angiography venous phase shows multiple hyperfluorescent spots; (c) late phase shows extensive areas of hyperfluorescence due to pooling of dye under the serous detachments

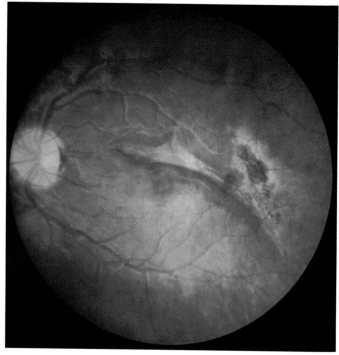

Fig. 6.176 Subretinal fibrosis in Harada disease

Differential diagnosis of bilateral exudative retinal detachments

- Metastatic carcinoma to the choroid.

- Uveal effusion syndrome.

- Posterior scleritis.

- Eclampsia.

- Central serous retinopathy.

FURTHER READING

Bouchenaki N, Herbort CP. The contribution of indocyanine green angiography to the appraisal and management of Vogt-Koyanagi-Harada disease. *Ophthalmology* 2001;108:54–64.

Kahn M, Pepose JS, Green WR, et al. Immunocytologic findings in a case of Vogt-Koyanagi-Harada syndrome. *Ophthalmology* 1993;100:1191–1198.

Kohno T, Miki T, Shiraki K, et al. Subtraction ICG angiography in Harada's disease. *Br J Ophthalmol* 1999;83:822–833.

Moorthy RS, Inomata H, Rao NA. Vogt-Koyanagi-Harada syndrome. *Surv Ophthalmol* 1995;39:265–292.

Perry HD, Font RL. Clinical and histopathologic observations in severe Vogt-Koyanagi-Harada syndrome. *Am J Ophthalmol* 1997;83:242–254.

Rajendram R, Evans M, Rao NA. Vogt-Koyanagi-Harada disease. *Int Ophthalmol Clin* 2005;45:115–134.

Read RW, Holland GN, Rao NA, et al. Revised diagnostic criteria for Vogt-Koyanagi-Harada disease: report of an international committee on nomenclature. *Am J Ophthalmol* 2001;131:647–652.

Rubasamen PE, Gass JDM. Vogt-Koyanagi-Harada syndrome; clinical course, therapy, and long-term outcome. *Arch Ophthalmol* 1991;109:682–687.

Russell WR, Holland GN, Rao NA, et al. Revised diagnostic criteria for Vogt-Koyanagi-Harada disease: report of an International Committee on Nomenclature. *Am J Ophthalmol* 2001;131:647–652.

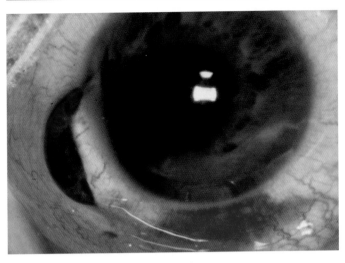

Fig. 6.177 Scleral laceration with iris prolapse

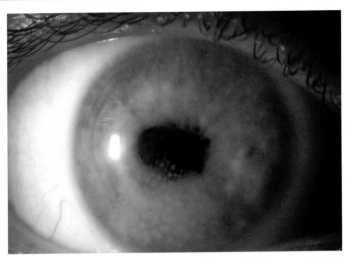

Fig. 6.178 Severe granulomatous anterior uveitis in sympathetic ophthalmitis

Sympathetic ophthalmitis

Sympathetic ophthalmitis (SO) is a rare bilateral granulomatous panuveitis occurring after penetrating trauma, often associated with uveal prolapse (Fig. 6.177), or, less frequently, following intraocular surgery, most commonly multiple vitreoretinal procedures. The traumatised eye is referred to as the *exciting* eye, and the fellow eye, which also develops uveitis, is the *sympathising* eye. Since histological proof is frequently lacking, the diagnosis is mostly presumptive.

Diagnosis

1. **Presentation** in 65% of cases is between 2 weeks and 3 months after initial injury and 90% of all cases occur within the first year.

2. **Signs**, in chronological order:

- The exciting eye shows evidence of the initial trauma and is frequently very red and irritable.

- The sympathising eye then becomes photophobic and irritable.

- Both eyes develop anterior uveitis, which may be mild or severe and granulomatous (Fig. 6.178). Because the severity of uveitis may be asymmetric, mild involvement in one eye may be missed.

- Multifocal choroidal infiltrates in the midperiphery (Fig. 6.179) and sub-RPE infiltrates, corresponding to Dalen–Fuchs nodules seen on histology (Fig. 6.180).

- Exudative retinal detachment may occur in severe cases.

- Residual chorioretinal scarring may cause visual loss when involving the macula.

- 'Sunset-glow' appearance, similar to VKH.

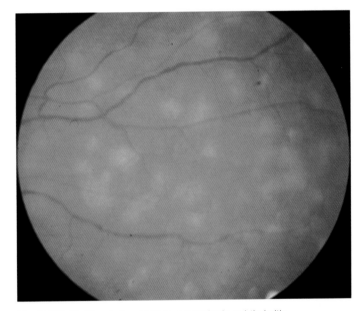

Fig. 6.179 Multifocal choroiditis in sympathetic ophthalmitis

3. **FA** shows multiple foci of leakage at the level of RPE, with subretinal pooling in the presence of exudative retinal detachment.

4. **ICG** shows dark spots in the choroid, indicating the presence of active disease, which tend to disappear if treated aggressively in the early stages, but will leave permanent damage if allowed to progress (dark spots will persist in late phases of the ICG).

5. **Ultrasonography** may show choroidal thickening and retinal detachment.

6. **Systemic manifestations** may be the same as in VKH (headache, pleocytosis in the CSF, dysacousis, tinnitus, alopecia, poliosis and vitiligo) but are less common.

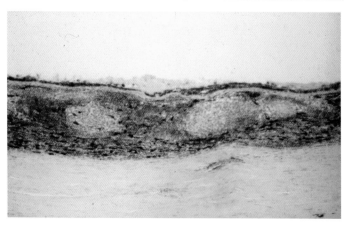

Fig. 6.180 Histology of sympathetic ophthalmitis, showing diffuse Dalen–Fuchs nodules consisting of epithelioid cells between the RPE and Bruch membrane

Treatment

1. **Enucleation** within the first 10 days following trauma should be considered only in eyes with a hopeless visual prognosis, because the exciting eye may eventually have better vision than the sympathising eye.

> **NB:** Evisceration does not seem to protect against SO.

2. **Topical** treatment of the anterior uveitis with steroids and cycloplegics, but the inflammation tends to be resistant to this form of therapy (diagnostic clue).

3. **Systemic** steroids (1–1.5 mg/kg) are usually effective, although occasionally ciclosporin or azathioprine may be required. Treatment is often required for at least a year, with gradual tapering of the dose to reduce the risk of relapse.

Prognosis

With aggressive therapy, the prognosis is good, with 75% of eyes having a visual acuity of better that 6/12.

> **NB:** Long-term follow-up is mandatory because relapses occur in 50% of cases, which may be delayed for several years.

FURTHER READING

Bilyk JR. Enucleation, evisceration and sympathetic ophthalmia. *Curr Opin Ophthalmol* 2000;11:372–386.

Chan CC, Roberge FG, Whitcup SM, et al. 32 cases of sympathetic ophthalmia. *Arch Ophthalmol* 1995;113:597–600.

Kilmartin DJ, Dick A, Forrester JV. Prospective surveillance of sympathetic ophthalmia in the UK and Republic of Ireland. *Br J Ophthalmol* 2000;84:259–263.

Makey TA, Azar A. Sympathetic ophthalmia. *Arch Ophthalmol* 1978;96:257–262.

Rao N. Mechanisms of inflammatory response in sympathetic ophthalmia and VKH syndrome. *Eye* 1997;11:213–216.

Reynard M, Riffenburg RS, Maes EF. Effect of corticosteroid treatment and enucleation on the visual prognosis of sympathetic ophthalmia. *Am J Ophthalmol* 1983;96:290–294.

Vote BJ, Hall A, Cairns J, Buttery R. Changing trends in sympathetic ophthalmia. *Clin Experiment Ophthalmol* 2004;32:542–545.

Tuberculosis

Pathogenesis

Tuberculosis is a chronic granulomatous infection caused by the tubercule bacillus which is of the genus *Mycobacterium* (see Ch. 8). Tuberculous uveitis is rare in the developed world and may be difficult to diagnose because it may occur in patients without systemic manifestations of tuberculosis. The diagnosis is therefore often presumptive, based on indirect evidence such as intractable uveitis unresponsive to steroid therapy, a positive history of contact, a positive skin test and negative findings for other causes of uveitis.

Signs

1. **Chronic anterior uveitis**, usually granulomatous, but occasionally non-granulomatous, is the most frequent feature.

2. **Choroiditis** is caused by direct infection.

- Unilateral focal (Fig. 6.181) or, less frequently, multifocal.

- Extensive diffuse choroiditis may occur in patients with AIDS (Fig. 6.182).

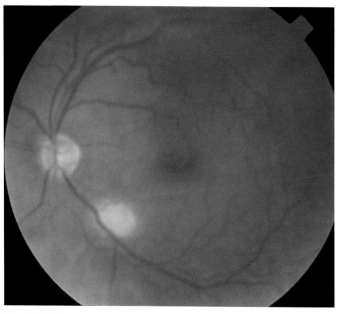

Fig. 6.181 Solitary tuberculous choroiditis (Courtesy of A Curi)

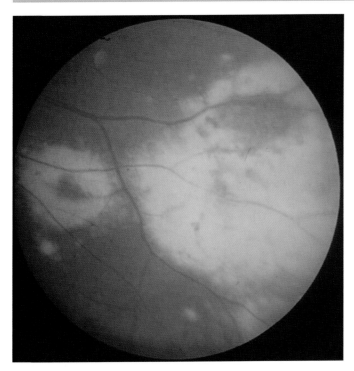

Fig. 6.182 Severe diffuse tuberculous choroiditis in AIDS

- Choroiditis may occasionally resemble serpiginous choroidopathy (Fig. 6.183).

3. **Large solitary choroidal granulomas** are uncommon.

4. **Periphlebitis** is often bilateral and represents a manifestation of hypersensitivity to the bacillus.

- Occlusive periphlebitis (Fig. 6.184a) is associated with retinal capillary closure seen on FA (Fig. 6.184b).

- Retinal neovascularisation may occur in eyes with extensive capillary non-perfusion (Fig. 6.185).

Treatment

Treatment is initially with at least three drugs (isoniazid, rifampicin, pyrazinamide or ethambutol) and then with isoniazid and rifampicin. Quadruple therapy is sometimes necessary in resistant cases, more frequently seen in highly endemic areas such as India. Concomitant systemic steroid therapy is also frequently necessary. The steroid dose needs to be adjusted when given with rifampicin.

FURTHER READING

Biswas J, Madhaven HN, Lingham G, et al. Intraocular tuberculosis, clinicopathologic study of five cases. *Retina* 1995;15:461–468.

Demirci H, Shields CL, Shields JA, et al. Ocular tuberculosis masquerading as ocular tumors. *Surv Ophthalmol* 2004;49:78–89.

Gupta V, Gupta A, Arora S, et al. Presumed tubercular serpiginous-like choroiditis: clinical presentations and management. *Ophthalmology* 2003;110:1744–1749.

Helm CJ, Holland GN. Ocular tuberculosis. *Surv Ophthalmol* 1993;38:229–256.

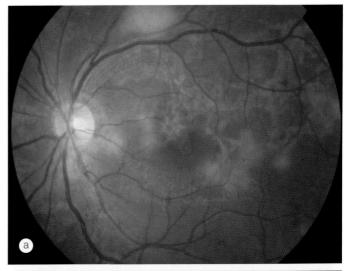

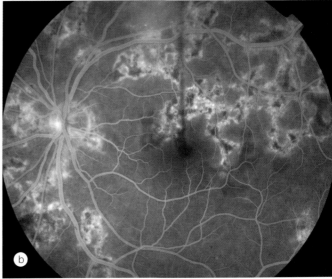

Fig. 6.183 Tuberculous choroiditis resembling serpiginous choriodopathy. (a) Colour image; (b) fluorescein angiography shows extensive hyperfluorescence due to window defects associated with spotty hypofluorescence due to blockage by RPE hyperplasia

Morimura Y, Okada AA, Kawahara S, et al. Tuberculin skin testing in uveitis patients and treatment of presumed intraocular tuberculosis. *Ophthalmology* 2002;109:851–857.

Rosen PH, Spalton DJ, Graham EM. Intraocular tuberculosis. *Eye* 1990;4:486–492.

Sheu SJ, Shyu JS, Chen LM, et al. Ocular manifestations of tuberculosis. *Ophthalmology* 2001;108:1580–1585.

Syphilis

Syphilis is a sexually transmitted disease caused by the spirochaete *Treponema pallidum* (see Ch. 8). Ocular syphilis is uncommon and there are no pathognomonic signs. Eye involvement typically occurs during the secondary and tertiary stages, although occasionally it may be seen during primary syphilis. The disease must therefore be suspected in any case of intraocular inflammation resistant to conventional therapy.

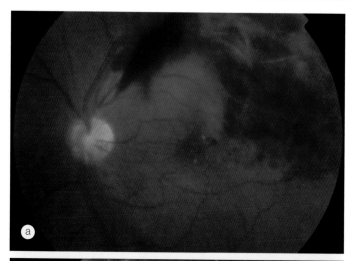

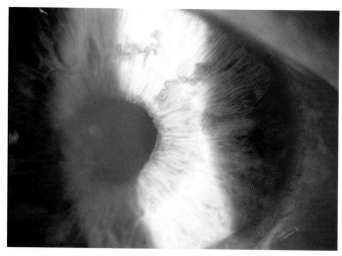

Fig. 6.186 Dilated iris vessels (roseolae) in syphilitic anterior uveitis

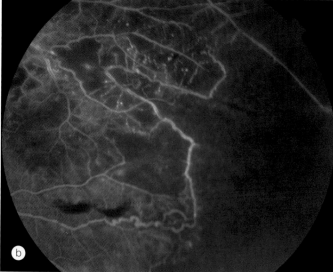

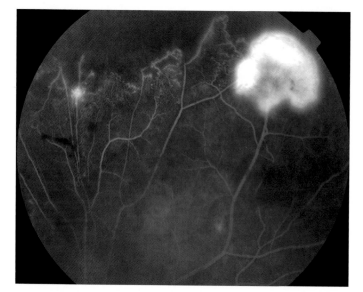

Fig. 6.184 (a) Venous occlusion associated with tuberculous periphlebitis; (b) fluorescein angiography shows extensive hypofluorescence due to capillary non-perfusion

Fig. 6.185 Fluorescein angiography shows extensive capillary non-perfusion and two areas of intense hyperfluorescence due to leakage of dye from retinal neovascularisation in tuberculous occlusive periphlebitis

Anterior uveitis

Iridocyclitis occurs in about 4% of patients with secondary syphilis and is bilateral in 50%. The inflammation is usually acute, and unless appropriately treated, becomes chronic. In some cases, iritis is first associated with dilated iris capillaries (roseolae) (Fig. 6.186) which may develop into more localised papules and subsequently into larger yellowish nodules. Various types of postinflammatory iris atrophy may ensue.

Posterior uveitis

The absence of pathognomonic signs and the ability of syphilis to mimic any ocular and systemic inflammatory disease often leads to misdiagnosis and delay in appropriate treatment.

1. **Chorioretinitis**

- Focal lesions are less common than multifocal and are often located near the disc or macula (Fig. 6.187); bilateral involvement is common.

- Acute posterior placoid chorioretinitis is characterised by bilateral, large, solitary, placoid, pale-yellowish subretinal lesions (Fig. 6.188).

2. **Neuroretinitis** (Fig. 6.189), unless treated, gives rise to secondary optic atrophy and replacement of retinal vessels by white strands.

3. **Periphlebitis** may be associated with central retinal vein occlusion.

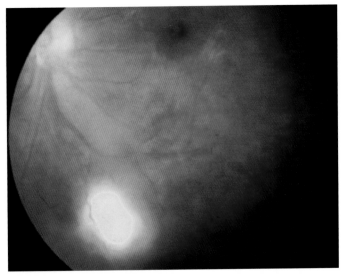

Fig. 6.187 Solitary syphilitic chorioretinitis (Courtesy of C de A Garcia)

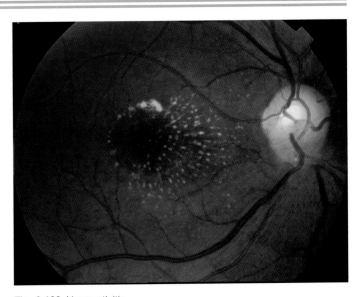

Fig. 6.189 Neuroretinitis

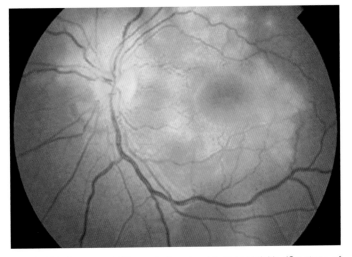

Fig. 6.188 Acute syphilitic posterior placoid chorioretinitis (Courtesy of C de A Garcia)

Syphilis in HIV-positive patients

Syphilis is an uncommon cause of uveitis in HIV-infected patients. Because syphilis may pursue a more aggressive course in HIV patients and respond less well to conventional therapy, it seems reasonable to test all patients with ocular syphilis for HIV and vice versa.

Treatment

Conventional doses of penicillin are inadequate; the therapeutic regimen is the same as for neurosyphilis (which should be ruled out by lumbar puncture). One of the following regimens may be used:

1. **Intravenous aqueous penicillin G** 12–24 mega units (MU) daily for 10–15 days.

2. **Intramuscular procaine benzylpenicillin** 2.4 MU daily, supplemented with oral probenecid (2 g daily), for 10–15 days.

3. **Oral amoxicillin** 3 g b.d. for 28 days.

NB: Penicillin-allergic patients can be treated with oral tetracycline or erythromycin 500 mg q.i.d. for 30 days.

FURTHER READING

Gass JDM, Braunstein RA, Chenoweth RG. Acute syphilitic posterior placoid chorioretinitis. *Ophthalmology* 1990;97:1288–1297.

Levy JH, Liss RA, Maguire AM. Neurosyphilis and ocular syphilis in patients with concurrent human immunodeficiency virus infection. *Retina* 1989;9:175–180.

McCarron MJ, Albert DM. Iridocyclitis and an iris mass associated with secondary syphilis. *Ophthalmology* 1998;91:1264–1268.

Margo CE, Hamed LM. Ocular syphilis. *Surv Ophthalmol* 1992;37:203–220.

Shalaby IA, Dunn JP, Semba RD, et al. Syphilitic uveitis in human immunodeficiency virus-infected patients. *Arch Ophthalmol* 1997;115:469–473.

Tamesis RR, Foster CS. Ocular syphilis. *Ophthalmology* 1990;97:1281–1287.

Lyme disease

Lyme disease (borreliosis) is an infection caused by a flagellated spirochaete, *Borrelia burgdorferi*, transmitted through the bite of a hard-shelled tick of the genus *Ixodes* which feeds on a variety of large mammals, particularly deer (see Ch. 8).

Ocular features

1. **Uveitis** is uncommon and may take the following forms: anterior, intermediate, peripheral multifocal choroiditis, retinal periphlebitis and neuroretinitis.

2. Other manifestations include follicular conjunctivitis, episcleritis, keratitis, scleritis, orbital myositis, optic neuritis, ocular motor nerve palsies and reversible Horner syndrome.

Treatment

1. Uveitis is treated with steroids.

2. Systemic disease

a. Acute disease is treated with oral doxycycline or amoxicillin.

b. Chronic cardiac, joint or neurological disease requires intravenous ceftriaxone 2 g daily for 14–28 days. Prophylaxis with doxycycline should be given within 72 hours of the tick bite.

FURTHER READING

Bergloff J, Gasser R, Feigl B. Ophthalmic manifestations in Lyme borreliosis. *J Neuro-Ophthalmol* 1994;14:15–20.

Breeveld J, Rothova A, Kuiper H. Intermediate uveitis and Lyme borreliosis. *Br J Ophthalmol* 1992;76:181–182.

Carvounis PE, Mehta AP, Geist CE. Orbital myositis associated with Borrelia burgdorferi (Lyme disease) infection. *Ophthalmology* 2004;111:1023–1028.

Flach AJ, Lavoie PE. Episcleritis, conjunctivitis and keratitis as ocular manifestations of Lyme disease. *Ophthalmology* 1990;97:973–975.

Huppertz H-I, Munchmeier D, Lieb W. Ocular manifestations in children and adolescents with Lyme arthritis. *Br J Ophthalmol* 1999;83:1149–1152.

Karma A, Seppala I, Mikkila H, et al. Diagnosis and clinical characteristics of ocular Lyme borreliosis. *Am J Ophthalmol* 1995;119:127–135.

Kornmehl EW, Lesser RL, Jaros P, et al. Bilateral keratitis in Lyme disease. *Ophthalmology* 1989:96:1194–1197.

Krist D, Wenkel H. Posterior scleritis associated with Borrelia burgdorferi (Lyme disease) infection. *Ophthalmology* 2002;109:143–145.

Mikkila HO, Seppala IJT, Viljanen MK, et al. The expanding clinical spectrum of ocular Lyme disease. *Ophthalmology* 2000;107:581–587.

Winterkorn JM. Lyme disease: neurologic and ophthalmic manifestations. *Surv Ophthalmol* 1990;35:191–204.

Zaidman GW. The ocular manifestations of Lyme disease. *Int Ophthalmol Clin* 1997;37:13–28.

Familial juvenile systemic granulomatosis syndrome

Familial juvenile systemic granulomatosis (Blau syndrome, Jabs disease) is a rare autosomal dominant disorder characterised by childhood onset of granulomatous disease of skin, eyes and joints. It is associated with CARD15/Nod2 mutation.

1. Systemic features, which develop in the first decade of life, include painful cystic joint swelling, an intermittent rash, cranial neuropathies and vasculopathy.

2. Ocular manifestations include panuveitis and multifocal choroiditis. Complications include cataract, band keratopathy and CMO.

3. Differential diagnosis includes juvenile idiopathic arthritis and sarcoidosis.

FURTHER READING

Blau EB. Familial granulomatous arthritis, iritis, and rash. *J Pediatrics* 1985;107:689–693.

Jabs DA, Houk JL, Bias WB, et al. Familial granulomatosis, synovitis, uveitis, and cranial neuropathies. *Am J Med* 1985;78:801–804.

Kurokawa T, Kikuchi T, Ohta K, et al. Ocular manifestations in Blau syndrome associated with a CARD15/Nod2 mutation. *Ophthalmology* 2003;110:2040–2044.

Latkany PA, Jabs DA, Smith JR, et al. Multifocal choroiditis in patients with familial juvenile systemic granulomatosis. *Am J Ophthalmol* 2002;134:897–904.

Pastores GM, Michels VV, Stickler GB, et al. Autosomal dominant granulomatous arthritis, uveitis, skin rashes, and synovial cysts. *J Pediatr* 1990;117:403–408.

Brucellosis

Zoonoses are human diseases caused by a pathogen that has an animal reservoir. Brucellosis is a zoonotic disease caused by the Gram-negative bacteria *Brucella melitensis* or *Brucella abortis*. It is transmitted from animals to man through the ingestion of unpasteurised milk products or uncooked meat.

1. Systemic features include fever, arthralgia, myalgia, anorexia, sweating, headache and malaise. The onset of symptoms may be acute or insidious, generally beginning within 2 to 4 weeks after inoculation.

2. Treatment involves tetracycline for 6 weeks and streptomycin for 2 weeks. Doxycycline and rifampicin is an alternative.

3. Ocular involvement usually develops after the acute phase and may be characterised by chronic anterior uveitis, multifocal choroiditis and, rarely, endogenous endophthalmitis. Other manifestations include dacryoadenitis, episcleritis, nummular keratitis and optic neuritis.

FURTHER READING

al-Kaff AS. Ocular brucellosis. *Int Ophthalmol Clin* 1995;35:139–145.

Rabinowitz R, Schneck M, Levy J, et al. Bilateral multifocal choroiditis with serous retinal detachment in a patient with *Brucella* infection: case report and review of the literature. *Arch Ophthalmol* 2005;123:116–118.

Tabbara KF. Brucellosis and nonsyphilitic treponemal uveitis. *Int Ophthalmol Clin* 1990;30:294–296.

Walker J, Sharma OP, Rao NA. Brucellosis and uveitis. *Am J Ophthalmol* 1992;114:374–375.

Primary intraocular lymphoma

Primary intraocular lymphoma (PIOL) is a rare, highly malignant, large B-cell (non-Hodgkin) lymphoma that represents a subset of primary central nervous system lymphoma (PCNSL). It arises from within the brain (Fig. 6.190), spinal cord and leptomeninges, and has a very poor prognosis. Onset is in the sixth and seventh decades with a higher incidence in women. About 20% of patients with PCNSL have ocular disease, and approximately 20–40% of patients with PIOL do

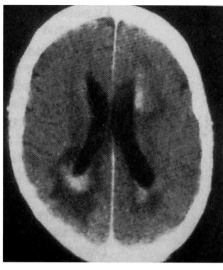

Fig. 6.190 Axial computed tomography showing cerebral lymphoma

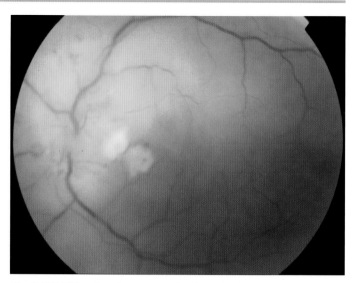

Fig. 6.192 Diffuse lymphomatous retinal infiltration

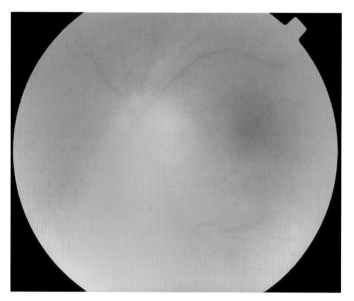

Fig. 6.191 Lymphomatous vitreous involvement (Courtesy of A Singh)

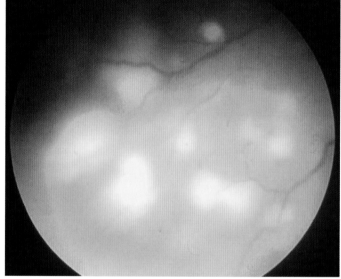

Fig. 6.193 Sub-RPE lymphomatous deposits (Courtesy of D Charteris)

not have CNS involvement at presentation. Although PIOL is not strictly a uveitis, it is included here because it may be mistaken for an inflammatory process. The increased incidence of PIOL and PCNSL over the last two decades is partially attributed to patients with AIDS and iatrogenic immunosuppression.

Ocular features

1. **Presentation** is with unilateral floaters or blurred vision, which frequently becomes bilateral after a variable interval.

2. **Signs**

- Mild anterior chamber reaction.

- Vitritis (Fig. 6.191) is very common and is characterised by the homogenous infiltrate (cells are all of the same small size), without the characteristic clumping seen in inflammatory conditions. On careful biomicroscopy, sheets of cells infiltrating the vitreous can be seen.

- Vasculitis, which angiographically manifests as continuous staining of the vessel wall, as opposed to the typical skipping seen in inflammatory cases (e.g. sarcoidosis).

- Diffuse retinal infiltration (Fig. 6.192) may resemble viral necrotising retinitis.

- Multifocal, large, yellowish, solid sub-RPE infiltrates that progress to involve the choroid, are seen in 60% of cases (Fig. 6.193).

- Occasionally, coalescence of sub-RPE deposits may form a ring encircling the equator (Fig. 6.194).

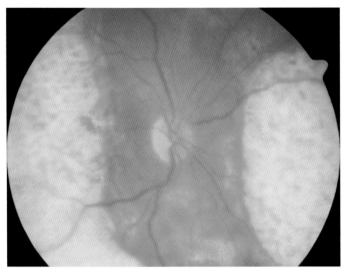

Fig. 6.194 Coalescent sub-RPE lymphoma (Courtesy of B Damato)

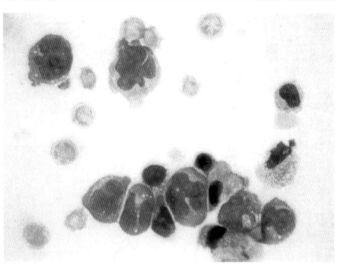

Fig. 6.195 Vitreous biopsy specimen in primary ocular lymphoma showing lymphoma cells with large nuclei (Courtesy of P Smith)

NB: Lack of CMO is an important diagnostic clue, since in true uveitis significant vitritis is almost always accompanied by CMO.

Investigations

1. **FA** shows blockage with a granular characteristic, due to the presence of sub-RPE accumulation of lymphomatous cells ('leopard-skin' spots).

2. **Cytology.** Vitreous biopsy may have to be repeated to obtain a positive sample (Fig. 6.195). Fine-needle biopsy of a subretinal nodule may produce a better yield. Cytological examination gives a 30% false negative result. The inadvertent use of steroids contributes to misdiagnosis of cell identification. Steroids are lymphotoxic and should be discontinued at least 6 weeks before a sample is taken.

3. **Immunohistochemistry** based on cell-surface markers allows identification of monoclonal proliferation of B cells.

4. **Molecular techniques** involving PCR detection of gene rearrangements is useful for B-cell lymphomas and is highly sensitive, but clinical experience is limited.

Treatment

1. **Radiotherapy** to the posterior two-thirds of the globe may be effective in short-term control but may be complicated by radiation retinopathy, optic neuropathy, cataract and glaucoma.

2. **Systemic chemotherapy** with high-dose methotrexate may not only control ocular disease but also increase survival.

3. **Intravitreal** methotrexate with thiotepa or dexamethasone is the treatment of choice for recurrent disease, but recurrences are still likely to occur and close monitoring is needed.

4. **Biologic agents** involving specific anti-B-cell monoclonal antibodies (such as rituximab) may represent an interesting alternative.

FURTHER READING

Akpek EK, Ahmed I, Hochberg FH, et al. Intraocular-central nervous system lymphoma. Clinical features, diagnosis and outcomes. *Ophthalmology* 1999;106:1805–1810.

Chan CC, Buggage RR, Nussenblatt RB. Intraocular lymphoma. *Curr Opin Ophthalmol* 2002;13:411–418.

Davis JL. Diagnosis of intraocular lymphoma. *Ocul Immunol Inflamm* 2004;12:7–16.

Johnston RL, Tufail A, Lightman S, et al. Retinal and choroidal biopsies are helpful in unclear uveitis of suspected infectious or malignant origin. *Ophthalmology* 2004;111:522–528.

Whitcup SM, de Smet MD, Rubin BI, et al. Itraocular lymphoma: clinical and histopathologic diagnosis. *Ophthalmology* 1993;100:1399–1406.

Zaldivar RA, Martin DF, Holden JT, et al. Primary intraocular lymphoma: clinical, cytologic, and flow cytometric analysis. *Ophthalmology* 2004;111:1762–1767.

PRIMARY INFLAMMATORY CHORIOCAPILLAROPATHIES

Acute posterior multifocal placoid pigment epitheliopathy (APMPPE)

APMPPE is an uncommon, idiopathic, usually bilateral condition, which typically affects individuals in the third to sixth decades of life. It affects both sexes equally and is associated with HLA-B7 and HLA-DR2. In about one-third of patients, APMPPE follows a flu-like illness, and occasionally it may be the initial manifestation of a CNS angiitis. APMPPE has been described in association with a variety of systemic conditions, including tuberculosis, anti-hepatitis B vaccination, mumps,

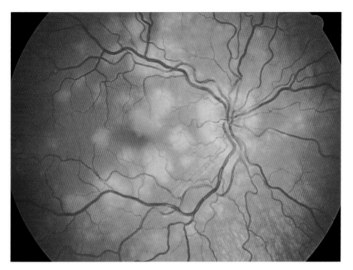

Fig. 6.196 *Active acute posterior multifocal placoid pigment epitheliopathy (Courtesy of C Barry)*

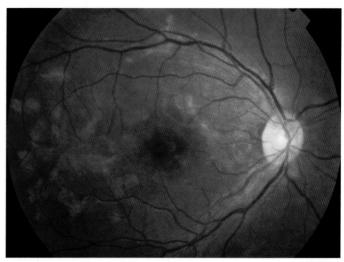

Fig. 6.197 *Resolved acute posterior multifocal placoid pigment epitheliopathy showing mild RPE changes*

Wegener granulomatosis, polyarteritis nodosa, ulcerative colitis, sarcoidosis and Lyme disease.

Diagnosis

1. **Presentation** is with subacute visual impairment associated with central and paracentral scotomas and often photopsia. Within a few days to several weeks, the fellow eye becomes affected.

2. **Signs**

- Multiple, large, cream-coloured or greyish-white placoid lesions at the level of the RPE, which typically begin at the posterior pole and then extend to the post-equatorial fundus (Fig. 6.196).

- After a few days, the lesions begin to fade centrally, but this is not accompanied by immediate improvement of vision.

- Within 2 weeks, the majority of acute lesions are replaced by RPE changes of varying severity (Figs 6.197 and 6.198).

- New lesions may appear, so different stages of evolution may be seen.

- Recurrences are rare.

- Mild vitritis.

- Rare associations include central retinal vein occlusion, retinal vasculitis and papillitis.

3. **FA** of active lesions shows early dense hypofluorescence associated with non-perfusion of the choriocapillaris (Fig. 6.199b) and late hyperfluorescence due to staining (Fig. 6.199c).

4. **ICG** is superior to FA in demonstrating non-perfusion of the choriocapillaris (Fig. 6.200).

5. **EOG** may be subnormal.

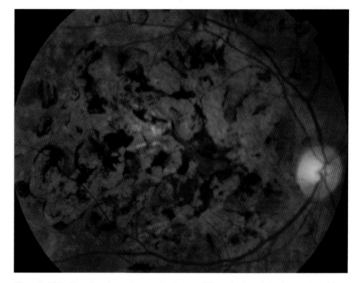

Fig. 6.198 *Resolved acute posterior multifocal placoid pigment epitheliopathy showing unusually severe RPE changes*

Treatment

Systemic steroids do not affect the natural course of APMPPE although they may be required for patients with CNS disease.

Prognosis

In the majority of patients, visual acuity returns to normal, but this may take up to 6 months, and occasionally, disturbing paracentral scotomas may persist.

Differential diagnosis

1. **Early serpiginous choroidopathy** may occasionally be confused with APMPPE but it tends to affect an older age group, runs a recurrent course and has a poor prognosis.

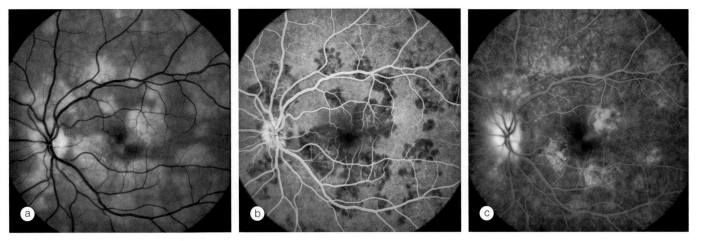

Fig. 6.199 Active acute posterior multifocal placoid pigment epitheliopathy. (a) Red-free image; (b) fluorescein angiography early phase shows dense hypofluorescence; (c) late phase shows hyperfluorescence (Courtesy of P Saine)

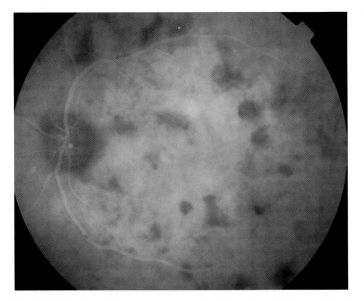

Fig. 6.200 Indocyanine green angiography of acute posterior multifocal placoid pigment epitheliopathy

2. **MEWDS** can also cause acute visual loss in healthy young adults. However, the lesions are smaller, unilateral and at the level of the outer retina and RPE. FA shows early hypofluorescence and late staining of the lesions, which are much more numerous than clinically observed. The ERG is usually abnormal.

3. **Harada disease** is characterised by diffuse choroidal infiltrates during the acute stage and similar residual RPE changes to APMPPE. However, it typically affects specific ethnic groups and is characterised by exudative retinal detachment.

4. **Other causes** of multifocal deep lesions include DUSN, multifocal choroiditis with panuveitis, sarcoidosis, secondary syphilis, sympathetic ophthalmitis and metastatic choroidal infiltrates.

FURTHER READING

Jones NP. Acute posterior multifocal placoid pigment epitheliopathy. *Br J Ophthalmol* 1995;79:384–389.

Kersten DH, Lessell S, Carlow TJ. Acute posterior multifocal placoid epitheliopathy and late-onset meningoencephalitis. *Ophthalmology* 1987;94:393–396.

Laatikainen LT, Immonen IJR. Acute posterior multifocal placoid pigment epitheliopathy in connection with acute nephritis. *Retina* 1988;8:122–124.

Pagliarini S, Piguet B, ffytche TJ, et al. Foveal involvement and lack of visual recovery in APMPPE associated with uncommon features. *Eye* 1995;9:42–47.

Park D, Schatz H, McDonald R, et al. Indocyanine green angiography of acute multifocal posterior placoid pigment epitheliopathy. *Ophthalmology* 1995;102:1877–1883.

Quillen DA, Davis JB, Gottlieb JL, et al. The white dots syndromes. *Am J Ophthalmol* 2004;137:538–550.

Williams DF, Mieler WF. Long-term follow up of acute multifocal placoid pigment epitheliopathy. *Br J Ophthalmol* 1989;73:985–990.

Serpiginous choroidopathy

Serpiginous choroidopathy (SC) is an uncommon, chronic, recurrent disease that is usually bilateral but the extent of involvement is frequently asymmetric. It affects individuals in the fourth to sixth decades of life. It affects men more than women and is associated with HLA-B7. SC has a chronic, recurrent evolution, which is variable between individuals and may remain inactive for months or years.

Diagnosis

1. **Presentation** is with unilateral blurring of central vision, scotoma or metamorphopsia as a result of macular involvement. After a variable period of time, the fellow eye is also affected, although it is not uncommon to find evidence of inactive asymptomatic disease in one eye at presentation.

2. **Signs**

- Active lesions are grey–white to yellow in appearance, located at the level of the RPE or inner choroid (Figs 6.201a and b).

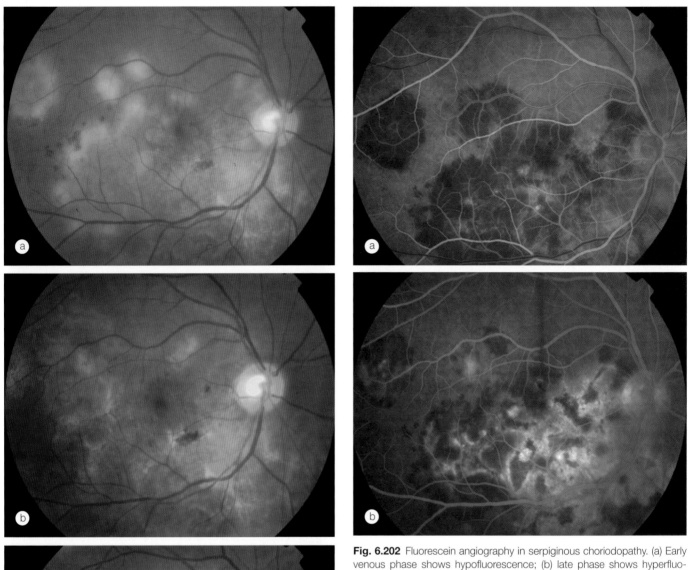

Fig. 6.201 Progression of serpiginous choroidopathy. (a) Active stage; (b) partial resolution of some lesions; (c) inactive stage

Fig. 6.202 Fluorescein angiography in serpiginous choriodopathy. (a) Early venous phase shows hypofluorescence; (b) late phase shows hyperfluorescence

- They develop first around the optic disc and then gradually spread in a serpentine-like manner towards the macula and peripheral fundus. Rarely, the initial lesion involves the macula.

- Inactive lesions are characterised by scalloped, atrophic, 'punched-out' areas of choroidal and RPE atrophy (Fig. 6.201c).

- Mild vitritis is present in up to 50% of eyes and mild anterior uveitis may occur.

3. **FA** of active lesions shows early hypofluorescence due to non-perfusion of the choriocapillaris (Fig. 6.202a) and late hyperfluorescence due to staining (Fig. 6.202b).

4. **ICG** of active lesions reveals marked hypofluorescence throughout all phases of the angiogram. It may also show localised areas of hyperfluorescence outside these areas

which do not correspond to clinically visible changes, which might represent areas of subclinical involvement.

5. ERG may be abnormal in eyes with extensive retinal damage.

Course

The course lasts many years in an episodic and recurrent fashion and disease activity may recur after several months of remission. Recurrences are characterised by yellow–grey extensions, contiguous or as satellites to existing areas of chorioretinal atrophy. Subretinal fibrosis occurs in a minority of cases.

Treatment

- Currently there is no definitive treatment strategy for serpiginous choroidopathy, although long-term immunosuppression appears to prolong remission. Treatment options include triple therapy with systemic steroids, azathioprine and ciclosporin, although early monotherapy with ciclosporin may be adequate. Cyclophosphamide has also been used.

- Loss of vision can be caused by either macular involvement by the disease (Fig. 6.203) or secondary CNV (Fig. 6.204). The latter develops in about 25% of cases and may be amenable to argon laser photocoagulation, photodynamic therapy or intravitreal injection of triamcinolone.

Prognosis

The prognosis is poor and 50–75% of patients will eventually develop visual loss in one or both eyes despite treatment.

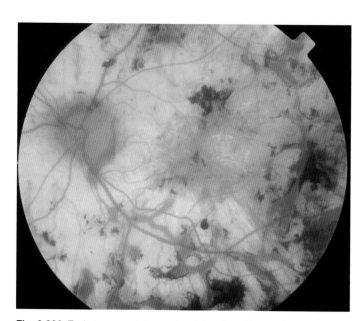

Fig. 6.203 End-stage serpiginous choroidopathy with macular involvement

FURTHER READING

Akpek EK, Jabs DA, Tessler HH, et al. Successful treatment of serpiginous choroiditis with alkylating agents. *Ophthalmology* 2002;109:1506–1513.

Akpek EK, Ilhan-Sarac O. New treatments for serpiginous choroiditis. *Curr Opin Ophthalmol* 2003;14:128–131.

Araujo AAQ, Wells AP, Dick AD, et al. Early treatment with cyclosporin in serpiginous choroidopathy maintains remission and good visual outcome. *Br J Ophthalmol* 2000;84:979–982.

Christmas NJ, Oh KT, Oh DM, et al. Long-term follow-up of patients with serpiginous choroiditis. *Retina* 2002;22:550–556.

Hooper PL, Kaplan HJ. Triple agent immunosuppression in serpiginous choroiditis. *Ophthalmology* 1991;98:944–952.

Mansour AM, Jampol LM, Packo KH, et al. Macular serpiginous choroidopathy. *Retina* 1988;8:125–131

Navajas EV, Costa RA, Farah ME, et al. Indocyanine green-mediated photothrombosis combined with intravitreal triamcinolone for the treatment of choroidal neovascularization in serpiginous choroiditis. *Eye* 2003;17:563–566.

Secchi AG, Tognon MS, Maselli C. Cyclosporine-A in the treatment of serpiginous choroiditis. *Int Ophthalmol* 1990;14:395–399.

Wu JS, Lewis H, Fine SL, et al. Clinicopathologic findings in a patient with serpiginous choroidopathy and treated choroidal neovascularization. *Retina* 1989;9:292–301.

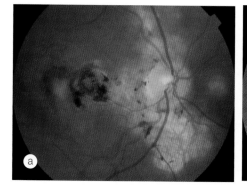
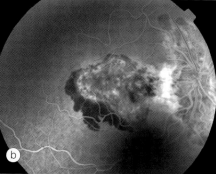
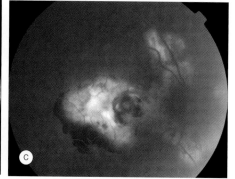

Fig. 6.204 Choroidal neovascularisation in old serpiginous choroidopathy. (a) Colour image shows a disciform scar at the macula associated with blood; (b) fluorescein angiography early venous phase shows spotty hyperfluorescence of the scar and hyperfluorescence corresponding to blood; (c) late phase shows intense hyperfluorescence of the scar and less intense hyperfluorescence of old serpiginous lesions

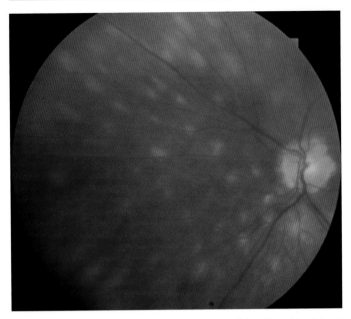

Fig. 6.205 Active birdshot chorioretinopathy involving the midperipheral fundus

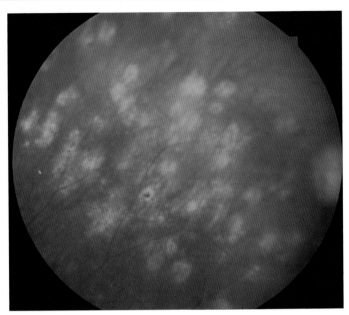

Fig. 6.207 Inactive birdshot lesions

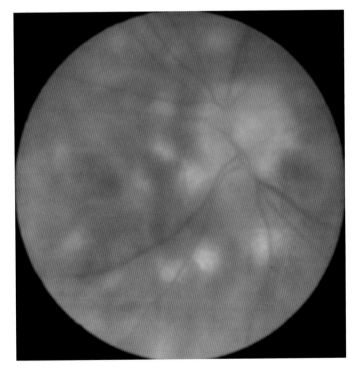

Fig. 6.206 Large active birdshot lesions

Birdshot retinochoroidopathy

Birdshot retinochoroidopathy is an uncommon, idiopathic, chronic, recurrent, bilateral disease which typically affects individuals in the fifth to seventh decades of life, predominantly females. Over 90% of patients are positive for HLA-A29.

Diagnosis

1. **Presentation** is with insidious impairment of central vision associated with photopsia and floaters, or night blindness and impairment of colour vision. The severity of visual disturbance is frequently out of proportion to the measured visual acuity, indicating diffuse retinal dysfunction.

2. **Signs** are usually bilateral but may be asymmetric.

- Moderate vitritis without snowballs or snowbanking.

- Retinal vasculitis involving large and small vessels.

- Multiple, small, ill-defined, cream-coloured choroidal spots with a typical radial distribution, along choroidal vessels (Fig. 6.205).

- One of the following patterns may be seen: (a) involving the macula and midperiphery; (b) with relative macular sparing; and (c) with macular predominance.

- These lesions may not be present at the onset of symptoms and may take several years to appear. CMO and vitreous cells may be the only signs detected at this early stage of the disease.

- Over several years, new spots may appear and old lesions may enlarge (Fig. 6.206).

- Inactive lesions consist of well-delineated, atrophic spots, which show no tendency to become hyperpigmented (Fig. 6.207).

3. **FA** shows early hypofluorescence and late mild hyperfluorescence. The disc may show hyperfluorescence due to

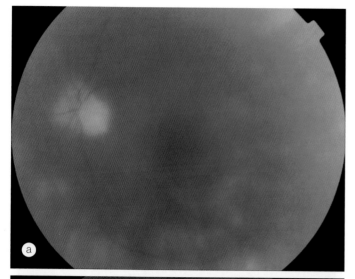

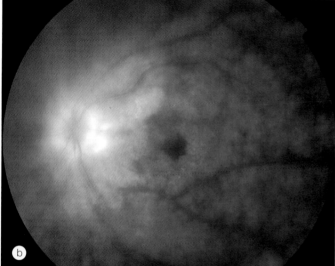

Fig. 6.208 (a) Active birdshot retinochoroidopathy; (b) late-phase fluorescein angiography shows disc hyperfluorescence and cystoid macular oedema

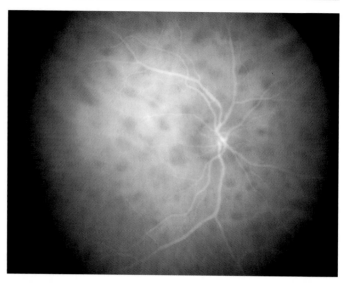

Fig. 6.209 Early-phase indocyanine green angiography in birdshot retinochoroidopathy, showing numerous hypofluorescent lesions (Courtesy of P Gili)

Treatment

- Until recently, the decision to start treatment was based on the level of visual acuity, but it is now apparent that ERG findings are much more important, because ERG abnormalities can be reversed by early treatment (i.e. before reduction of visual acuity).

- Although good response may be achieved with systemic steroids, maintenance of good retinal function with this therapy alone needs further observation.

- Optimal treatment may involve a steroid-sparing agent such as azathioprine or mycophenolate mofetil. Discontinuation of therapy should not be attempted while ERG abnormalities are still present, as this will lead to deterioration. The minimal period of stability necessary to allow tapering and discontinuation of treatment is unknown.

- Periocular steroids are useful for treatment of CMO but do not seem to offer the same level of benefit for global retinal function, and further deterioration is likely to occur.

Prognosis

The prognosis is guarded. About 20% of patients have a self-limited course and maintain normal visual acuity at least in one eye. The remainder have variable impairment of visual acuity in one or both eyes, with approximately 40% reaching levels of 6/60 after 10 years of follow-up. This usually happens as a result of one or more of the following:

1. **Macular involvement** by CMO, pucker, serous detachment or, rarely, CNV.

2. **Progressive retinal degeneration** leading to arteriolar narrowing, optic atrophy and night blindness (Fig. 6.210).

leakage, and CMO may be present (Fig. 6.208b). Fewer lesions are seen on FA than clinically, because they disappear after the choroidal flush and only become apparent when the RPE is involved.

4. **ICG** reveals well-defined hypofluorescent spots in the early phases (Fig. 6.209), becoming hyperfluorescent later. Many more spots can be seen by ICG than either clinically or on FA.

5. **ERG** is normal in early disease, but with time, the b-wave amplitude and then oscillatory potentials become decreased. A delay in implicit time of the 30 Hz flicker ERG is the most sensitive change. ERG findings seem to reflect intraretinal oedema and for this reason correlate well with the severity of retinal vasculopathy rather than choroidal involvement.

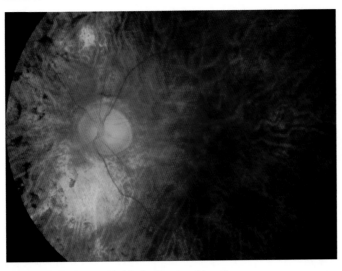

Fig. 6.210 End-stage birdshot retinochoroidopathy

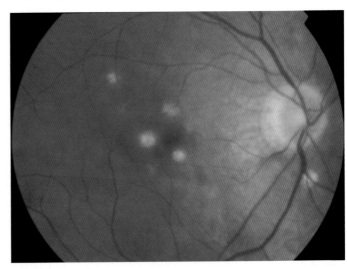

Fig. 6.211 Active punctate inner choroidopathy

NB: The introduction of early therapy based on ERG findings may significantly impact on the prognosis of this condition.

Punctate inner choroidopathy (PIC)

PIC is an uncommon, idiopathic disease which typically affects young myopic women. Both eyes are frequently involved but not simultaneously.

Diagnosis

1. **Presentation** is with blurring of central vision or paracentral scotomas which may be associated with photopsia.

2. **Signs**

- Absent or minimal intraocular inflammation.

- Multiple, small, yellow–white spots with fuzzy borders at the level of the inner choroid and retina. The lesions are all of the same age and principally involve the posterior pole (Fig. 6.211).

- Plentiful lesions occasionally may be associated with an overlying serous sensory retinal detachment which often resolves spontaneously.

- Large visual field defects, probably caused by acute damage to retinal receptors.

- After a few weeks, the acute lesions resolve, leaving sharply demarcated atrophic scars that may subsequently become pigmented (Fig. 6.212).

- CNV (type 2 – under the sensory retina) develops in up to 40% of patients.

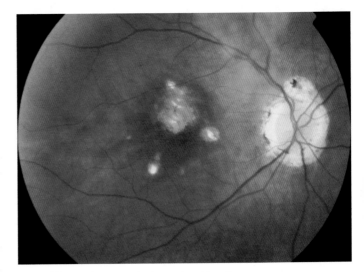

Fig. 6.212 Inactive punctate inner choroidopathy

- After a variable period of time, the fellow eye frequently becomes similarly involved.

3. **FA** of PIC lesions shows early hyperfluorescence and late staining. FA is of particular value in detecting CNV because it may be amenable to treatment (Fig. 6.213).

4. **ERG** is normal.

Treatment of CNV

There is no medical treatment for PIC and treatment is reserved for CNV. The following options may be considered:

1. **Argon laser photocoagulation**, usually under steroid cover, for extrafoveal CNV, particularly if there is evidence of progression towards the fovea.

2. **Systemic steroids** may be used for subfoveal CNV in order to reduce subretinal vascular leakage, but the

Fig. 6.213 Choroidal neovascularisation (CNV) in punctate inner choroidopathy. (a) Colour image; (b) fluorescein angiography arterial phase shows several hyperfluorescent spots associated with hypofluorescent edges, and mild lacy hyperfluorescence at the fovea, indicative of CNV; (c) venous phase shows increasing foveal hyperfluorescence; (d) late phase shows increase in size and intensity of foveal hyperfluorescence due to leakage from CNV (Courtesy of M Westcott)

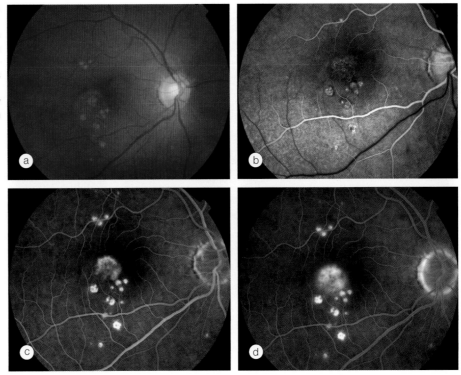

response to steroids is unpredictable for CNV larger than 200 μm in diameter.

3. **Photodynamic therapy**, also under steroid cover, may be considered in cases that have failed to respond to oral steroids.

4. **Surgical excision** of subfoveal CNV may be appropriate in selected cases, taking into account the timing of surgery and location of the membrane. Surgery is usually not indicated for CNV of less than 3 months' duration, especially in the presence of good visual acuity, since spontaneous resolution may occur. However, if treatment is delayed too long, fibrosis will develop and surgery will not be beneficial. Unfortunately, recurrences are common, restricting long-term visual outcome.

Prognosis

The prognosis is guarded because central vision may become compromised by either foveal involvement by a lesion or CNV, which usually occurs within the first year of presentation. Subfoveal CNV may undergo spontaneous involution, with or without recovery of central vision. Small, well-defined subfoveal areas of CNV carry a reasonable prognosis and many patients retain a visual acuity of 6/18 or better.

Differential diagnosis

1. **Multifocal choroiditis and panuveitis** is characterised by similar lesions when they affect the posterior pole, and, in contrast to PIC, is associated with intraocular inflammation and involvement of the peripheral fundus.

2. **Ocular histoplasmosis** is characterised by 'punched-out' chorioretinal scars, CNV and absence of intraocular inflammation. However, there is also peripapillary atrophy as well as linear peripheral streaks and peripheral lesions.

3. **Myopic maculopathy** may have similar macular changes, CNV and absence of intraocular inflammation. However, the severity of myopic changes may be greater with the presence of more extensive degenerative changes. Axial length of the eye and refraction will establish the diagnosis.

Multifocal choroiditis with panuveitis (MCP)

MCP is an uncommon, usually bilateral, chronic, recurrent, frequently asymmetric disease. It typically affects individuals in the third and fourth decades of life, predominantly myopic females.

Diagnosis

1. **Presentation** is usually with blurring of central vision, which may be associated with floaters and photopsia.

2. **Signs**

- Vitritis of variable intensity is universal and anterior uveitis is present in 50% of cases.

- Bilateral, multiple, discrete, round or ovoid, yellowish-grey lesions located at the level of the RPE and choriocapillaris.

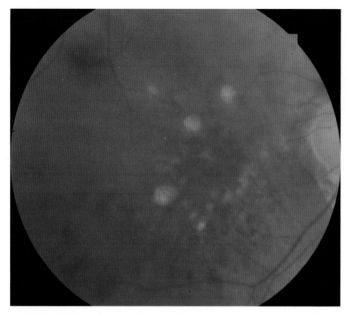

Fig. 6.214 Multifocal choroiditis involving the posterior pole in which small lesions form a linear streak (Schlagel line)

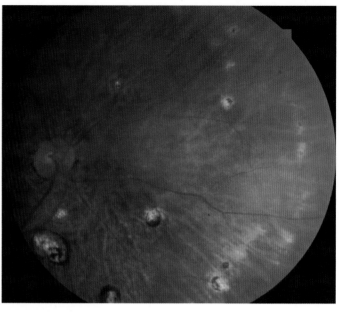

Fig. 6.215 Old pigmented peripheral lesions in multifocal choroiditis

- The lesions involve the posterior pole and/or periphery and may be arranged in clumps or linear streaks (Schlagel lines) (Fig. 6.214).

- Occasionally, in older patients, the lesions are confined to the periphery.

- Peripapillary atrophy may be present.

- Mild disc oedema and blind spot enlargement may be present.

- CMO affects more than 40% of patients with prolonged disease.

- Inactive lesions have sharp 'punched-out' margins and pigmented borders resembling POHS (Fig. 6.215).

- The course may last many months, with the development of new lesions and recurrent inflammatory episodes.

- Subretinal fibrosis develops in a minority.

3. **FA** of active lesions shows early hypofluorescence due to blockage and late hyperfluorescence due to staining. Old inactive lesions show RPE window defects.

4. **ICG** shows hypofluorescent acute lesions which may not be clinically apparent. Old lesions remain hypofluorescent throughout and correspond to atrophic chorioretinal scars seen on fundus examination.

5. **ERG** remains normal until there is advanced retinal atrophy and substantial midperipheral field loss, at which time visual loss may be irreversible. Multifocal ERG shows moderate to severe depression of retinal function.

6. **Large visual field defects** may appear acutely and are not explained on the basis of fundus abnormalities.

Treatment

Systemic and periocular steroids are effective when administered early and prior to the development of CNV or sub-retinal fibrosis. Steroid-resistant patients require immunosuppressive therapy. Eyes with CNV may require argon laser photocoagulation or photodynamic therapy, preferably under steroid cover.

Prognosis

The prognosis is variable because the disease has a wide spectrum, varying between patients with few lesions and short periods of activity to those with progressive scarring and visual loss due to one or more of the following:

- Direct involvement of the fovea, although some patients may have an apparently normal fovea and yet have very poor visual acuity.

- CNV, which develops in up to 50% of cases from an old scar.

- CMO.

- Diffuse subretinal fibrosis.

Differential diagnosis

1. **Sarcoidosis** may also present as multifocal choroiditis and panuveitis. However, the lesions are usually more numerous in the inferior fundus and CNV is less common.

2. **PIC** is also characterised by multifocal choroidal lesions affecting the posterior pole and CNV. However, there is absence of intraocular inflammation.

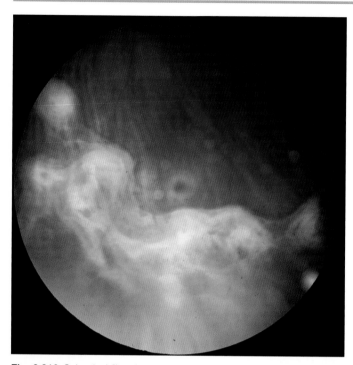

Fig. 6.216 Subretinal fibrosis

Progressive subretinal fibrosis and uveitis syndrome

Progressive subretinal fibrosis and uveitis syndrome is a rare, idiopathic, chronic, bilateral condition which typically affects healthy young women who are frequently myopic. It belongs to the same group of conditions as MCP and PIC, which are characterised by multifocal lesions of the RPE and choroid.

Diagnosis

1. **Presentation** is with gradual unilateral blurring of vision, although both eyes are usually eventually involved.

2. **Signs**

* Mild anterior uveitis and vitritis.

* Yellow, indistinct subretinal lesions which coalesce into dirty-yellow mounds at the posterior pole and midperiphery.

* Eventually, large areas of subretinal fibrosis develop (Fig. 6.216).

3. **FA** reveals normal retinal and choroidal filling, early mottled hyperfluorescence and window defects with late hyperfluorescence along the edges of the lesions.

4. **ERG** may be decreased.

Treatment

Non-steroidal immunosuppressive agents may be beneficial. Systemic steroids are usually not effective once the fibrotic process is established but may be useful in the treatment of recurrences, CNV and CMO.

Prognosis

The course is prolonged and recurrences common, with poor visual prognosis.

Differential diagnosis

Early stages may mimic other entities belonging to this group. The late stage of the subretinal fibrosis and uveitis syndrome has similar appearance to serpiginous choroidopathy and disciform age-related macular degeneration.

Multiple evanescent white dot syndrome (MEWDS)

MEWDS is an uncommon, idiopathic, usually unilateral, self-limiting disease which typically affects individuals between the ages of 20 to 40 years, particularly females. About one-third of patients have a preceding viral-like illness. MEWDS may form part of a spectrum of disease that includes acute idiopathic blind spot enlargement, acute zonal occult retinopathy and acute macular neuroretinopathy.

NB: Although uncommon, it is important to be aware of MEWDS because the subtle signs may be overlooked and a misdiagnosis made of a more serious disorder such as retrobulbar neuritis.

Diagnosis

1. **Presentation** is with sudden-onset decreased vision or paracentral scotomas which may be associated with photopsia, typically affecting the temporal visual field.

2. **Signs**

* Mild afferent pupillary defect.

* Mild vitritis.

* Numerous, very small, ill-defined white dots at the level of the outer retina and inner choroid, involving the posterior pole and midperiphery (Fig. 6.217).

* The macula is spared but has a granular appearance which renders the foveal reflex abnormal or absent.

* Optic disc oedema and enlargement of the physiological blind spot.

* Over several weeks to months, the dots and disc oedema fade and central vision returns to normal or near-normal levels. However, the foveal granularity may remain (Fig.

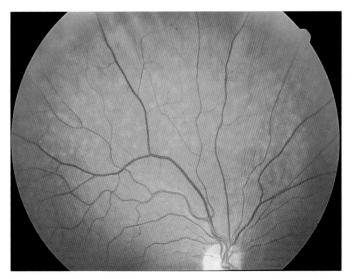

Fig. 6.217 Active multiple evanescent white dot syndrome (Courtesy of C Barry)

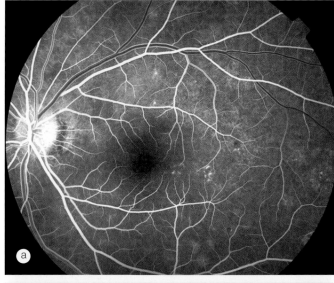

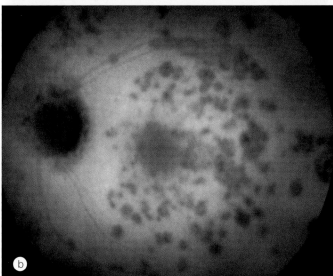

Fig. 6.219 Multiple evanescent white dot syndrome. (a) Fluorescein angiography (FA) early venous phase shows hyperfluorescent spots; (b) indocyanine green angiography shows hypofluorescent spots which are more numerous than on FA

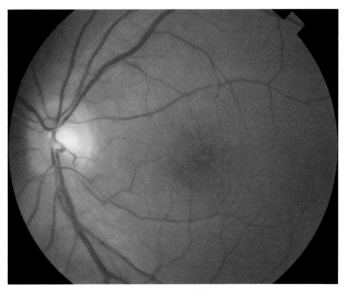

Fig. 6.218 Residual foveal granularity following resolution of multiple evanescent white dot syndrome

6.218) and blind spot enlargement may take much longer to diminish in size.

3. **FA** of active lesions shows early punctate hyperfluorescence expressed as a cluster or 'wreath-shaped' pattern (Fig. 6.219a) and late staining of these lesions and sometimes also of the optic nerve head.

4. **ICG** shows more numerous hypofluorescent spots than are apparent clinically or on FA (Fig. 6.219b). Peripapillary non-perfusion, as demonstrated by fluorescein and ICG angiography, explains the enlarged blind spot.

5. **ERG** shows a decrease in a-wave amplitude which returns to a normal pattern within a few weeks.

Prognosis

The prognosis is excellent and treatment is not appropriate. The course is short, with resolution of visual symptoms over several weeks, although occasionally photopsia may persist. Relapses occur in about 10% of cases and a very small minority of eyes develops chorioretinal scarring or CNV.

Acute idiopathic blind spot enlargement syndrome (AIBSE)

AIBSE is a rare condition which seems to exclusively affect women between the third and sixth decades of life. It shares common features with MEWDS and perhaps represents a different form of the same disease. It was first described as a neuro-ophthalmological condition in young patients, with enlarged blind spots and photopsia. However, further studies suggested a retinal origin for the enlarged blind spots.

Diagnosis

1. **Presentation** between the third and sixth decades of life with photopsia and decreased vision, which may be misdiagnosed as migraine or optic neuritis. Occasionally, photopsia may precede visual loss by several weeks.

2. **Signs**

* Visual acuity may be normal or reduced.

* Afferent pupillary defect may be present.

* Blind spot enlargement with steep margins but variable size is universal, showing a clustering of lesions around the optic nerve.

* Mild disc swelling or hyperaemia with peripapillary subretinal pigmentary changes in 50% of cases.

3. **FA** may show late staining of the optic nerve head.

Prognosis

Visual acuity improves spontaneously but blind spot enlargement may persist. Recurrence may occur in the same or fellow eye.

Differential diagnosis

Patients with multifocal choroiditis, MEWDS and acute macular neuroretinopathy may present with enlarged blind spots.

FURTHER READING

Barile GR, Reppucci VS, Schiff WM, et al. Circumpapillary chorioretinopathy in multiple evanescent white dot syndrome. *Retina* 1997;17:75–77.

Borruat FX, Auer CA, Piguet B. Choroidopathy in multiple evanescent white dot syndrome. *Arch Ophthalmol* 1995;113:1569–1570.

Brown J, Folk JC, Reddy CV, et al. Visual prognosis of multifocal choroiditis, punctate inner choroidopathy, and diffuse subretinal fibrosis syndrome. *Ophthalmology* 1996;103:1100–1105.

Brueggeman RM, Noffke AS, Jampol LM. Resolution of punctate inner choroidopathy lesions with oral prednisone therapy. *Arch Ophthalmol* 2002;120:996.

Bryant RG, Freund KB, Yannuzzi LA, et al. Multiple evanescent white dot syndrome in patients with multifocal choroiditis. *Retina* 2002;22:317–322.

Chatterjee S, Gibson JM. Photodynamic therapy: a treatment option in choroidal neovascularization secondary to punctuate inner choroidopathy. *Br J Ophthalmol* 2003;87:925–927.

Dunlop AAS, Cree IA, Hague S, et al. Multifocal choroiditis. Clinicopathologic correlation. *Arch Ophthalmol* 1998;116:801–803.

Gasch AT, Smith J, Whitcup SM. Birdshot retinochoroidopathy. *Br J Ophthalmol* 1999;83:241–249.

Gass JD. Overlap among acute idiopathic blind spot enlargement syndrome and other conditions. *Arch Ophthalmol* 2001;119:1729–1731.

Gaudio PA, Kaye DB, Crawford JB. Histopathology of birdshot retinochoroidopathy. *Br J Ophthalmol* 2002;86:1439–1441.

Jampol LM. MEWDS, MFC, PIC, AMN, AIBSE, and AZOOR: one disease or many? *Retina* 1995;15:373–378.

Lardenoye CWTA, Van der Lelij A, de Loos WS, et al. Peripheral multifocal choroiditis. A distinct clinical entity? *Ophthalmology* 1997;104:1820–1826.

Leslie T, Lois N, Christopoulou D, et al. Photodynamic therapy for inflammatory choroidal neovascularization unresponsive to immunosuppression. *Br J Ophthalmol* 2005;89:147–150.

Levinson RD, Rajalingam R, Park MS, et al. Human leukocyte antigen A29 subtypes associated with birdshot retinochoroidopathy. *Am J Ophthalmol* 2004;138:631–634.

Oh KT, Christmas NJ, Folk JC. Birdshot retinochoroiditis: long term follow-up of a chronically progressive disease. *Am J Ophthalmol* 2002;133:622–629.

Parnell J, Jampol LM, Yannuzzi LA, et al. Differentiation between presumed ocular histoplasmosis syndrome and multifocal choroiditis with panuveitis based on morphology of photographic fundus lesions and fluorescein angiography. *Arch Ophthalmol* 2002;119:208–212.

Reddy CV, Brown J Jr, Folk JC, et al. Enlarged blind spots in chorioretinal inflammatory disorders. *Ophthalmology* 1996;103:606–617.

Rothova A, Berendschot TT, Probst K, et al. Birdshot chorioretinopathy: long-term manifestations and visual prognosis. *Ophthalmology* 2004;111:954–959.

Ryan SJ, Maumenee AE. Birdshot retinochoroidopathy. *Am J Ophthalmol* 1980;89:31–45.

Spaide RF, Freund KB, Slakter J, et al. Treatment of subfoveal choroidal neovascularization associated with multifocal choroiditis and panuveitis. *Retina* 2002;22:545–549.

Volpe NJ, Rizzo JF III, Lessell S. Acute idiopathic blind spot enlargement syndrome. A review of 27 new cases. *Arch Ophthalmol* 2001;119:59–63.

Watzke RC, Shults WT. Clinical features and natural history of the acute idiopathic enlarged blind spot syndrome. *Ophthalmology* 2002;109:1326–1335.

TREATMENT OF COMPLICATIONS

Cataract

Cataract is a potential complication in every form of uveitis, the incidence depending on the type, duration, pattern and activity of intraocular inflammation. Prolonged breakdown of the blood–aqueous or blood–vitreous barrier, especially in chronic disease, combined with the use of corticosteroids, topically or systemically, represent the main risk factors.

Signs

Initially the opacity is central and posterior subcapsular (Fig. 6.220). If the intraocular inflammation continues, the opacity may progress (Fig. 6.221) and eventually become mature (Fig. 6.222). A very small pupil due to posterior synechiae may make surgery and assessment of the posterior segment difficult (Fig. 6.223).

Preoperative considerations

1. **Indications for surgery**

* Poor visual acuity.

* Difficulty in monitoring posterior segment disease.

* Lens-induced uveitis.

2. **Preoperative management**

* Identification of potential limitations for surgical success, such as band keratopathy, glaucoma and CMO.

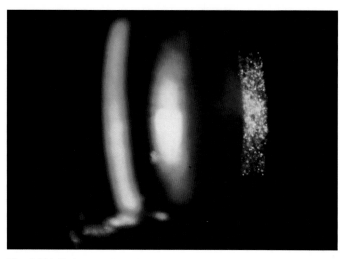

Fig. 6.220 Early posterior subcapsular cataract

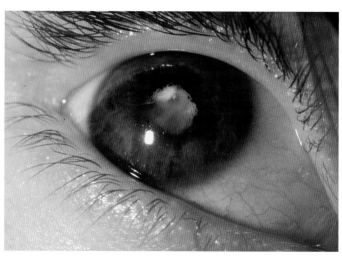

Fig. 6.222 Advanced cataract in a child with chronic anterior uveitis

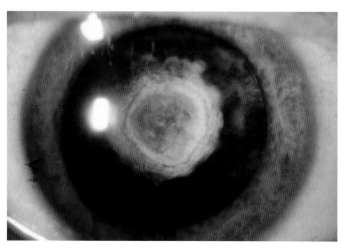

Fig. 6.221 Advanced posterior subcapsular cataract

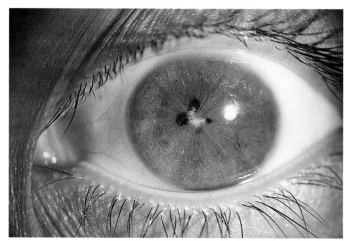

Fig. 6.223 Severe miosis due to posterior synechiae

- Ultrasonography in eyes with dense cataracts, to identify major posterior segment pathology such as retinal detachment.

- Control of the disease activity prior to surgery is crucial to minimise complications. Ideally, anterior chamber activity should be absent or minimal (+1 cells or less) for 3 months prior to surgery.

- CMO should be treated because cataract surgery may make it worse.

- Elevated IOP should be controlled medically. Combined glaucoma and cataract operation is more likely to result in failure of the filtering procedure, and it is advisable to perform glaucoma surgery first and operate on the cataract 6 months later (see below).

3. Steroid regimen

- In quiet eyes, topical steroids (prednisolone acetate 1% or dexamethasone sodium 0.1%) are used six times a day, starting 1 week before surgery. This may be combined with a topical NSAID q.i.d.

- Patients with significant posterior synechiae, previous history of CMO or on systemic therapy to control uveitis, require systemic steroid cover in addition to the topical therapy mentioned above. Prednisolone 0.5 mg/kg is started 3 days before surgery; another regimen starting the steroids 2 weeks preoperatively is also commonly used.

- Patients already receiving systemic steroids should have their dose increased.

- If systemic steroids are contraindicated, options include periocular steroid injection 2 weeks before surgery, another systemic anti-inflammatory agent (e.g. ciclosporin, tacrolimus or an antimetabolite), or intravit-

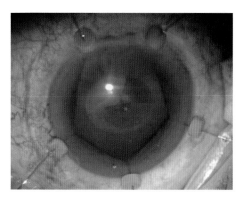

Fig. 6.224 Dilating hooks can be used in eyes with small pupils

real injection of triamcinolone acetonide (4 mg in 0.1ml) at the end of the operation. There is no evidence regarding the efficacy of these strategies.

Surgery

1. Techniques

- Extracapsular cataract extraction has been largely abandoned in favour of phacoemulsification.

- Pars plana vitreo-lensectomy is indicated for children with chronic anterior uveitis which may be associated with JIA, although phacoemulsification with or without primary posterior capsulorhexis and anterior vitrectomy may also be used.

2. Management of a small pupil

- Injection of a viscoelastic substance between the iris and lens may be sufficient to break mild posterior synechiae.

- Blunt dissection is often required to break the tough synechiae.

- Pupillary membranes should be stripped from the pupillary margin using forceps or excised with Vannas scissors.

- Other methods of dealing with small pupils include sphincterotomies, iridotomy, dilating rings or hooks (Fig. 6.224).

3. Capsulorhexis

- Ideally, the capsulorhexis should cover the entire optic of the intraocular lens (IOL), about 5 mm in diameter.

- A larger rhexis, extending beyond the IOL edge, may lead to posterior capsule opacification.

- An undersized rhexis may result in contraction of the anterior capsule (capsulophimosis) which may facilitate the development of synechiae between the pupillary margin and the capsule. A small rhexis can always be enlarged at the end of the procedure with scissors and forceps.

4. IOL implantation

- Posterior chamber IOLs are used in most cases, with the exception of children with chronic anterior uveitis. This is because the IOL with an intact posterior capsule may act as a 'scaffold' for cyclitic membrane formation and result in ciliary body detachment and hypotony.

- Other complications of implantation include exacerbation of uveitis, posterior synechiae and pupillary membrane formation.

- IOL should be placed within the posterior chamber, preferably inside the capsular bag, since sulcus fixation may cause an increase in aqueous flare, probably due to rubbing between the iris and the IOL optic, and may result in inflammation and CMO.

5. Type of IOL

- The design of the IOL, with sharp edges, is a key factor in the prevention of posterior capsule opacification.

- IOL biocompatibility is inversely related to inflammation.

- Hydrophilic acrylic material has good uveal but worse capsular biocompatibility.

- Hydrophobic acrylic material has lower uveal but better capsular biocompatibility.

6. Specific operative complications

- Zonular dehiscence may be more common than in age-related cataract, due to a possible weakening of zonules by longstanding inflammation.

- Intraoperative filiform haemorrhages occur in patients with Fuchs uveitis syndrome (Amsler sign).

- Intraoperative bleeding may be induced by procedures used to enlarge a small pupil.

Postoperative considerations

1. Steroids

- Topical steroids are used hourly for at least 1 week and then tapered.

- Systemic steroid dose is not changed for 1 week and then tapered by 5 mg/week until reaching baseline levels.

- A flare meter is a sensitive way of monitoring postoperative recovery.

2. Complications

- Severe postoperative inflammation with or without fibrinous reaction may occur despite appropriate steroid cover. Intracameral injection of recombinant tissue plasminogen activator (rTPA) (12.5 mg in 0.05 ml) should be considered in eyes with a very severe fibrinous reaction.

- Transient hypotony may occur as a result of diminished aqueous secretion associated with inflammation of the secretory ciliary epithelium. Treatment involves aggressive anti-inflammatory therapy and cycloplegia.

- Prolonged hypotony and phthisis may be associated with cyclitic membrane formation and ciliary body traction or detachment. Surgical excision of the membranes must be considered and removal of an IOL may eventually be necessary.

- Removal of an IOL may also be required in eyes with severe treatment-resistant uveitis.

- Elevated IOP is often transient and innocuous and is caused by the viscoelastic substance used during surgery. Occasionally, cataract surgery may provoke the onset of glaucoma or worsen the course of pre-existing glaucoma.

- Posterior capsular opacification is common, particularly in young patients. YAG-laser capsulotomy should be delayed for 4–6 months. Ideally, the eye should be quiet at the time of capsulotomy and topical steroids should be used after the intervention.

- Synechiae between the iris and anterior capsule may develop when the rhexis is too small.

- Pre-existing CMO may be aggravated by surgery, or CMO may develop for the first time.

- Macular epiretinal membrane formation is relatively common.

FURTHER READING

Dana MR, Chatzistefanou K, Schaumberg DA, et al. Posterior capsule opacification after cataract surgery in patients with uveitis. *Ophthalmology* 1997;104:1387–1393.

Estafanous MF, Lowder CY, Meisler DM, et al. Phacoemulsification cataract extraction and posterior chamber lens implantation in patients with uveitis. *Am J Ophthalmol* 2001;131:620–625.

Flynn HW Jr, Davis JL, Culbertson WW. Pars plana lensectomy and vitrectomy for complicated cataracts in juvenile rheumatoid arthritis. *Ophthalmology* 1998;95:1114–1119.

Fox JGM, Flynn HW, Davis JL Jr. Causes of reduced visual acuity on long-term follow-up after cataract extraction in patients with uveitis and juvenile rheumatoid arthritis. *Am J Ophthalmol* 1992;114:708–714.

Holland GN. Intraocular lens implantation in patients with juvenile rheumatoid arthritis-associated uveitis: an unresolved management issue. *Am J Ophthalmol* 1996;122:255–257.

Holland GN, Van Horn SD, Margolis TP. Cataract surgery with ciliary sulcus fixation of intraocular lenses in patients with uveitis. *Am J Ophthalmol* 1999;128:21–30.

Hooper PL, Rao NA, Smith RE. Cataract extraction in uveitis patients. *Surv Ophthalmol* 1990;35:120–144.

Kanski JJ. Lensectomy for complicated cataract in juvenile chronic iridocyclitis. *Br J Ophthalmol* 1992;76:72–75.

Lam LA, Lowder CY, Baerveldt G, et al. Surgical management of cataracts in children with juvenile rheumatoid arthritis-associated uveitis. *Am J Ophthalmol* 2003;135:772–778.

Meacock WR, Spalton DJ, Bender L, et al. Steroid prophylaxis in eyes with uveitis undergoing surgery. *Br J Ophthalmol* 2004;88:1122–1124.

Meier FM, Tuft SJ, Pavesio CE. Cataract surgery in uveitis. *Ophthalmol Clin North Am* 2002;15:365–373.

Okhravi N, Lightman S, Towler HMA. Assessment of visual outcome after cataract surgery in patients with uveitis. *Ophthalmology* 1999;106:710–722.

Rahman I, Jones NP. Long-term results of cataract extraction with intraocular lens implantation in patients with uveitis. *Eye* 2005;19:191–197.

Rauz S, Stavrou P, Murray PI. Evaluation of foldable intraocular lenses in patients with uveitis. *Ophthalmology* 2000;107:909–919.

Schauersberger J, Kruger A, Abela C, et al. Course of postoperative inflammation after implantation of 4 types of foldable intraocular lenses. *J Cataract Refract Surg* 1999;25:1116–1120.

Suresh PS, Jones NP. Phacoemulsification with intraocular lens implantation in patients with uveitis. *Eye* 2001;15:621–628.

Glaucoma

Elevation of IOP secondary to intraocular inflammation frequently presents a diagnostic and therapeutic challenge. The elevation of IOP may be transient and innocuous, or persistent and severely damaging. The prevalence of secondary glaucoma increases with chronicity and severity of disease. Secondary glaucoma is particularly common in Fuchs uveitis syndrome and chronic anterior uveitis associated with JIA. Posterior uveitis is less likely to affect the aqueous outflow pathway and consequently less likely to lead to IOP elevation. In eyes with chronic uveitis, trabecular meshwork function is reduced by chronic inflammation and steroid therapy.

Diagnostic problems

1. **Fluctuation of IOP** may be dramatic in uveitic glaucoma and phasing may be helpful in patients with borderline IOP.

2. **Ciliary body shutdown** caused by acute exacerbation of chronic anterior uveitis is frequently associated with lowering of IOP that may mask the underlying tendency to glaucoma.

- Even eyes with considerably elevated IOP (30–35 mmHg) may become hypotonous during acute exacerbations of uveitis.

- Return of ciliary body function with subsidence of uveitis may be associated with a rise in IOP in the presence of permanently compromised outflow facility. It is therefore important to continue monitoring the IOP as the inflammation resolves.

3. **The pathogenesis** of elevation of IOP may be uncertain; multiple mechanisms may be involved. Steroid responders often represent a therapeutic challenge.

4. **Assessment of glaucomatous damage** may be hampered by a miotic pupil or opacities in the media. Poor visual acuity may also compromise accurate perimetry.

Angle-closure glaucoma

ANGLE CLOSURE WITH PUPIL BLOCK

1. Pathogenesis

- Secondary angle closure is caused by posterior synechiae extending for 360° (seclusio pupillae) which obstruct aqueous flow from the posterior to the anterior chamber.

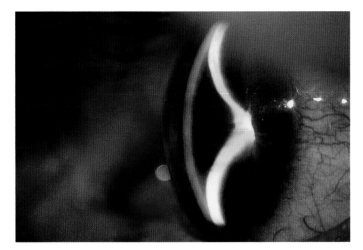

Fig. 6.225 Seclusio pupillae and iris bombe

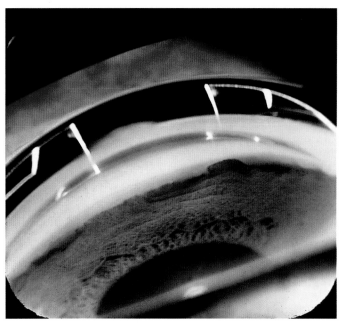

Fig. 6.226 Gonioscopy showing broad peripheral anterior synechiae

- The resultant increased pressure in the posterior chamber produces anterior bowing of the peripheral iris (iris bombe), with shallowing of the anterior chamber and apposition of the peripheral iris to the trabeculum and peripheral cornea.

- Such an inflamed iris easily sticks to the trabeculum; and the iridocorneal contact becomes permanent with the development of peripheral anterior synechiae (PAS).

> **NB:** Angle-closure glaucoma with pupil block is uncommon; most eyes with seclusio pupillae exhibit a normal or subnormal IOP due to concomitant chronic ciliary body shutdown. In some cases, the IOP may subsequently become elevated as ciliary function returns.

2. Signs

- Slit-lamp biomicroscopy shows seclusio pupillae, iris bombe and a shallow anterior chamber (Fig. 6.225).

- Gonioscopy shows angle closure from iridotrabecular contact. Indentation gonioscopy with a Zeiss four-mirror goniolens, or equivalent, may be used to assess the extent of appositional as opposed to synechial angle closure.

ANGLE CLOSURE WITHOUT PUPIL BLOCK

1. Pathogenesis

- Chronic anterior uveitis causes the deposition of inflammatory debris in the angle, subsequent organisation and contraction of which pulls the peripheral iris over the trabeculum, thereby causing gradual and progressive synechial angle closure with eventual elevation of IOP.

- The eye with a pre-existing narrow angle may be at higher risk, as may one with granulomatous inflammation with inflammatory nodules in the angle.

- Forward rotation of the iris–lens diaphragm as a result of choroidal effusions.

2. Signs

- The anterior chamber is deep but gonioscopy shows extensive angle closure by PAS (Fig. 6.226).

- In eyes with choroidal effusions, the anterior chamber will be shallow without PAS.

Open-angle glaucoma

IN ACUTE ANTERIOR UVEITIS

In acute anterior uveitis, the IOP is usually normal or subnormal due to concomitant ciliary shutdown. Occasionally, however, secondary open-angle glaucoma develops due to obstruction of aqueous outflow, most commonly as the acute inflammation is subsiding and ciliary body function is returning. This effect, which is often transient and innocuous, may be steroid-induced or caused by a combination of the following mechanisms:

1. **Trabecular obstruction** by inflammatory cells and debris, which may be associated with increased aqueous viscosity due to leakage of proteins from the inflamed iris blood vessels.

2. **Acute trabeculitis** involving inflammation and oedema of the trabecular meshwork with secondary diminution of intertrabecular porosity may result in a reduction in outflow facility. It is thought that this is relevant in anterior uveitis associated with herpes zoster and herpes simplex as well as in toxoplasma retinitis.

IN CHRONIC ANTERIOR UVEITIS

1. **Trabecular scarring** and/or sclerosis secondary to chronic trabeculitis. The exact incidence and importance of this

mechanism is difficult to determine, however, as most eyes also have some degree of synechial angle closure.

2. **Mechanical blockage and cellular depletion** of the trabecular meshwork associated with deposition of pigment and cellular debris.

Steroid glaucoma

- In genetic steroid responders, the IOP elevation observed on topical steroid treatment classically occurs within 4 weeks of exposure.

- In steroid non-responders, a chronic steroid-induced IOP elevation may develop over longer periods of time as a result of long-term therapy.

- Though less common, elevation of IOP may also occur with periocular or systemic steroid therapy. A chronic steroid response may also last for many weeks after termination of steroid therapy.

Treatment

MEDICAL

- Medical control of IOP is more likely to be achieved if the angle is completely open, and there are no PAS or pigment deposits.

- The aim of therapy in terms of IOP level to be attained depends on the health of the optic nerve head; eyes with advanced damage require a low target IOP to prevent further damage.

- In steroid reactors, it is important not to sacrifice control of inflammation for fear of steroid-induced IOP elevation. Long-acting depot preparations should be used with great caution in patients with a history of a steroid response.

- The IOP-lowering effect of ocular hypotensive drugs is less predictable in uveitis and some cases may be unexpectedly sensitive to topical carbonic anhydrase inhibitors (CAIs).

- The use of prostaglandin agonists (e.g. latanoprost) as first-line agents in uveitic glaucoma is tempered by the small but finite risk of precipitating a uveitic episode or CMO.

- A topical beta blocker (e.g. timolol) is therefore usually the first drug of choice.

- The choice of a second-line agent often depends on the IOP level. If the IOP is very high, a systemic CAI (e.g. acetazolamide) may be required in the short term. On the other hand, if elevation of IOP is moderate (e.g. less than 35 mmHg on a beta blocker) in the absence of significant glaucomatous damage, an alpha-adrenergic agonist (e.g. brimonidine), a topical CAI (e.g. dorzolamide) or prostaglandin analogue might be appropriate.

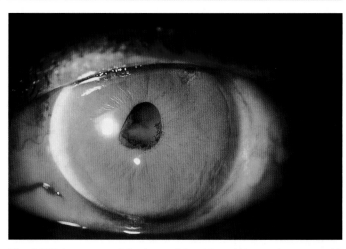

Fig. 6.227 Appearance following peripheral laser iridotomy in an eye with chronic anterior uveitis (Courtesy of J Salmon)

NB: Miotics are contraindicated, as they increase vascular permeability and may induce inflammation, and the miosis enhances the formation of posterior synechiae.

LASER IRIDOTOMY

- Laser iridotomy is performed to re-establish communication between the posterior and anterior chambers in eyes with pupil-block angle-closure glaucoma. The resulting hole is usually quite small and likely to become occluded in the presence of an active uveitis (Fig. 6.227).

- It is important to bear in mind that correction of pupil block may not control the IOP if there is insufficient open angle for drainage. In cases of progressive angle closure, iridotomy may nevertheless prevent further PAS formation.

- Intensive topical steroid therapy should be used to minimise post-laser inflammation.

- Surgical iridectomy is the definitive method for preventing further pupil block.

SURGERY

As in any type of glaucoma, the decision to operate is based on the level of the IOP, the response to medication and the health of the optic nerve head.

1. **Preoperative preparation**

- Control of uveitis for a minimum of 3 months before surgery is ideal but often impractical, as glaucoma surgery is rarely an elective procedure.

- Preoperative topical steroids should be used, not only as prophylaxis against recurrent inflammation but also to reduce the conjunctival inflammatory cell population and enhance the success rate of a filtration procedure.

- In patients with particularly labile inflammatory disease, systemic steroids should be considered (0.5 mg/kg/day of oral prednisolone).

2. **Trabeculectomy** is the procedure of choice.

- Combined cataract and glaucoma surgery is not appropriate. Ideally, cataract surgery should be performed about 6 months after trabeculectomy, because the results are better.

- Adjunctive antimetabolites, particularly mitomycin C, are required since these eyes carry a high risk of failure.

- Postoperative hypotony is a risk where a delicate balance may exist between reduced aqueous production and severely restricted aqueous outflow. If production drops in the early postoperative period, any filtration may be excessive. It is therefore imperative to perform tight scleral suturing in order to prevent early hypotony.

- After trabeculectomy, steroids are tapered according to the level of inflammation and the appearance of the filtering bleb, and usually discontinued after 2–3 months, although earlier tapering may be necessary in cases of overfiltration.

3. **Glaucoma drainage devices (GDD)** should be considered in cases where trabeculectomy, even with adjunctive antimetabolites, has a poor success rate. This includes aphakic eyes, children with chronic anterior uveitis, or a previously failed trabeculectomy.

- While the exact role of GDD has yet to be clearly defined, it is widely accepted that the threshold for using these devices is lower in uveitic glaucoma than in other types.

- GDD implantation generally produces better IOP control in uveitic eyes than in other glaucomas, probably because it also reduces aqueous secretion. For this reason, implants with smaller surface areas for drainage, such as the Ahmed valve (Fig. 6.228), single plate Molteno and 250 Baerveldt, are preferred.

- Post-operative hypotony is a problem with these devices and a two-step procedure is recommended, using a suture fed inside the tube, which is later removed.

5. **Cyclodestructive** procedures (Fig. 6.229) should be used with caution because they may not only exacerbate the intraocular inflammation but also result in profound hypotony which may proceed to phthisis bulbi. Even eyes with seemingly intractable uveitic glaucoma may paradoxically develop ciliary body insufficiency in the longer term.

6. **Angle procedures** including trabeculodialysis and goniotomy may be successful in children. The former procedure involves making an incision along Schwalbe line in order to establish communication between the anterior chamber and Schlemm canal (Fig. 6.230).

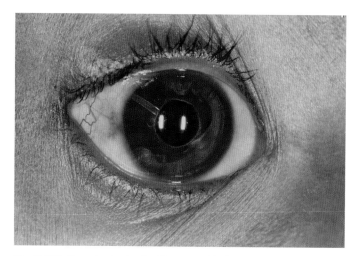

Fig. 6.228 Ahmed valve in situ (Courtesy of U Raina)

Fig. 6.229 Diode laser cycloablation (Courtesy of J Salmon)

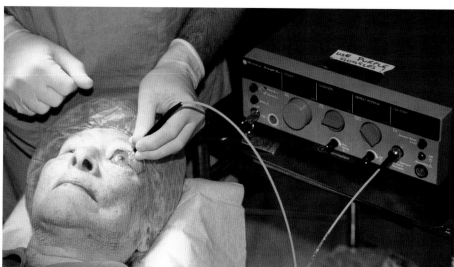

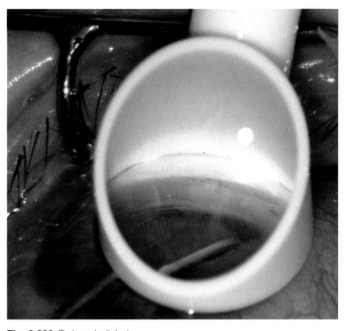

Fig. 6.230 Trabeculodialysis

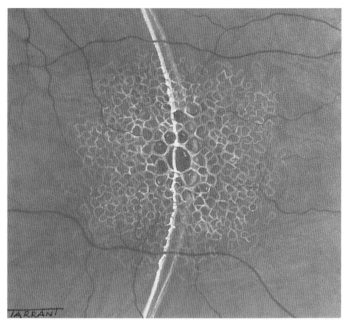

Fig. 6.231 Cystoid macular oedema as seen on slit-lamp biomicroscopy

FURTHER READING

Freedman SF, Rodriguez-Rosa RE, Rojas MC, et al. Goniotomy for glaucoma secondary to chronic childhood uveitis. *Ophthalmology* 2002;133:617–621.

Hill RA, Nguyen QH, Baerveldt G, et al. Trabeculectomy and Molteno implantation for glaucoma associated with uveitis. *Ophthalmology* 1993;100:903–908.

Jampel HD, Jabs DA, Quigley HA. Trabeculectomy with 5-fluorouracil for adult inflammatory glaucoma. *Am J Ophthalmol* 1990;109:168–173.

Jones NP. Glaucoma in Fuchs' heterochromic cyclitis; aetiology, management and outcome. *Eye* 1991;5:662–667.

Kanski JJ, McAllister JA. Trabeculodialysis for inflammatory glaucoma in children and young adults. *Ophthalmology* 1985;92:927–930.

La Hey E, de Vries J, Langerhorst CT, et al. Treatment and prognosis of secondary glaucoma in Fuchs' heterochromic cyclitis. *Am J Ophthalmol* 1993;116:327–340.

Moorthy RS, Mermoud A, Baerveldt G, et al. Glaucoma associated with uveitis. *Surv Ophthalmol* 1997;41:361–394.

Neri P, Azuara-Blanco A, Forrester JV. Incidence of glaucoma in patients with uveitis. *J Glaucoma* 2004;13:461–465.

Panek WC, Holland GN, Lee DA, et al. Glaucoma in patients with uveitis. *Br J Ophthalmol* 1990;74:223–227.

Prata JA Jr, Neves RA, Minckler DS, et al. Trabeculectomy with mitomycin C in glaucoma associated with uveitis. *Ophthal Surg* 1994;25:616–620.

Sung VC, Barton K. Management of inflammatory glaucomas. *Curr Opin Ophthalmol* 2004;15:136–140.

Valimaki J, Airaksinen PJ, Tuulonen A. Molteno implantation for secondary glaucoma in juvenile rheumatoid arthritis. *Arch Ophthalmol* 1997;115:1253–1256.

Cystoid macular oedema

CMO is the result of accumulation of fluid in the outer plexiform layer at the fovea and the formation of cyst-like changes. CMO is the most important cause of visual loss in uveitis, and, if longstanding, may result in permanent impairment of central vision as a result of lamellar hole formation or RPE degeneration. CMO is a common problem in intermediate uveitis and posterior uveitis.

Pathogenesis

- Breakdown of the blood retinal barrier at the level of the RPE or capillary endothelial cells.

- Inflammatory response and the pro-inflammatory mediators affecting vascular permeability at the macula.

- RPE disturbance resulting in accumulation of subretinal fluid and retinal oedema.

- Macular epiretinal membrane formation may cause CMO by distorting the retinal capillaries.

- Vitreomacular traction is another important mechanism.

Diagnosis

1. **Slit-lamp biomicroscopy** shows loss of the foveal depression, retinal thickening and multiple cystoid areas at the fovea (Fig. 6.231). In early cases, cystoid changes may be difficult to discern and the main finding is a small yellow spot.

2. **FA** (see Fig. 6.11).

3. **OCT** is as effective as FA at detecting CMO (see Fig. 6.14), and produces highly reproducible measurements. However, unlike FA, it is useful in detecting vitreoretinal traction.

Treatment

STEROIDS

1. **Topical** steroids are of limited value because of lack of penetration of the posterior segment.

2. **Periocular** injections have the advantage over topical therapy as they allow administration of a large bolus of drug whilst minimising the systemic side effects and also allow a more sustained release of the drug. Posterior sub-Tenon injections are of particular value in eyes with CMO.

3. **Systemic** steroids may be used in bilateral cases or unilateral cases resistant to periocular injections. An additive effect may be achieved by using a combination of systemic and posterior sub-Tenon injection.

4. **Deep intramuscular** methylprednisolone may be considered as an alternative to oral and periocular injections. It avoids potential hazards of periocular injections and ensures patient compliance with fewer systemic side effects.

5. **Intravitreal** triamcinolone produces a very rapid response, with complete resolution of CMO within 1 week and with a duration of about 4 months in non-vitrectomised eyes.

OTHER FORMS OF THERAPY

1. **Topical NSAIDs** may be beneficial, especially when used in combination with steroids.

2. **Systemic CAIs** may alter the polarity of the ionic transport systems in the RPE, and as a result, there is increased fluid transport across the RPE from the subretinal space to the choroid, with a reduction in the oedema.

- CAIs may be beneficial in the treatment of CMO associated with intermediate uveitis but the effect is frequently transient.

- The starting dose is 500 mg daily, which should be continued for at least 1 month.

- Long-term use of CAIs is often limited by bothersome side effects.

3. **Hyperbaric oxygen** may be beneficial in longstanding CMO caused by uveitis. The mechanism, which results in reduction of leakage, is probably associated with the vasoconstrictive effect of oxygen. The therapeutic effect seems to be stable and may lead to a significant improvement in visual acuity.

4. **Interferon alfa-2a** may be useful in CMO associated with steroid-resistant autoimmune uveitis, although discontinuation may provoke a relapse of inflammation. Side effects include arrhythmias and disturbances in blood pressure.

5. **Pars plana vitrectomy** may be useful in the management of refractory uveitic CMO, and it should probably be considered earlier in the course of the disease. Vitrectomy may also reduce the severity of the uveitis and the need for systemic therapy. It may also increase intraocular penetration of systemic drugs.

Vitrectomy may also eliminate vitreoretinal macular traction or epiretinal membranes responsible for CMO.

FURTHER READING

Antcliff RJ, Stanford MR, Chauhan DS, et al. Comparison between optical coherence tomography and fundus fluorescein angiography for the detection of cystoid macular edema in patients with uveitis. *Ophthalmology* 2000;107:593–599.

Antcliff RJ, Spalton DJ, Stanford MR, et al. Intravitreal triamcinolone for uveitic cystoid macular edema: an optical coherence tomography study. *Ophthalmology* 2001;108:765–772.

Durrani OM, Tehrani NN, Marr JE, et al. Degree, duration, and causes of visual loss in uveitis. *Br J Ophthalmol* 2004;88:1159–1162.

Freeman G, Matos KT, Pavesio CE. Cystoid macular edema in uveitis: an unsolved problem. *Eye* 2001;15:12–17.

Jaffe GJ, Ben-Nun J, Guo H, et al. Fluocinolone acetonide sustained drug delivery device to treat severe uveitis. *Ophthalmology* 2000;107:2024–2033.

Kiryu J, Kita M, Tanabe T, et al. Pars plana vitrectomy for cystoid macular edema secondary to sarcoid uveitis. *Ophthalmology* 2001;108:1140–1144.

Markomichelakis NN, Halkiadakis J, Pantelia E, et al. Patterns of macular edema in patients with uveitis. *Ophthalmology* 2004;111:946–953.

Nussenblatt RB, Kauffman SC, Palestine AG, et al. Macular thickening and visual acuity: measurement in patients with cystoid macular edema. *Ophthalmology* 1987;94:1134–1139.

Sonoda K-H, Enaida H, Ueno A, et al. Pars plana assisted by triamcinolone acetonide for refractory uveitis: a case series study. *Br J Ophthalmol* 2003;87:1010–1014.

Tehrani NN, Saeed T, Murray PI. Deep intramuscular methylprednisolone for the treatment of cystoid macular edema in uveitis. *Eye* 2000;14:691–694.

Whitcup SM, Csaky KG, Podgor MJ, et al. A randomized, masked, cross-over trial of acetazolamide for cystoid macular edema in patients with uveitis. *Ophthalmology* 1996;103:1054–1062.

Yoshikawa K, Kotake S, Ichiishi A, et al. Posterior sub-Tenon injections of repository corticosteroids in uveitis patients with cystoid macular edema. *Jpn J Ophthalmol* 1995;39:71–76.

Choroidal neovascularisation

CNV is a potentially blinding complication of posterior uveitis. The membranes are type 2, in which neovascular growth occurs beneath the sensory retina and anterior to the RPE, with bridging vessels connecting to the underlying choroidal circulation. Uveitic entities commonly associated with CNV include presumed ocular histoplasmosis, multifocal choroiditis and punctate inner choroidopathy. Treatment options, depending on the location of CNV, include anti-inflammatory therapy, argon laser photocoagulation, photodynamic therapy and surgical excision.

FURTHER READING

Berger AS, Conway MD, Del Priore LV, et al. Submacular surgery for subfoveal choroidal neovascular membranes in presumed ocular histoplasmosis. *Arch Ophthalmol* 1997;115:991–996.

Chatterjee S, Gibson JM. Photodynamic therapy: a treatment option in choroidal neovascularization secondary to punctate inner choroidopathy. *Br J Ophthalmol* 2003;87:925–927.

Dees C, Arnold JJ, Forrester JV, et al. Immunosuppressive treatment of choroidal neovascularization associated with endogenous posterior uveitis. *Arch Ophthalmol* 1998;116:1456–1461.

Eckstein M, Wells JA, Aylward B, et al. Surgical removal of non-age-related subfoveal choroidal neovascular membranes. *Eye* 1998;12:775–780.

Gass JD. Biomicroscopic and histopathologic considerations regarding the feasibility of surgical excision of subfoveal neovascular membranes. *Am J Ophthalmol* 1994;118:285–298.

Kilmartin DJ, Forrester JV, Dick AD. Cyclosporine-induced resolution of choroidal neovascularization associated with sympathetic ophthalmia. *Arch Ophthalmol* 1998;116:249–250.

Lewis ML, Van Newkirk, Gass D. Follow-up study of presumed ocular histoplasmosis syndrome. *Ophthalmology* 1980;87:390–398.

Macular Photocoagulation Study Group. Five-year follow-up of fellow eyes of individuals with ocular histoplasmosis and unilateral extrafoveal or juxtafoveal choroidal neovascularization. *Arch Ophthalmol* 1996;114:677–688.

Pavan PR, Margo CE. Submacular neovascular membrane and focal granulomatous inflammation. *Ophthalmology* 1996;103:586–589.

Chapter **7**

Endophthalmitis

ACUTE POSTOPERATIVE BACTERIAL ENDOPHTHALMITIS

Pathogenesis

Acute endophthalmitis is a devastating complication of intraocular surgery. The estimated incidence following cataract surgery is approximately 0.15%. This has reduced over the last decade despite a great increase in the volume of cataract surgery. Toxins produced by the infecting bacteria and the host inflammatory responses cause rapid and irreversible photoreceptor damage. These effects can continue long after the ocular contents have been rendered sterile.

1. **Risk factors** include age over 80 years, diabetes, secondary lens implantation, posterior capsule rupture, and cataract surgery combined with other procedures.

2. **Pathogens.** About 90% of isolates are Gram-positive and 10% Gram-negative. In order of frequency they include:

- Coagulase-negative staphylococci (e.g. *Staph. epidermidis*).

- Other Gram-positive organisms (e.g. *Staph. aureus* and *Streptococcus* sp.).

- Gram-negative organisms (e.g. *Pseudomonas* and *Proteus* sp.).

3. **The source of infection** usually cannot be identified with certainty. It is thought that the flora of the eyelids and conjunctiva are the most frequent source. Other potential sources of infection include contaminated solutions and instruments, the air in theatre, and the surgeon or operating room personnel.

Prophylaxis

Because of the low rate of endophthalmitis, it is very difficult to prove that any method of prophylaxis is effective or superior to any other. Prophylaxis reduces the colony counts of organisms on the surface of the eye, but it cannot sterilise the surface. The following measures may be beneficial:

1. **Treatment of pre-existing infections** such as blepharitis, conjunctivitis, chronic dacryocystitis and infection in the contralateral eye or socket (Fig. 7.1).

2. **Povidone–iodine** is instilled preoperatively as follows:

- A 5% solution is prepared by diluting commercially available 10% aqueous solution with an equal volume of balanced salt solution.

- The solution is instilled into the conjunctival sac prior to surgery (Fig. 7.2) and is also used to paint the skin of the eyelids prior to draping (Fig. 7.3).

NB: Chlorhexidine is a suitable alternative for patients sensitive to iodine.

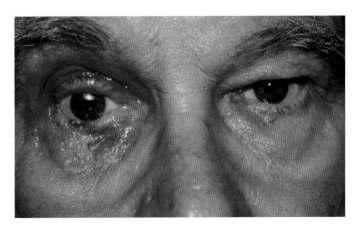

Fig. 7.1 Infected right ocular prosthesis and socket is a risk factor for postoperative endophthalmitis

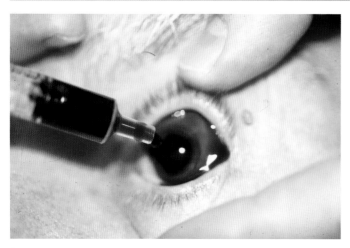

Fig. 7.2 Preoperative instillation of povidone–iodine

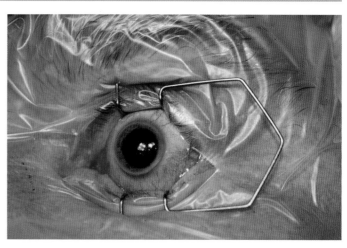

Fig. 7.4 Drapes isolating the lids and lashes from the operating field

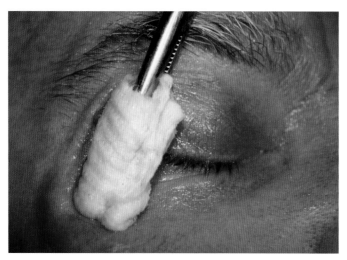

Fig. 7.3 Preparation of the skin with povidone–iodine

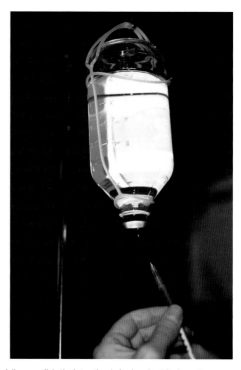

Fig. 7.5 Adding antibiotic into the infusion bottle is not recommended

3. **Careful draping** ensuring that the lashes and lid margins are isolated from the surgical field (Fig. 7.4).

4. **Prophylactic antibiotics**

- Preoperative topical fluoroquinolone antibiotics are frequently given from 1 hour to 3 days before surgery.

- Intracameral cefuroxine injected behind the implant at the end of surgery.

- Postoperative subconjunctival injection of antibiotics is commonly performed and can achieve bactericidal levels in the anterior chamber for 1 to 2 hours.

NB: Intraoperative perfusion of the anterior chamber by adding vancomycin or gentamicin to the infusion fluid (Fig. 7.5) is unlikely to be effective, as bactericidal levels are lost almost immediately after the end of surgery. This may also encourage emergence of vancomycin-resistant strains of bacteria.

5. **Surgical technique**

- Phacoemulsification reduces risk compared with extracapsular surgery.

- It is possible that the risk of infection is greater with a self-sealing temporal clear corneal incision compared with superior scleral tunnel incisions.

- Injectable intraocular lenses (IOLs) may reduce the risk by preventing contamination of the implant from the surface of the eye.

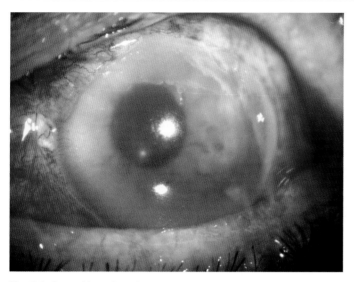

Fig. 7.6 Corneal haze in early postoperative endophthalmitis

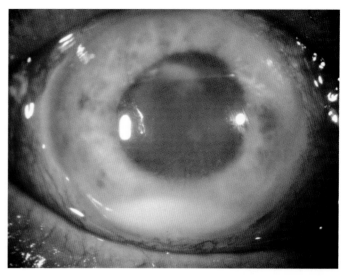

Fig. 7.8 Severe corneal haze and hypopyon in postoperative endophthalmitis

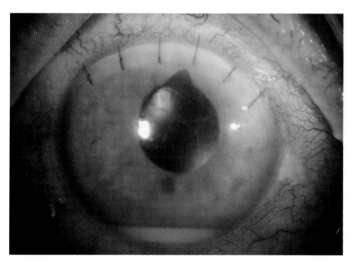

Fig. 7.7 Fibrinous exudate and small hypopyon in postoperative endophthalmitis

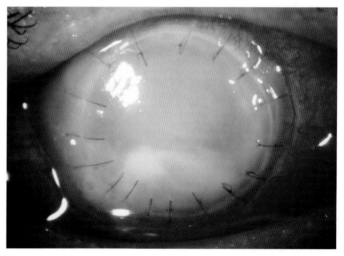

Fig. 7.9 Very advanced endophthalmitis following penetrating keratoplasty

Diagnosis

The diagnosis relies on clinical suspicion and microbiological confirmation.

1. **Symptoms** are pain and visual loss.

2. **Signs** vary according to severity.

* Chemosis, conjunctival injection and discharge.

* Relative afferent pupil defect.

* Corneal haze (Fig. 7.6).

* Fibrinous anterior uveitis and small hypopyon (Fig. 7.7).

* Enlarging hypopyon (Figs 7.8 and 7.9).

* Vitreous cells and debris (Fig. 7.10).

* Loss of the red reflex and impaired view of the fundus (Fig. 7.11).

* Retinal periphlebitis is present but seldom clinically visible.

Differential diagnosis

If there is any doubt about the diagnosis, treatment should be that of infectious endophthalmitis.

1. **Retained lens material** in the anterior chamber (Fig. 7.12) or vitreous may precipitate a severe uveitis, corneal oedema and raised intraocular pressure.

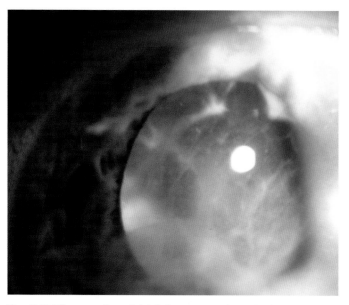

Fig. 7.10 Vitreous cells and debris in postoperative endophthalmitis

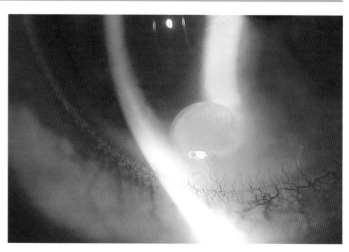

Fig. 7.12 Retained lens matter in the anterior chamber

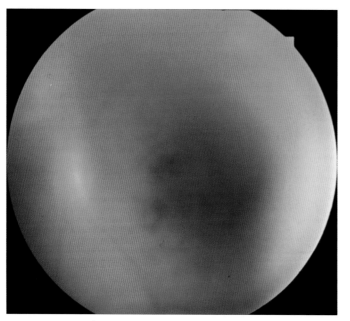

Fig. 7.11 Impaired view of the fundus in postoperative endophthalmitis

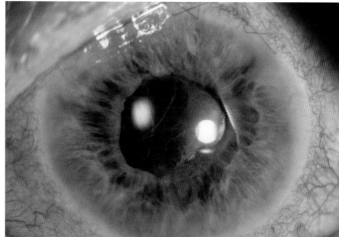

Fig. 7.13 Sterile fibrinous exudate

2. **Vitreous haemorrhage**, especially if blood in the vitreous is depigmented.

3. **Postoperative uveitis.** A confident diagnosis of infection can be difficult in patients with a prior history of uveitis. If signs of inflammation are mild, a trial of topical steroid therapy and early review (<6 hours) is appropriate. If there is not substantial improvement, management should be that of endophthalmitis.

4. **Toxic reaction** to the use of inappropriate or contaminated irrigating fluid or viscoelastic. An intense fibrinous reaction (Fig. 7.13) with corneal oedema may develop although other signs of infectious endophthalmitis are

absent. Treatment is with intensive topical steroids and mydriatics. Corneal decompensation may be permanent.

5. **Complicated or prolonged surgery** may result in corneal oedema and uveitis.

Identification of pathogens

Samples for culture should be obtained from aqueous and vitreous to confirm the diagnosis. However, negative culture does not necessarily rule out infection and treatment should be continued. The samples can be taken in a minor procedures operating room, making sure that all equipment is available prior to starting.

1. **Antibiotics.** Because of the risk of dilution errors, pharmacy-prepared packs should be used if possible.

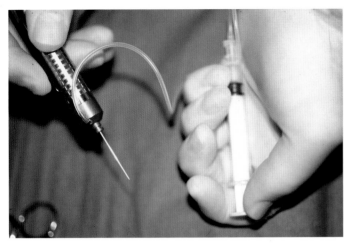

Fig. 7.14 Mini vitrector used to obtain vitreous samples in bacterial endophthalmitis

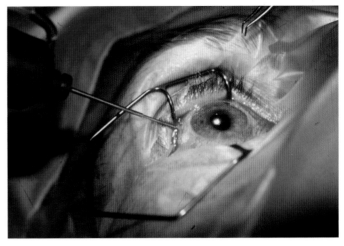

Fig. 7.15 Vitreous biopsy using a mini vitrector

2. Preparation

- Povidone–iodine 5% is instilled and the eye draped.

- Topical and subconjunctival or peribulbar anaesthesia is administered.

3. Aqueous samples

- Between 0.1 ml and 0.2 ml of aqueous is aspirated via a limbal paracentesis using a 25-gauge needle on a tuberculin syringe.

- The syringe is capped and labelled.

4. Vitreous samples are more likely to yield a positive culture than are aqueous.

- A 2-ml syringe and a 23-gauge needle may be used or a special disposable vitrector (Fig. 7.14).

- The needle or a mini vitrector is inserted 4 mm (phakic eye) or 3 mm (aphakic eye) behind the limbus, into the mid-vitreous cavity, and 0.2–0.4 ml aspirated (Fig. 7.15).

- The syringe is capped and labelled.

Treatment

1. **Intravitreal antibiotics** are the key to management. They achieve levels above the minimal inhibitory concentration of most pathogens, and these are maintained for days. They should be administered immediately after culture specimens have been obtained.

- Amikacin or ceftazidime will kill most Gram-negative organisms.

- Vancomycin will kill coagulase-negative and coagulase-positive cocci.

- Amikacin (0.4 mg in 0.1 ml) and vancomycin (1 or 2 mg in 0.1 ml); ceftazidime (2.2 mg in 0.1 ml) may be used as

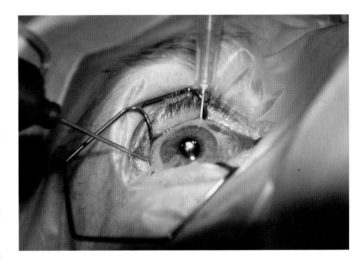

Fig. 7.16 Intravitreal antibiotic injection

an alternative to amikacin because it carries a lesser risk of retinal toxicity.

- The antibiotics are injected slowly into the mid-vitreous cavity using a 25-gauge needle (Fig. 7.16).

- After the first injection has been given, the syringe is disconnected but the needle is left inside the vitreous cavity so that the second injection can be given through the same needle. Alternatively, a second needle entry can be used.

2. **Periocular antibiotic injections** are often given but are of doubtful additional benefit if intravitreal antibiotics have been used. Suggested doses are vancomycin 25 mg, ceftazidime 100 mg, or ceftriaxone 100 mg.

3. **Topical antibiotics** are of limited benefit in the absence of associated infectious keratitis. Vancomycin (50 mg/ml) or ceftazidime (50 mg/ml) applied intensively may penetrate the cornea in therapeutic levels.

4. **Oral antibiotics** are of uncertain benefit. Fluoro-quinolones penetrate the eye and ciprofloxacin 750 mg b.d. for 10 days is recommended; clarithromycin 500 mg b.d. may be helpful for culture-negative infections.

5. **Oral steroids.** The rationale for the use of steroids is to limit the destructive complications of the inflammatory process. Prednisolone 60 mg daily should be started in severe cases after 12 hours, provided fungal infection has been excluded from examination of smears.

6. **Periocular steroids.** Dexamethasone (12 mg) or triam-cinolone (1.0 mg) should be considered if systemic therapy is contraindicated.

7. **Topical dexamethasone** 0.1% q.i.d. for anterior uveitis.

8. **Intravitreal steroid** (dexamethasone 400 µg) is contro-versial. Although it reduces inflammation in the short term, it does not influence the final visual outcome. Some studies even suggest a detrimental effect. Conversely, improvement in outcome in some bacterial subgroups has been reported.

9. **Pars plana vitrectomy.** The Endophthalmitis Vitrectomy Study (EVS) showed a benefit for immediate pars plana vitrectomy for eyes with a visual acuity of perception of light (NOT hand movements vision or any better acuity level) at presentation, with a 50% reduction in severe visual loss. However, in practice, many retinal surgeons consider that the risks of causing severe iatrogenic retinal damage by performing vitrectomy 'blind' in such eyes may outweigh the potential benefits. Although vitrectomy may debulk the eye of inflammatory material, it may also increase clearance of intravitreal antibiotics.

> **NB:** The conclusions of the EVS cannot be extrapolated to other forms of endophthalmitis that have a different microbiological spectrum.

Microbiology

The syringes should be sent directly to the laboratory during working hours even if they appear to be empty (do not send needles).

1. **Culture media**

- Blood agar.

- Cooked meat broth.

- Brain–heart infusion.

- Slide for Gram stain if sufficient sample is available.

> **NB:** A standard blood culture bottle is an alternative for culture if specific media are unavailable.

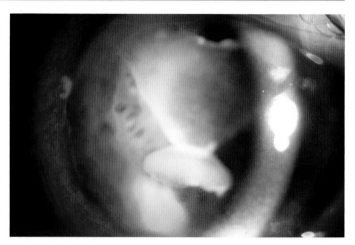

Fig. 7.17 Contraction of hypopyon and fibrinous exudate following successful treatment

2. **Polymerase chain reaction** (PCR) can be helpful in iden-tifying unusual organisms, the cause of culture-negative disease, and organisms after antibiotic treatment has been started. The great sensitivity means that contamination can lead to false positive results.

Subsequent management

Subsequent management is partly determined by culture results and clinical findings.

1. **Signs of improvement** include reduction of anterior chamber cellular activity and hypopyon, and contraction of fibrinous exudate (Fig. 7.17). In this situation, treat-ment is not modified irrespective of culture results.

2. **If the clinical signs are worsening** after 48 hours, antibi-otic sensitivities should be reviewed and therapy modified accordingly. A vitrectomy should be considered if not pre-viously performed. Intravitreal antibiotics can be repeated after 2 days, preferably without using amikacin, to reduce the risk of retinal toxicity.

3. **Outcome** is related to the duration of the infection prior to treatment and the virulence of the organisms.

- If visual acuity at presentation is light perception, 30% of eyes achieve 6/12 following treatment. If visual acuity is better than light perception, this figure increases to 60%.

- Infection with *Bacillus cereus* and streptococci has a poor visual outcome despite aggressive and appropriate therapy, with 70% and 55%, respectively, achieving a final visual acuity of 6/60 or less. The poor visual outcome is proba-bly related to early retinopathy from exotoxins released by some organisms.

Complications

Severe visual loss may occur in patients presenting with any level of visual acuity. The severity of endophthalmitis reflects the virulence of the offending organism. Streptococcal, *Staph. aureus* and enterococcal infections tend to be aggressive with a poor visual outcome despite early treatment. Endophthalmitis caused by *Staph. epidermidis* has a more gradual onset with milder disease. The main causes of visual loss are:

• Chronic uveitis, macular oedema and macular ischaemia.

• Secondary glaucoma.

• Retinal detachment.

• Phthisis.

• Panophthalmitis or perforation requiring evisceration.

DELAYED-ONSET POSTOPERATIVE BACTERIAL ENDOPHTHALMITIS

Pathogenesis

Delayed-onset endophthalmitis develops following cataract surgery when an organism of low virulence becomes trapped within the capsular bag.

It has an onset ranging from 4 weeks to years (mean of 9 months) postoperatively and typically follows uneventful cataract extraction with a posterior chamber IOL. It may rarely be precipitated by YAG-laser capsulotomy, which releases the sequestrated organism from the posterior capsule into the vitreous. The infection is caused most frequently by *P. acnes* and occasionally by *Staph. epidermidis*, *Actinomyces israelii*, *Corynebacterium* sp. or *Candida parapsilosis*.

Diagnosis

1. **Presentation** is with painless, mild, progressive visual deterioration which may be associated with floaters.

2. **Signs**

• Low-grade anterior uveitis, sometimes with 'mutton-fat' keratic precipitates (Fig. 7.18).

• Vitritis is common but hypopyon infrequent.

• An enlarging white capsular plaque composed of organisms sequestered in residual cortex within the peripheral capsular bag is characteristic (Fig. 7.19).

NB: It is important to perform gonioscopy under mydriasis so as not to miss an equatorial plaque.

3. **Investigations.** The diagnosis should be confirmed by cultures of the aqueous and vitreous with growth of the organism. Anaerobic culture should be requested if *P. acnes* infection is suspected, and isolates may take 10–14 days to grow. Detection rate of pathogens can be greatly improved with PCR.

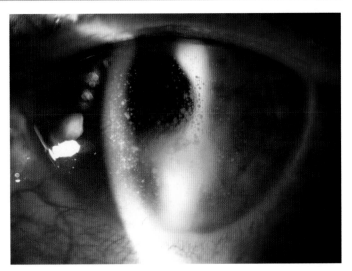

Fig. 7.18 Granulomatous uveitis in delayed-onset postoperative endophthalmitis

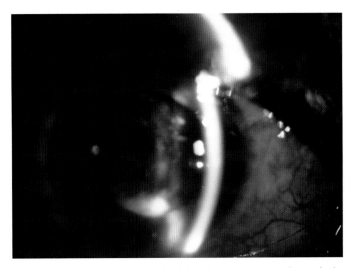

Fig. 7.19 White capsular plaque in delayed-onset postoperative endophthalmitis

4. **Clinical course.** Without antibiotic treatment, the inflammation initially responds well to topical steroids but recurs when treatment is stopped and eventually becomes steroid-resistant.

Treatment

Because the sequestered organisms are isolated from host defences and antibiotics, antibiotic treatment alone is unlikely to be successful.

1. **Removal** of the capsular bag, residual cortex and IOL is recommended. This may require pars plana vitrectomy. Secondary IOL implantation may be considered at a later date.

2. **Intravitreal vancomycin** (1 mg in 0.1 ml) is the antibiotic of choice. This can also be irrigated into any capsular remnant.

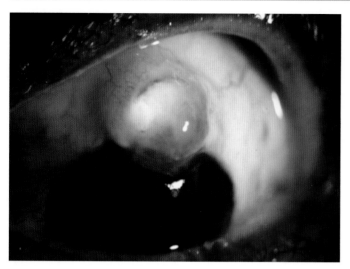

Fig. 7.20 Thin bleb is a risk factor for infection

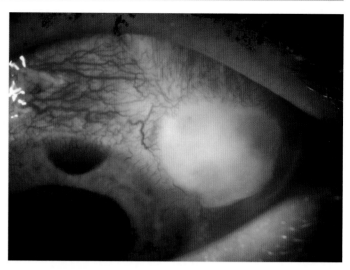

Fig. 7.21 Bleb infection ('blebitis') following trabeculectomy

BLEB-ASSOCIATED BACTERIAL INFECTION AND ENDOPHTHALMITIS

Glaucoma filtration-associated infection is classified as limited to the bleb (blebitis) or endophthalmitis, although there is some overlap. The incidence of blebitis following trabeculectomy with mitomycin is estimated to be 5% per year and endophthalmitis about 1% per year.

Pathogenesis

Adjunctive antifibrotic agents (mitomycin C, 5-fluorouracil) are frequently used to increase the success of glaucoma filtration surgery. The use of these agents can lead to a very thin-walled drainage bleb (Fig. 7.20) that significantly increases the risk of late-onset infection. The infection presumably gains access directly through the thin and avascular wall of the drainage bleb. All patients with such blebs should be warned of the possibility of late infection and strongly advised to report immediately should they develop a red and sticky eye, or blurred vision (RSVP – red, sticky, visual loss, pain).

1. **Risk factors** include blepharitis, long-term topical antibiotic use, an inferior or nasally placed bleb, and bleb leak. Late bleb leaks should be treated aggressively to reduce the risk of infection.

2. **Pathogens.** The most frequent are *H. influenzae*, *Streptococcus* sp. and *Staphylococcus* sp. The often poor visual prognosis is related the virulence of these organisms.

Blebitis

Blebitis describes infection without vitreous involvement.

1. **Presentation** is with mild discomfort and redness.

2. **Signs**

- A white bleb that appears to contain inflammatory material (Fig. 7.21).

- Anterior uveitis is absent.

- The red reflex is normal.

3. **Investigation.** A conjunctival swab should be taken.

NB: Do not try to aspirate a sample from within the bleb.

4. **Treatment**

- Topical ofloxacin and cefuroxime (or vancomycin 50 mg/ml) hourly.

- Oral augmentin 625 mg three times daily and ciprofloxacin 750 mg b.d. for 5 days; azithromycin 500 mg daily for 5 days is an alternative to augmentin.

Bleb-associated endophthalmitis

1. **Presentation** is with a short history of rapidly worsening vision, pain and redness.

2. **Signs**

- White milky bleb.

- Severe anterior uveitis that may be associated with hypopyon (Fig. 7.22).

- Vitritis and impairment of the red reflex.

3. **Treatment** involves topical and systemic therapy as for blebitis and intravitreal antibiotics (e.g. amikacin, vancomycin) as for acute postoperative endophthalmitis (see above).

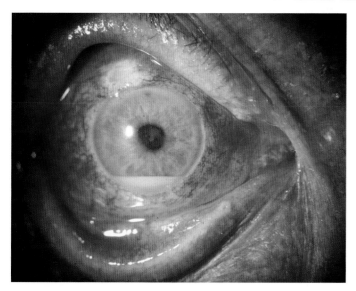

Fig. 7.22 Bacterial endophthalmitis with hypopyon following trabeculectomy

NB: Successfully treated eyes remain at risk of recurrent infection.

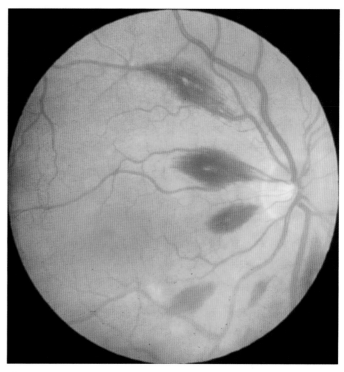

Fig. 7.23 Retinal haemorrhages with white centres (Roth spots) in bacteraemia

POST-TRAUMATIC BACTERIAL ENDOPHTHALMITIS

Pathogenesis

Endophthalmitis develops in about 8% of cases of penetrating trauma with retained foreign body.

1. **Risk factors** include delay in primary repair, retained intraocular foreign body, and the position and extent of the laceration. Clinical signs are the same as acute postoperative endophthalmitis (see above).

2. **Pathogens.** *Staphylococcus* sp. and *Bacillus* sp. are isolated from about 90% of culture-positive cases.

Management

1. **Prophylaxis**

- Ciprofloxacin 750 mg b.d. is given for open globe injuries.

- Prompt removal of retained intraocular foreign bodies.

- Intravitreal antibiotics for high-risk cases requiring vitrectomy (e.g. agricultural injuries).

2. **Culture** of removed intraocular foreign bodies (do not stick them in the clinical notes!).

3. **Treatment** for established cases is the same as for acute bacterial endophthalmitis (see above).

ENDOGENOUS BACTERIAL ENDOPHTHALMITIS

Pathogenesis

Endogenous (metastatic) endophthalmitis occurs when organisms enter the eye through the blood–eye barrier from the bloodstream. However, no ocular infection occurs in the vast majority of cases of bacteraemia, although Roth spots develop in about 1% of cases (Fig. 7.23). Both eyes are involved in about 12% of cases.

1. **Risk factors** are diabetes, cardiac disease and malignancy. Other risks include indwelling catheters, intravenous drug abuse, liver abscess, pneumonia, endocarditis, cellulitis, urinary tract infection (*E. coli*), meningitis, septic arthritis and abdominal surgery.

2. **Pathogens.** The most common is *Klebsiella* species although a wide variety of organisms may be responsible, notably *Staph. aureus*, *Streptococcus* sp., *E. coli*, *P. aeruginosa*, *N. meningitidis* and *B. cereus*. *N. meningitides* and *H. influenzae* can cause endogenous endophthalmitis secondary to septicaemia in the absence of systemic disease. Immunosuppressed (but not HIV-positive) patients are particularly susceptible.

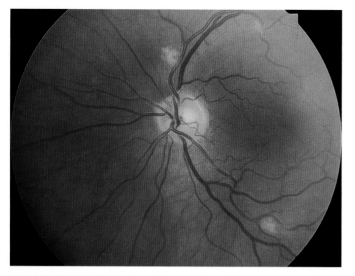

Fig. 7.24 Retinal infiltrates in endogenous bacterial endophthalmitis

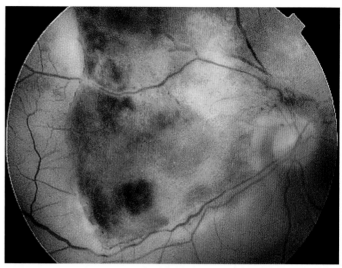

Fig. 7.25 Retinal necrosis in endogenous bacterial endophthalmitis

Clinical signs

Misdiagnosis as uveitis, conjunctivitis or acute glaucoma is common, and this may delay treatment. Diagnosis and management may be difficult if the patient is immobile or moribund.

1. Symptoms

- Pain, blurred vision, floaters, photophobia and headache.
- The patient is usually systemically unwell with fever and rigors.

2. Anterior segment

- Proptosis, chemosis, swollen lids and corneal oedema.
- Discrete iris nodules or plaques, anterior fibrinous uveitis and hypopyon in severe cases.

3. Posterior segment

- Vitreous haze or abscess.
- White or yellow retinal infiltrates (Fig. 7.24).
- Retinal necrosis in severe cases (Fig. 7.25).
- Spread to the orbital may occur.

Investigations

1. Systemic

- Search for septic foci (skin, joints); collaboration with a physician or intensive care specialist is essential.
- Blood and urine cultures in all patients.
- Appropriate cultures from other sites, depending on the clinical features (e.g. catheter tips, cerebrospinal fluid, skin wounds, abscesses and joints) (Fig. 7.26).

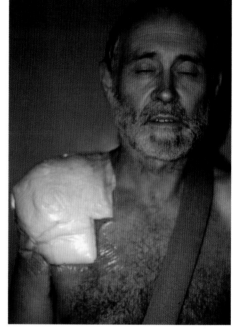

Fig. 7.26 A patient with endogenous bacterial endophthalmitis associated with septic arthritis

- Investigations for endocarditis (chest X-ray, ECG and echocardiography).
- Abdominal ultrasound.

> **NB:** Exclude meningitis in children, using PCR on blood for *N. meningitidis*.

2. Ocular

- Aqueous and vitreous samples should be taken (see above).
- Fine-needle biopsy of a focal abscess should be considered.

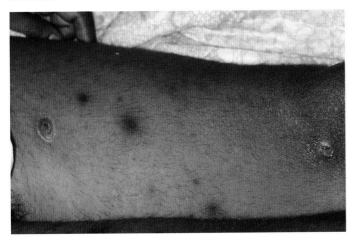

Fig. 7.27 Foci of skin infection at sites of drug injection in a drug addict

Table 7.1 Comparison of exogenous and endogenous endophthalmitis

	Postoperative	Metastatic
Ocular cultures	Yes	Yes
Blood culture	No	Yes
Systemic investigation	No	Yes
Topical antibiotic	Yes	Yes
Systemic antibiotic	Oral fluoroquinolone	Intravenous (various)
Intravitreal antibiotics	Yes	Yes
Corticosteroid	Yes	No proven value
Visual outcome	70% > 6/60	70% < count fingers
Mortality	None	10%

Treatment

1. **Systemic infection** is treated with intravenous antibiotics. The choice is based on culture and sensitivity results and should continue for 2–3 weeks, or longer if there is endocarditis. Patients without an evident source of infection should be treated with a combination of ceftazidime 1 g every 12 hours and vancomycin 1 g every 12 hours. If an organism is identified, specialist microbiological advice should be obtained.

2. **Endophthalmitis** is treated with oral ciprofloxacin and intravitreal antibiotics, although the benefits of the latter are less clear than for acute postoperative bacterial endophthalmitis, which presents much earlier.

Prognosis

The prognosis is poor, with 70% of eyes reduced to light perception, probably as a result of delay in presentation and the virulence of the organism. Phthisis or evisceration occurs in 25%.

NB: There is a mortality of 5% to 10% from associated systemic disease.

ENDOGENOUS FUNGAL ENDOPHTHALMITIS

Pathogenesis

The major source of fungal infection within the eye is metastatic spread from a septic focus associated with catheters, intravenous drug abuse (Fig. 7.27), parenteral nutrition or chronic lung disease such as cystic fibrosis. Neutropenia following immunosuppression and AIDS are also major risk factors. Approximately 75% of isolates are *Candida* species (*C. albicans*, *C. parapsilosis*). Other pathogens include *Cryptococcus* species, *Sporothrix schenckii* and *Blastomyces* species.

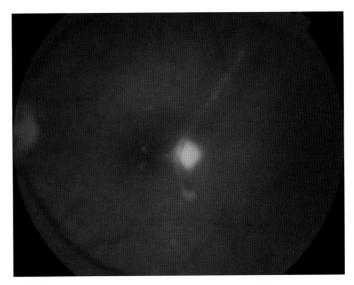

Fig. 7.28 Fungal retinitis

Diagnosis

1. **Presentation** is dependent on the location of the inflammatory focus. Peripheral lesions may cause little or no visual symptoms, while central lesions or those resulting in severe vitritis will manifest earlier. The progression is, however, much slower than in bacterial endophthalmitis.

2. **Signs**

- Anterior uveitis is uncommon in the early stages but may become prominent later.

- Creamy white retinal lesions with overlying vitritis (Fig. 7.28).

- Extension into the vitreous (Fig. 7.29).

- Floating vitreous 'cotton-ball' colonies (Fig. 7.30).

- Chronic endophthalmitis characterised by severe vitreous infiltration and abscess formation (Fig. 7.31).

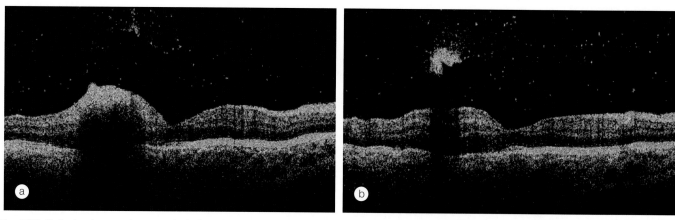

Fig. 7.29 Optical coherence tomography in fungal endophthalmitis. (a) Inflammatory focus is confined to the retina; (b) extension into the vitreous

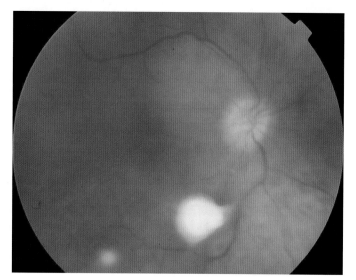

Fig. 7.30 Vitreous 'cotton-ball' colonies in fungal endophthalmitis

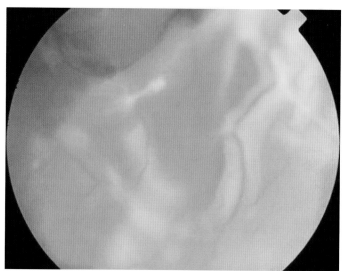

Fig. 7.32 Retinal detachment associated with fungal endophthalmitis

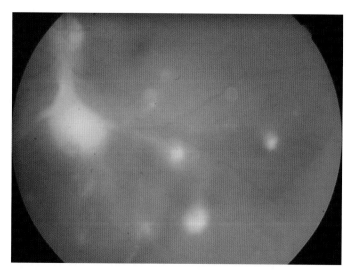

Fig. 7.31 Severe vitreous involvement in fungal endophthalmitis

3. **Course** is relatively chronic and may result in the development of retinal necrosis and retinal detachment associated with severe proliferative vitreoretinopathy (Fig. 7.32).

4. **Investigations** involving vitreous biopsy and smears and cultures may be required to confirm the diagnosis and test sensitivity of the organisms to antifungal agents.

Treatment

1. **Medical** treatment is indicated for systemic disease and ocular disease without vitreous involvement.

• Intravenous amphotericin 5% dextrose; the initial dose is 5 mg and after a few days can be increased to 20 mg.

• Oral fluconazole 100–200 mg/day (400–800 mg for disseminated disease) for 3 to 6 weeks. It can be used in conjunction with flucytosine (100 mg/kg/day).

- Oral voriconazole can be used to treat *Aspergillus*, *Fusarium*, *Scedosporium* and *Candida* species resistant to fluconazole.

NB: Systemic steroids are contraindicated in fungal infections.

2. **Pars plana vitrectomy** combined with intravitreal injection of amphotericin 5–10 µg in 0.1 ml is indicated in the presence of vitreous involvement.

FURTHER READING

Benz MS, Scott IU, Flynn HW Jr, et al. Endophthalmitis isolates and antibiotic sensitivities: a 6-year review of culture-proven cases. *Am J Ophthalmol* 2004;137:38–42.

Breit SM, Hariprasad SU, Mieler WF, et al. Management of endogenous fungal endophthalmitis with voriconazole and caspofungin. *Am J Ophthalmol* 2005;139:135–140.

Busbee BG, Recchia FM, Kaiser R, et al. Bleb-associated endophthalmitis. Clinical characteristics and visual outcomes. *Ophthalmology* 2004;111:1495–1503.

Chignell AH. Endogenous candidiasis. *J Royal Soc Med* 1992;85:721–724.

Ciulla TA. Update on acute and chronic endophthalmitis. *Ophthalmology* 1999;106:2237–2238.

Clark WL, Kaiser PK, Flynn HW Jr, et al. Treatment strategies and visual acuity outcomes in chronic postoperative P. acnes endophthalmitis. *Ophthalmology* 1999;106:1665–1670.

DeBry PW, Perkins TW, Heatley G, et al. Incidence of late-onset bleb-related complications following trabeculectomy with mitomycin. *Arch Ophthalmol* 2002;120:297–300.

Donahue SP, Greven CM, Zuravleff JJ, et al. Intraocular candidiasis in patients with candidemia. Clinical implications derived from a prospective multicenter study. *Ophthalmology* 1994;101:1302–1309.

Endophthalmitis Vitrectomy Study Group. Results of the Endophthalmitis Vitrectomy Study. A randomized trial of immediate vitrectomy and of intravenous antibiotics for the treatment of postoperative bacterial endophthalmitis. *Arch Ophthalmol* 1995;113:1479–1496.

Endophthalmitis Vitrectomy Study Group. Microbiologic factors and visual outcome in the Endophthalmitis Vitrectomy Study. *Am J Ophthalmol* 1996;122:830–846.

Ferguson AW, Scott JA, McGavigan J, et al. Comparison of 5% povidone-iodine solution against 1% povidone-iodine solution in preoperative cataract surgery antisepsis: a prospective randomized double-blind study. *Br J Ophthalmol* 2003;87:163–167.

Flynn HW Jr, Scott IU, Brod RD, et al. Current management of endophthalmitis. *Int Ophthalmol Clin* 2004;44:115–137.

Fox GM, Joondeph BC, Flynn HW Jr, et al. Delayed onset pseudophakic endophthalmitis. *Am J Ophthalmol* 1991;111:163.

Jackson TL, Eykyn SJ, Graham EM, et al. Endogenous bacterial endophthalmitis: a 17-year prospective series and review of 267 reported cases. *Surv Ophthalmol* 2003;48:403–423.

Jampel HD, Quigley HA, Kerrigan-Baumrind LA, et al. The Glaucoma Surgical Outcomes Study Group. Risk factors for late-onset infection following glaucoma filtration surgery. *Arch Ophthalmol* 2001;119:1001–1008.

Kamalarajah S, Silvestri G, Sharma N, et al. Surveillance of endophthalmitis following cataract surgery in the UK. *Eye* 2004;18:580–587.

Kunimoto DY, Das T, Sharma S, et al. Microbiologic spectrum and susceptibility of isolates: part 1. Postoperative endophthalmitis. Endophthalmitis Research Group. *Am J Ophthalmol* 1999;128:240–242.

Luttrull JK, Wan WL, Kubak BM, et al. Treatment of ocular fungal infections with oral fluconazole. *Am J Ophthalmol* 1995;119:477–481.

Mayer E, Cadman D, Ewings P, et al. A 10-year retrospective survey of cataract surgery and endophthalmitis in a single eye unit: injectable lenses lower the incidence of endophthalmitis. *Br J Ophthalmol* 2003;87:867–869.

Mieler WF, Ellis MK, Williams DF, et al. Retained intraocular foreign bodies and endophthalmitis. *Ophthalmology* 1990;97:1532.

Okada AA, Johnson RP, Liles C, et al. Endogenous bacterial endophthalmitis. *Ophthalmology* 1994;101:832–838.

Olson RJ. Reducing the risk of postoperative endophthalmitis. *Surv Ophthalmol* 2004;49:S55–S61.

Rao NA, Hidayat AA. Endogenous mycotic endophthalmitis: variations in clinical and histopathologic changes in candidiasis compared with aspergillosis. *Am J Ophthalmol* 2001;132:244–251.

Roth DB, Flynn HW Jr. Antibiotic selection in the treatment of endophthalmitis: the significance of combinations and synergy. *Surv Ophthalmol* 1997;41:395–401.

Samiy N, D'Amico DJ. Endogenous fungal endophthalmitis. *Int Opthalmol Clin* 1996;36:147–162.

Schiedler V, Scott IU, Flynn HW Jr, et al. Culture-proven endogenous endophthalmitis: clinical features and visual acuity outcomes. *Am J Ophthalmol* 2004;137:725–731.

Soltau JB, Rothman RF, Budenz DL, et al. Risk factors for glaucoma filtering bleb infections. *Arch Ophthalmol* 2000;118:338–342.

Song A, Scott IU, Flynn HW Jr, et al. Delayed-onset bleb-associated endophthalmitis. Clinical features and visual acuity outcomes. *Ophthalmology* 2002;109:985–991.

Thompson WS, Rubsamen PE, Flynn HW Jr, et al. Endophthalmitis after penetrating trauma. Risk factors and visual acuity outcomes. *Ophthalmology* 1995;102:1696–1701.

Waheed S, Ritterband DC, Greenfield DS, et al. New patterns of infecting organisms in late bleb-related endophthalmitis: a ten year review. *Eye* 1998;12:910–915.

Weishar PD, Flynn HW Jr, Murray TG, et al. Endogenous Aspergillus endophthalmitis. Clinical features and treatment outcomes. *Ophthalmology* 1998;105:57–65.

Winward KE, Pflugfelder SC, Flynn HW Jr, et al. Postoperative Propionibacterium endophthalmitis: treatment strategies and long term results. *Ophthalmology* 1993;100:447–451.

Wong JS, Chan TK, Lee HM, et al. Endogenous bacterial endophthalmitis: an East Asian experience and a reappraisal of a severe ocular affliction. *Ophthalmology* 2000;107:1483–1491.

Chapter **8**

Systemic diseases

This chapter describes the systemic diseases mentioned in the previous chapters. Ocular manifestations are indicated briefly because they are covered in the other chapters. Their importance is indicated by their order when listed.

CONNECTIVE TISSUE DISEASES

Rheumatoid arthritis (RA)

RA is an autoimmune disease characterised by a destructive, deforming, inflammatory polyarthropathy, in association with a spectrum of extra-articular manifestations and circulating antiglobulin antibodies, termed rheumatoid factors. It is much more common in females than males.

1. **Presentation** is in the fourth decade with joint swelling (Fig. 8.1).

2. **Signs**

   - Symmetric arthritis of the small joints of the hands and feet. Inflammation typically involves the proximal interphalangeal and spares the distal interphalangeal joints. The metacarpophalangeal and wrist joints are also commonly involved (Fig. 8.2).

   - Less frequent involvement of the shoulders, elbows, hips and cervical spine.

   - Joint instability secondary to chronic inflammation may result in subluxation and deformities, such as ulnar deviation of the metacarpophalangeal joints (Fig. 8.3).

   - Skin involvement includes subcutaneous 'rheumatoid' nodules over bony prominences (Fig. 8.4), vasculitis which may cause ulceration (Fig. 8.5), and, occasionally, pyoderma gangrenosum.

3. **Complications**

   - Pulmonary nodules and fibrosis (Fig. 8.6).

   - Multifocal neuropathy.

   - Septic arthritis.

   - Secondary amyloidosis.

   - Carpal tunnel syndrome.

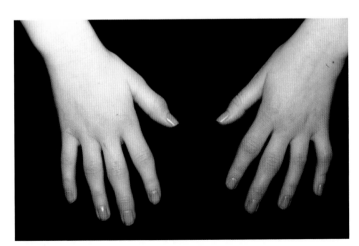

Fig. 8.1 Swelling of the fingers in early active rheumatoid arthritis

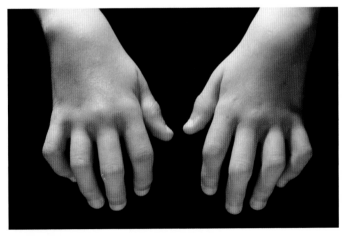

Fig. 8.2 More advanced involvement of the wrists and fingers in rheumatoid arthritis

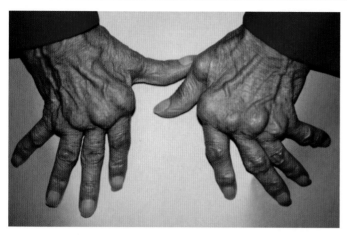

Fig. 8.3 Ulnar deviation of the hands in longstanding rheumatoid arthritis

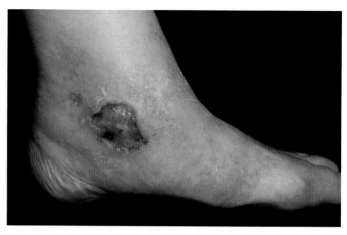

Fig. 8.5 Severe vasculitis resulting in ulceration

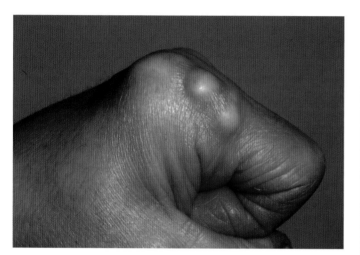

Fig. 8.4 'Rheumatoid' nodules

4. **Treatment** options include non-steroidal anti-inflammatory drugs (NSAIDs), gold salts, D-penicillamine, hydroxychloroquine, sulfasalazine, steroids and cytotoxic agents.

5. **Ocular features:** keratoconjunctivitis sicca (secondary Sjögren syndrome), scleritis, ulcerative keratitis and, rarely, acquired superior oblique tendon sheath syndrome.

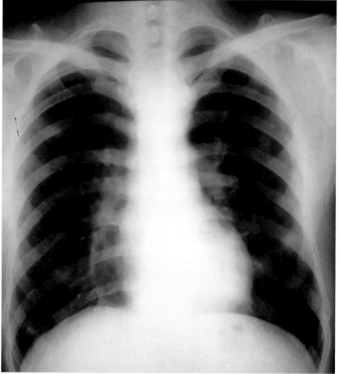

Fig. 8.6 Pulmonary fibrosis in rheumatoid disease

Juvenile idiopathic arthritis (JIA)

JIA is arthritis of at least 6 weeks' duration occurring before the age of 16 years when all other causes, such as infection, metabolic disorders and neoplasms, have been excluded. Females are affected more commonly by a 3:2 ratio. JIA is by far the most common disease associated with childhood anterior uveitis.

NB: JIA is not the same as juvenile rheumatoid arthritis (JRA); the former is negative for rheumatoid arthritis whereas the latter is positive. JRA is the same disease as RA except that it occurs before the age of 16 years.

1. **Presentation** is based on the onset and the extent of joint involvement during the first 6 months. Three types of presentation are recognised:

a. Pauciarticular-onset JIA involves four or fewer joints and accounts for about 60% of cases.

- Girls are affected five times as often as boys, with a peak age of onset around 2 years.

- The arthritis involves most commonly the knees (Fig. 8.7), although the ankles and wrists may also be affected.

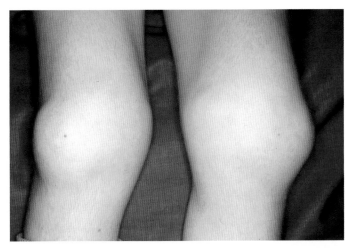

Fig. 8.7 Severe involvement of the knees in pauciarticular juvenile idiopathic arthritis

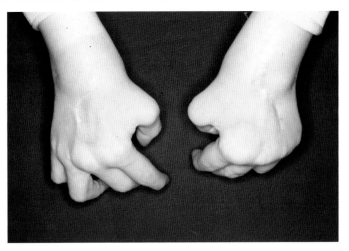

Fig. 8.9 Symmetric involvement of the hands in severe polyarticular juvenile idiopathic arthritis

Fig. 8.8 Early-onset juvenile idiopathic arthritis, which is a risk factor for chronic anterior uveitis

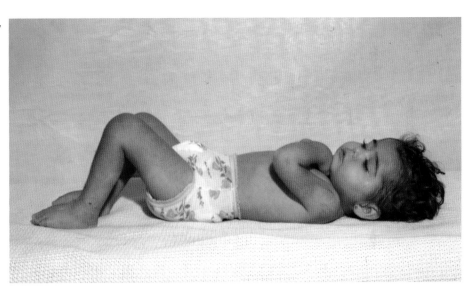

- Some patients in this subgroup remain pauciarticular, others subsequently develop a polyarthritis.

- About 75% of children are positive for antinuclear antibodies (ANA).

- Uveitis is common in this group and affects about 20% of children.

- Risk factors for uveitis are early onset of JIA (Fig. 8.8), and positive findings for ANA and HLA-DR5.

b. Polyarticular-onset JIA affects five or more joints and accounts for a further 20% of cases.

- Girls are affected about three times as often as boys and the disease may commence at any age throughout childhood.

- The arthritis involves both small (Fig. 8.9) and large joints symmetrically.

- Systemic features such as fever and rash are mild or absent.

- About 40% of children are ANA-positive.

- Uveitis occurs in about 5% of cases.

c. Systemic-onset JIA accounts for about 20% of cases.

- The disease occurs with equal frequency in boys and girls and may occur at any age throughout childhood.

- Systemic features include a high remittent fever, transient maculopapular rash (Fig. 8.10), generalised lymphadenopathy, hepatosplenomegaly and serositis.

- Initially, arthralgia or arthritis may be absent or minimal and a minority of patients subsequently develop progressive polyarthritis.

- The vast majority are negative for ANA.

- Uveitis does not occur.

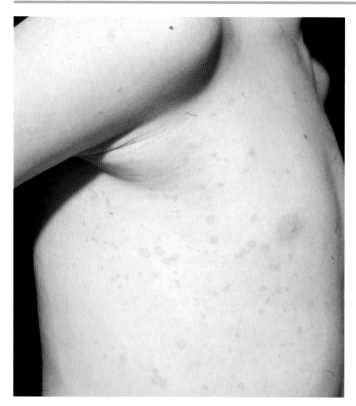

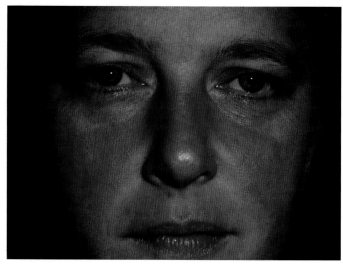

Fig. 8.11 'Butterfly' facial skin rash in systemic lupus erythematosus

Fig. 8.10 Maculopapular skin rash in systemic-onset juvenile idiopathic arthritis

NB: The term 'Still disease' is reserved for patients in this subgroup.

2. **Treatment** options include physiotherapy, NSAIDs, intraarticular triamcinolone hexacetonide injection and low-dose methotrexate.

3. **Ocular feature:** chronic anterior uveitis.

Systemic lupus erythematosus (SLE)

SLE is an autoimmune, non-organ-specific disease characterised by numerous autoantibodies and circulating immune complexes which mediate widespread vasculitis and tissue damage. It predominantly affects young females.

1. **Presentation** is in the third to fifth decades with fatigue without specific organ involvement. Alternatively, the disease may present with symmetric arthralgia.

2. **Signs**

* Mucocutaneous features include a 'butterfly' facial rash (Fig. 8.11), discoid rash, vasculitis, telangiectasia, photosensitivity, alopecia, oral ulceration and Raynaud phenomenon (Fig. 8.12).

* Arthritis, myositis and tendonitis.

* Glomerulonephritis.

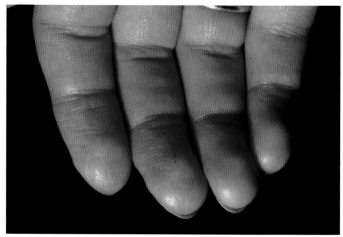

Fig. 8.12 Raynaud phenomenon involving the fingertips in systemic lupus erythematosus

* Pericarditis, endocarditis, myocarditis, and arterial and venous occlusion.

* Pleurisy, atelectasis and 'shrinking lungs'.

* Anaemia, thrombocytopenia, lymphopenia and leucopenia.

* Splenomegaly and lymphadenopathy.

* Polyneuritis, cranial nerve palsies, spinal cord lesions, epilepsy, stroke and psychosis.

3. **Diagnostic tests**

* The erythrocyte sedimentation rate (ESR) is raised, but C-reactive protein is usually not.

* A variety of autoantibodies, including lupus anticoagulant (Fig. 8.13), antiphospholipid and antinuclear, may be present.

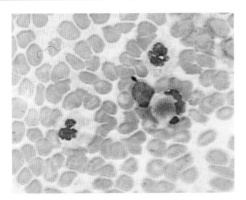

Fig. 8.13 'LE' cells

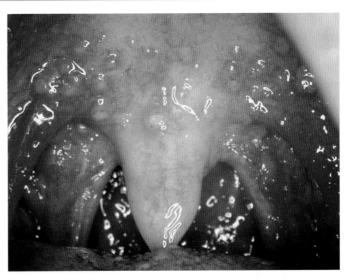

Fig. 8.15 Necrotising granulomas of the upper respiratory tract in Wegener granulomatosis (Courtesy of M A Mir, from *Atlas of Clinical Diagnosis*, Saunders, 2003)

4. **Treatment** options include antimalarials, NSAIDs, steroids and cytotoxic agents.

5. **Ocular features:** madarosis, keratoconjunctivitis sicca, scleritis, peripheral ulcerative keratitis, retinal vasculitis and optic neuropathy.

Wegener granulomatosis

Wegener granulomatosis is an idiopathic, multisystem, granulomatous disorder characterised by generalised small vessel vasculitis (Fig. 8.14) affecting predominantly the respiratory tract and kidneys. It affects males more commonly than females. Because the disease can be localised to the eye and the orbit, without any systemic involvement, orbital biopsy may be required for diagnosis.

1. **Presentation** is in the fifth decade, often with pulmonary symptoms.

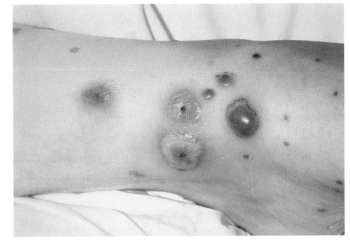

Fig. 8.16 Cutaneous vasculitis and bullae in Wegener granulomatosis (Courtesy of M A Mir, from *Atlas of Clinical Diagnosis*, Saunders, 2003)

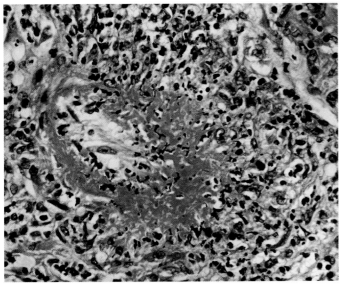

Fig. 8.14 Histology in Wegener granulomatosis, showing fibrinoid necrosis of the vessel wall and granulomatous inflammation (Courtesy of Watson, Hazleman, Pavésio and Green, from *The Sclera and Systemic Disorders*, 2nd edition, Butterworth-Heineman, 2004)

2. **Signs**

- Upper respiratory tract involvement by necrotising granulomatous inflammation (Fig. 8.15) may result in perforation of the nasal septum, 'saddle-shaped' nasal deformity and nasal–paranasal fistulae.

- Cutaneous vasculitis and bullae (Fig. 8.16).

- Lower respiratory tract involvement may result in nodular lesions, infiltrates and cavitation with fluid levels (Fig. 8.17).

- Necrotising glomerulonephritis, with renal failure.

- Focal vasculitis involving the spleen, heart and adrenals.

- Polyneuritis and meningoencephalitis.

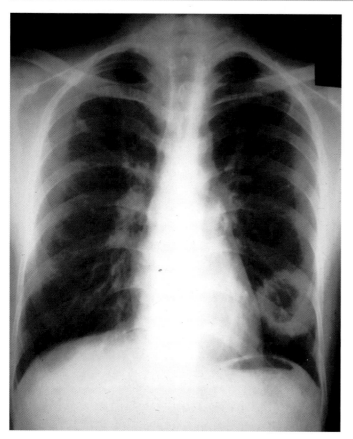

Fig. 8.17 Chest radiograph showing cavitation in Wegener granulomatosis

3. **Diagnostic tests.** Antineutrophil cytoplasmic antibodies (c-ANCA) are found in over 90% of patients with active disease.

4. **Treatment** is with systemic steroids and cyclophosphamide.

5. **Ocular features:** scleritis, peripheral ulcerative keratitis, occlusive retinal periarteritis, orbital pseudotumour, nasolacrimal obstruction and dacryocystitis.

Polyarteritis nodosa (PAN)

PAN is an idiopathic, potentially lethal disease affecting medium-sized and small arteries (Fig. 8.18). It is three times

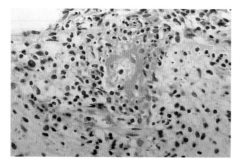

Fig. 8.18 Histology showing fibrinoid necrosis and an inflammatory infiltrate with polymorphs in polyarteritis nodosa (Courtesy of P-M G Bouloux, from *Clinical Medicine Assessment Questions in Colour*, Wolfe, 1993)

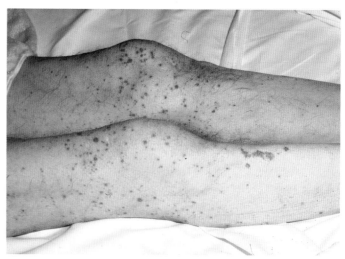

Fig. 8.19 Purpura in polyarteritis nodosa

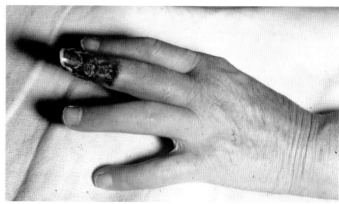

Fig. 8.20 Gangrene in polyarteritis nodosa

more common in males than in females. Ocular involvement may precede the systemic manifestations by several years.

1. **Presentation** is in the third to sixth decades with tachycardia, myalgia, arthralgia, fever and weight loss.

2. **Signs**

- Cutaneous signs include purpura (Fig. 8.19), gangrene (Fig. 8.20) and livedo reticularis (Fig. 8.21).

- Muscular weakness and tenderness.

- Renal involvement and hypertension.

- Coronary arteritis, which may lead to heart failure and myocardial infarction.

- Gastrointestinal bleeding or an acute abdominal crisis.

- Stroke or multifocal neuropathy.

3. **Diagnostic tests** show eosinophilia, hypergammaglobulinaemia and necrotising lesions on skin biopsy.

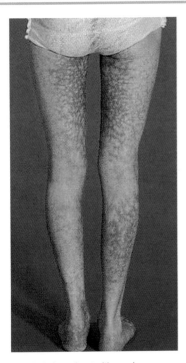

Fig. 8.21 Livedo reticularis in polyarteritis nodosa

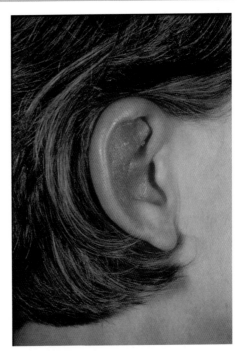

Fig. 8.22 Swelling of the pinna in relapsing polychondritis

4. **Treatment** is with systemic steroids and cytotoxic agents.

5. **Ocular features:** necrotising scleritis, peripheral ulcerative keratitis, orbital pseudotumour and occlusive retinal periarteritis.

Relapsing polychondritis

Relapsing polychondritis is a rare idiopathic condition characterised by small vessel vasculitis involving cartilage, resulting in recurrent, often progressive, inflammatory episodes involving multiple organ systems. It most frequently affects patients between the ages of 40 and 60 years.

1. **Signs**

* Recurrent swelling of the pinnae (Fig. 8.22).

* Involvement of the tracheobronchial cartilage may give rise to hoarse voice, cough and stridor.

* Collapse of the tip of the nose (Fig. 8.23).

* Cardiac valve dysfunction.

* Non-erosive inflammatory polyarthritis.

* Cochlear or vestibular damage resulting in neurosensory hearing loss, tinnitus or vertigo.

2. **Treatment.** Mild ear disease usually responds to systemic NSAIDs but major organ involvement requires high-dose systemic steroids in combination with cytotoxic drugs.

3. **Ocular features:** scleritis and acute anterior uveitis.

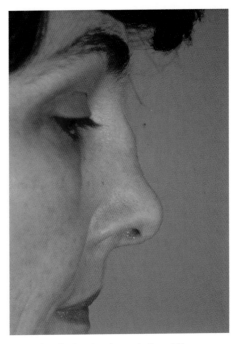

Fig. 8.23 Nasal deformity in relapsing polychondritis

Sjögren syndrome

Sjögren syndrome is characterised by autoimmune inflammation and destruction of lacrimal and salivary glands (Fig. 8.24). The condition is classified as primary when it exists in isolation, and secondary when associated with other diseases such as RA, SLE, systemic sclerosis, primary biliary cirrho-

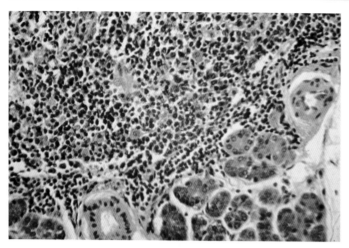

Fig. 8.24 Histology of a lacrimal gland in Sjögren syndrome, showing lymphocytic infiltration

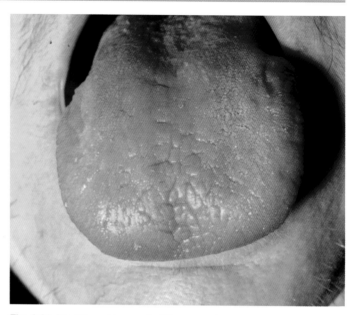

Fig. 8.26 Dry fissured tongue in Sjögren syndrome.

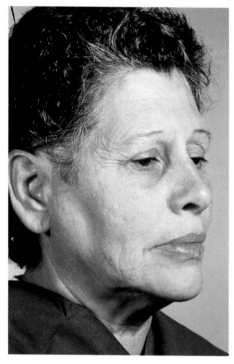

Fig. 8.25 Enlargement of the parotid gland in Sjögren syndrome (Courtesy of M A Mir, from *Atlas of Clinical Diagnosis*, Saunders, 2003)

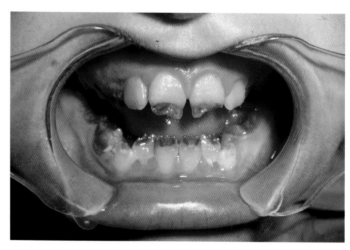

Fig. 8.27 Severe dental caries in Sjögren syndrome (Courtesy of M A Mir, from *Atlas of Clinical Diagnosis*, Saunders, 2003)

sis, chronic active hepatitis and myasthenia gravis. Primary Sjögren syndrome affects females more commonly than males.

1. **Presentation** is in adult life with grittiness of the eyes and dryness of the mouth.

2. **Signs**

- Enlargement of salivary glands (Fig. 8.25) and, occasionally, lacrimal glands, with secondary diminished salivary flow rate and a dry fissured tongue (Fig. 8.26).

- Dry nasal passages, diminished vaginal secretions and dyspareunia.

- Raynaud phenomenon and cutaneous vasculitis.

3. **Complications**

- Dental caries (Fig. 8.27).

- Reflux oesophagitis and gastritis.

- Malabsorption due to pancreatic failure.

- Pulmonary disease, renal disease and polyneuropathy.

4. **Diagnostic tests:** serum autoantibodies, Schirmer test, and biopsy of minor salivary glands.

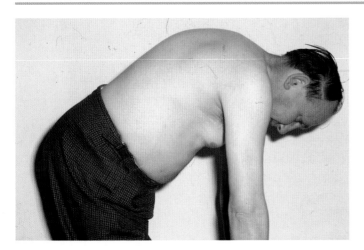

Fig. 8.28 Limitation of flexion in ankylosing spondylitis

5. **Treatment options** include systemic steroids and cytotoxic agents.

6. **Ocular features:** keratoconjunctivitis sicca and Adie pupil (rare).

SPONDYLOARTHROPATHIES

Ankylosing spondylitis (AS)

AS is characterised by inflammation, calcification and finally ossification of ligaments and capsules of joints with resultant bony ankylosis of the axial skeleton. It typically affects males, 90% of whom are HLA-B27-positive; some patients also have inflammatory bowel disease (enteropathic arthritis).

1. **Presentation** is in early adulthood with insidious onset of pain and stiffness in the lower back or buttocks. This is initially worse after inactivity, but may be aggravated by weight bearing.

2. **Signs**

a. *Arthritis.* In order of frequency, the joints most affected are the sacroiliac, spine, hips, ribs and shoulders. Progressive limitation of spinal movements occurs (Fig. 8.28); the spine characteristically becomes fixed in flexion (Fig. 8.29). Reduced mobility of the thoracic cage may predispose to pulmonary infection.

b. *Enthesopathy* characterised by inflammation and pain at ligamentous attachments to bone.

3. **Complications** include apical pulmonary fibrosis, aortic incompetence and cardiac conduction defects.

4. **Diagnostic tests.** The ESR is raised. Radiology of the sacroiliac joints reveals juxta-articular osteoporosis in the early stages, later followed by sclerosis and bony obliteration of the joint. The spinal ligaments may also manifest calcification ('bamboo spine') (Fig. 8.30), as may other joints involved by the inflammatory process.

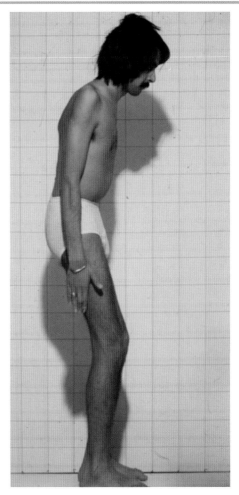

Fig. 8.29 Early flexion deformity in ankylosing spondylitis

NB: Radiological changes often predate clinical symptoms.

5. **Treatment** options include physiotherapy, NSAIDs, sulfasalazine and intra-articular steroid injections. Surgical correction of bony deformities may be necessary.

6. **Ocular features:** acute anterior uveitis and rarely scleritis.

Reiter syndrome (RS)

RS, also referred to as reactive arthritis, is characterised by the triad of non-specific (non-gonococcal) urethritis, conjunctivitis and arthritis. Although relatively rare, RS develops in 1–3% of men after non-specific urethritis, up to 4% of persons after enteric infections caused by *Shigella*, *Salmonella* and *Campylobacter*, and in a higher proportion of patients with *Yersinia* enteric infections. Post-dysenteric RS affects males and females equally, whereas post-venereal RS is more common in men. About 85% of patients with RS are positive for HLA-B27, but the diagnosis is clinical and is

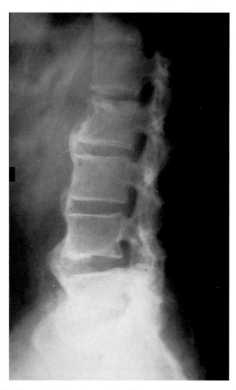

Fig. 8.30 Radiograph showing a 'bamboo spine' due to ossification of ligaments

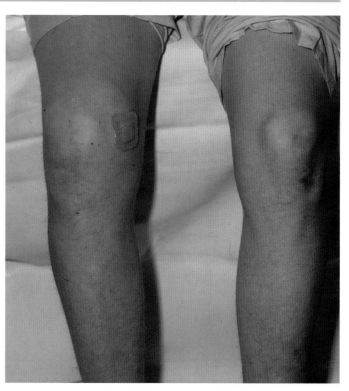

Fig. 8.31 Asymmetric arthritis of the knees in Reiter syndrome

based on the presence of arthritis and other characteristic manifestations.

1. **Presentation** is between the second and fourth decades with non-specific urethritis, conjunctivitis and arthritis, occurring within a short period of each other, classically a month after dysentery or sexual intercourse. However, presentation may be insidious.

2. **Signs**

a. ***Peripheral arthritis*** is typically acute in onset, asymmetric and migratory. Two to four joints tend to be involved, most commonly the knees (Fig. 8.31), ankles and toes. In some patients, peripheral arthritis may be recurrent or become chronic.

b. ***Spondyloarthritis*** (spondylitis and sacroiliitis) affects about 30% of patients with severe chronic RS and is related to the presence of HLA-B27.

c. ***Enthesopathy*** may manifest as plantar fasciitis, Achilles tenosynovitis (Fig. 8.32), bursitis and calcaneal periostitis; reactive bone formation in the latter may result in a calcaneal spur.

d. ***Mucocutaneous*** features include painless mouth ulceration, keratoderma blenorrhagica involving the palms and soles (Fig. 8.33), circinate balanitis (Fig. 8.34) and nail dystrophy.

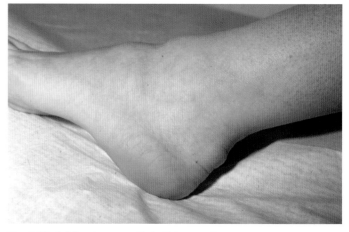

Fig. 8.32 Achilles tenosynovitis in Reiter syndrome

e. ***Genitourinary*** features include cystitis, cervicitis, prostatitis, epididymitis and orchitis.

f. ***Other manifestations*** include cardiac disease, amyloidosis, thrombophlebitis, pleurisy, diarrhoea, neuropathy and meningoencephalitis.

3. **Treatment** is with NSAIDs.

4. **Ocular features:** conjunctivitis, acute anterior uveitis, nummular keratitis, episcleritis, scleritis, papillitis and retinal vasculitis.

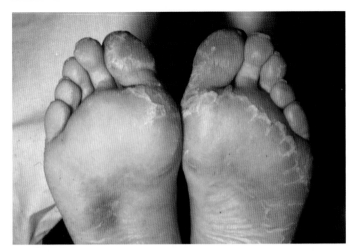

Fig. 8.33 Keratoderma blenorrhagica in Reiter syndrome

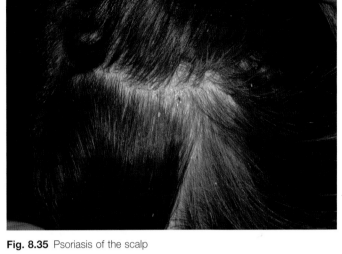

Fig. 8.35 Psoriasis of the scalp

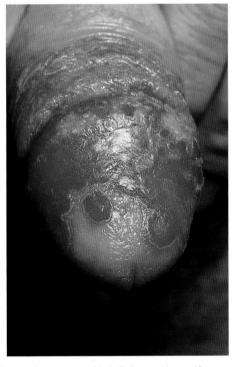

Fig. 8.34 Severe circinate balanitis in Reiter syndrome (Courtesy of Emond, Welsby and Rowland, from *Colour Atlas of Systemic Diseases*, Mosby, 2003)

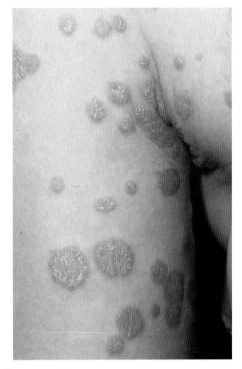

Fig. 8.36 Plaque psoriasis

Psoriatic arthritis

About 7% of patients with psoriasis develop arthritis. Psoriatic arthritis affects both sexes equally and is associated with an increased prevalence of HLA-B27 and HLA-B17.

1. **Presentation** is in the third to fourth decades.

2. **Signs**

a. Skin

- Plaque psoriasis (most common) is characterised by well-demarcated, salmon-pink areas covered with thick, silvery plaques (Figs 8.35 and 8.36).

- Flexural psoriasis is characterised by non-scaly pink lesions, usually affecting the groin and perineum.

b. Nail dystrophy is characterised by pitting, transverse depression and onycholysis (Fig. 8.37).

c. Arthritis may take one of the following patterns:

- Asymmetric involvement of the distal interphalangeal joints, which may give rise to sausage-shaped deformities (Fig. 8.38).

- Pauciarticular peripheral involvement.

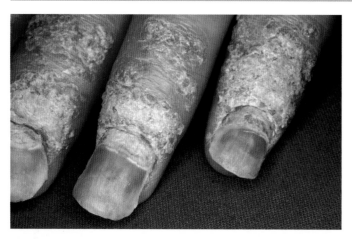

Fig. 8.37 Psoriatic nail dystrophy

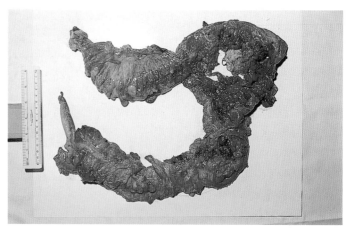

Fig. 8.39 Surgical specimen of ulcerative colitis

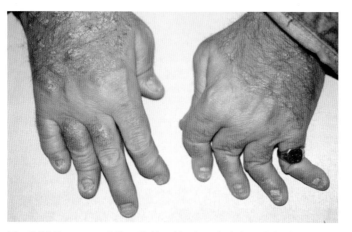

Fig. 8.38 Severe psoriatic arthritis with ulnar deviation of the fingers and severe nail dystrophy

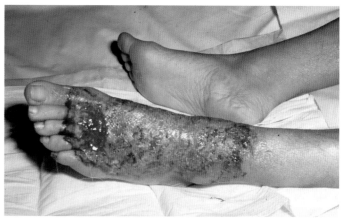

Fig. 8.40 Pyoderma gangrenosum in ulcerative colitis

- Symmetric peripheral involvement similar to rheumatoid arthritis.

- Arthritis mutilans affecting a few digits is rare.

- Associated AS.

3. **Treatment** involves NSAIDs, intra-articular steroids and cytotoxic drugs for severe disease.

4. **Ocular features:** anterior uveitis, conjunctivitis, marginal corneal infiltrates and secondary Sjögren syndrome.

INFLAMMATORY BOWEL DISEASE

Ulcerative colitis (UC)

UC is an idiopathic, chronic, relapsing inflammatory disease involving the rectum and extending proximally to involve part or all of the large intestine. The disease is characterised by diffuse surface ulceration of the mucosa, with the develop-ment of crypt abscesses and pseudopolyps (Fig. 8.39). Patients with longstanding disease carry an increased risk of developing carcinoma of the colon.

1. **Presentation** is in the second to third decades with bloody diarrhoea, lower abdominal cramps, urgency and tenesmus. Constitutional symptoms include tiredness, weight loss, malaise and fever.

2. **Extraintestinal manifestations**

a. *Mucocutaneous* features include oral aphthous ulceration, erythema nodosum and pyoderma gangrenosum (Fig. 8.40).

b. *Skeletal* manifestations include asymmetric lower limb arthritis of large joints; sacroiliitis and AS may develop in HLA-B27-positive patients.

c. *Hepatic disease* may be in the form of autoimmune hepatitis, sclerosing cholangitis and cholangiocarcinoma.

d. *Thromboses*, which may involve both arteries and veins.

e. *Secondary amyloidosis.*

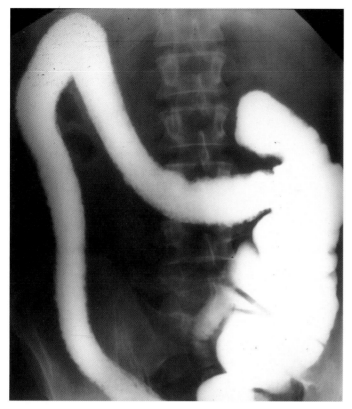

Fig. 8.41 Barium meal in ulcerative colitis, showing pseudopolyposis, lack of haustral markings and straightening of the ascending and transverse colon

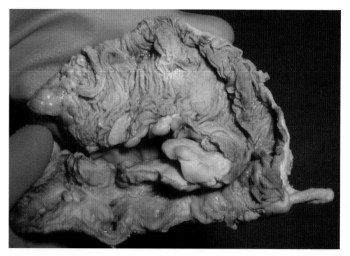

Fig. 8.42 Surgical specimen of Crohn disease involving the ileocaecal region

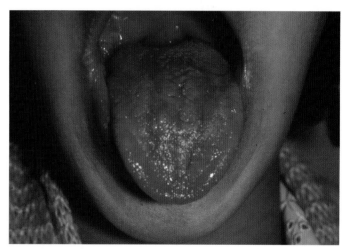

Fig. 8.43 Glossitis in Crohn disease

3. **Diagnostic tests** involve barium enema (Fig. 8.41), endoscopy and biopsy.

4. **Treatment** options include systemic steroids, sulfasalazine, immunosuppressive agents and colectomy.

5. **Ocular features:** acute anterior uveitis, peripheral corneal infiltrates, conjunctivitis, episcleritis, scleritis, papillitis and retinal vasculitis.

Crohn disease

Crohn disease (regional ileitis) is an idiopathic, chronic, relapsing disease characterised by multifocal, full-thickness, non-caseating granulomatous inflammation of the intestinal wall. It most frequently involves the ileocaecal region (Fig. 8.42) but any area of the bowel, including the mouth, may be affected.

1. **Presentation** is in the second to third decades with fever, weight loss, diarrhoea and abdominal pain.

2. **Extraintestinal manifestations**

a. *Oral* lesions include glossitis (Fig. 8.43) and aphthous ulceration.

b. *Cutaneous* lesions consist of erythema nodosum, pyoderma gangrenosum and psoriasis.

c. *Skeletal* findings include finger clubbing, acute peripheral arthritis, sacroiliitis and ankylosing spondylitis.

3. **Complications** include intestinal obstruction due to stricture formation (Fig. 8.44), perirectal fistulae, abscesses and fissures, and liver disease.

4. **Diagnostic tests** involve endoscopy and biopsy.

5. **Treatment** options include nutritional support, steroids, antibiotics, immunosuppressive agents and surgery.

6. **Ocular features:** acute anterior uveitis, conjunctivitis, episcleritis, peripheral corneal infiltrates and retinal periphlebitis.

Fig. 8.45 shows a summary of systemic manifestations of inflammatory bowel disease.

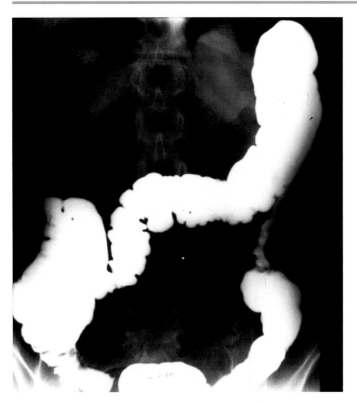

Fig. 8.44 Barium meal in Crohn disease, showing a stricture involving the descending colon

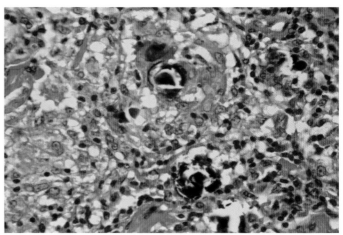

Fig. 8.46 Histology of sarcoid granuloma, showing many epithelioid cells, lymphocytes and a few multinucleated Langerhans type giant cells (Courtesy of P-M G Bouloux, from *Clinical Medicine Assessment Questions in Colour*, Wolfe, 1993)

NON-INFECTIOUS MULTISYSTEM DISEASES

Sarcoidosis

Sarcoidosis is a T-lymphocyte-mediated, non-caseating granulomatous inflammatory disorder of unknown cause (Fig. 8.46). It is most common in colder climates, although it also more frequently affects patients of African descent than Caucasians. The clinical spectrum of disease varies from mild single-organ involvement to potentially fatal multisystem disease that can affect almost any tissue. The tissues most commonly involved are the mediastinal and superficial lymph nodes, lungs, liver, spleen, skin, parotid glands, phalangeal bones and the eye (Fig. 8.47).

Presentation

1. **Acute-onset** sarcoidosis presents in one of the following ways:

a. **Löfgren syndrome** is characterised by erythema nodosum and bilateral hilar lymphadenopathy, often accompanied by fever and/or arthralgia.

b. **Heerfordt syndrome** (uveoparotid fever) is characterised by uveitis, parotid gland enlargement, fever and often facial nerve palsy.

2. **Insidious-onset** sarcoidosis typically occurs during the fifth decade with pulmonary involvement resulting in cough and dyspnoea, or extrapulmonary signs.

Pulmonary disease

Stage 1: Bilateral asymptomatic hilar lymphadenopathy (Fig. 8.48); spontaneous resolution occurs within 1 year in most cases.

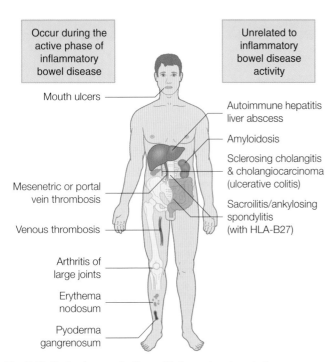

Occur during the active phase of inflammatory bowel disease

Unrelated to inflammatory bowel disease activity

Mouth ulcers

Autoimmune hepatitis liver abscess

Amyloidosis

Sclerosing cholangitis & cholangiocarcinoma (ulcerative colitis)

Mesenetric or portal vein thrombosis

Sacroilitis/ankylosing spondylitis (with HLA-B27)

Venous thrombosis

Arthritis of large joints

Erythema nodosum

Pyoderma gangrenosum

Fig. 8.45 Systemic complications of inflammatory bowel disease

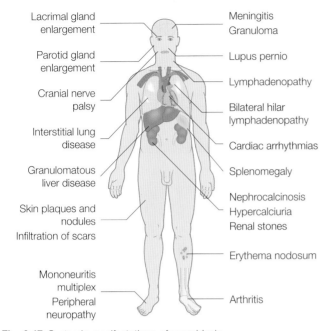

Lacrimal gland enlargement
Parotid gland enlargement
Cranial nerve palsy
Interstitial lung disease
Granulomatous liver disease
Skin plaques and nodules
Infiltration of scars
Mononeuritis multiplex
Peripheral neuropathy

Meningitis
Granuloma
Lupus pernio
Lymphadenopathy
Bilateral hilar lymphadenopathy
Cardiac arrhythmias
Splenomegaly
Nephrocalcinosis
Hypercalciuria
Renal stones
Erythema nodosum
Arthritis

Fig. 8.47 Systemic manifestations of sarcoidosis

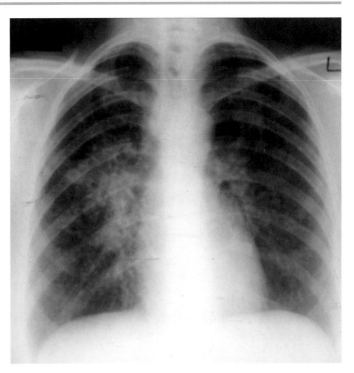

Fig. 8.49 Bilateral hilar lymphadenopathy and parenchymal infiltrates

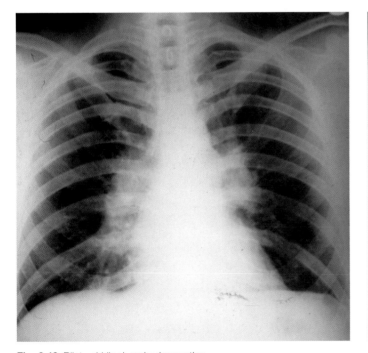

Fig. 8.48 Bilateral hilar lymphadenopathy

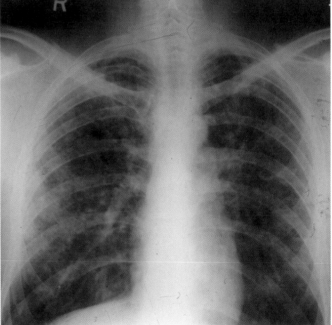

Fig. 8.50 Parenchymal infiltrates

Stage 2: Bilateral hilar lymphadenopathy and diffuse parenchymal reticulonodular infiltrates (Fig. 8.49); spontaneous resolution occurs in the majority.

Stage 3: Reticulonodular infiltrates alone (Fig. 8.50); spontaneous resolution is less common.

Stage 4: Pulmonary fibrosis, which may result in progressive ventilatory failure, pulmonary hypertension and cor pulmonale (Fig. 8.51).

Skin lesions

The skin is involved in about 25% of patients by one of the following:

1. **Erythema nodosum** are tender erythematous plaques, typically involving the shins (Fig. 8.52) and occasionally the thighs and forearms.

271

2. **Granulomas** are characterised by scattered papules, plaques or nodules (Fig. 8.53).

3. **Lupus pernio**, which is characterised by indurated, purple–blue lesions involving exposed parts of the body such as the nose, cheeks or ears (Fig. 8.54).

4. **Granulomatous deposits** (Fig. 8.55) in longstanding scars or tattoos.

Other manifestations

1. **Neurological** disease affects about 5–10% of patients. The most common lesion is unilateral facial nerve palsy (Fig. 8.56); less common manifestations include seizures, meningitis, peripheral neuropathy and psychiatric symptoms.

2. **Arthritis** in chronic sarcoidosis is typically symmetric and may involve both small and large joints.

NB: In children, the presentation can be very similar to that of JIA, because arthropathy tends to be more prominent than pulmonary disease.

3. **Renal disease** in the form of nephrocalcinosis, hypercalciuria and renal stones.

4. **Miscellaneous** involvement includes lymphadenopathy, granulomatous liver disease, splenomegaly and cardiac arrhythmias.

Diagnostic tests

1. **Chest radiographs** are abnormal in 90%.

2. **Biopsy**

- Biopsy of the lungs gives the greatest yield (90%), even in asymptomatic patients with normal chest radiograms.

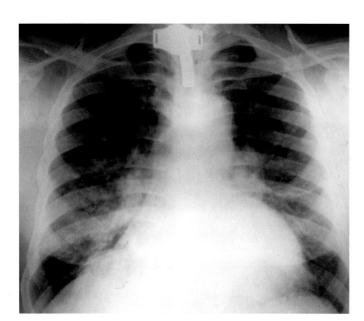

Fig. 8.51 Pulmonary fibrosis

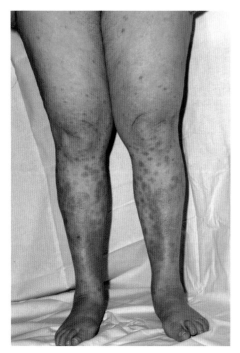

Fig. 8.52 Erythema nodosum

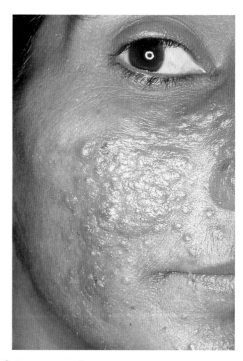

Fig. 8.53 Cutaneous granulomas

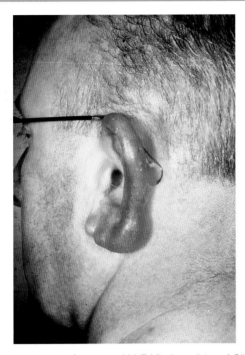

Fig. 8.54 Lupus pernio (Courtesy of M F Mir, from *Atlas of Clinical Diagnosis*, Saunders, 2003)

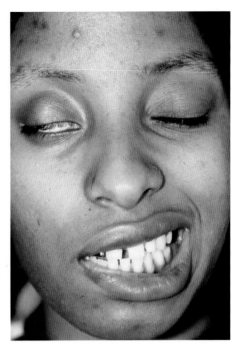

Fig. 8.56 Right facial palsy

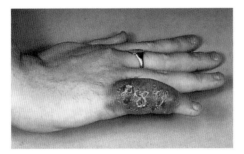

Fig. 8.55 Granulomatous sarcoid deposition (Courtesy of P-M G Bouloux, from *Clinical Medicine Assessment Questions in Colour*, Wolfe, 1993)

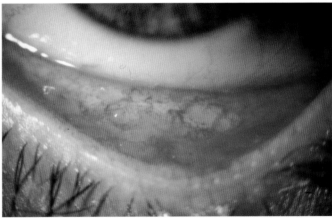

Fig. 8.57 Conjunctival sarcoid granulomas

- Biopsy of the conjunctiva is positive in about 70% of patients with granulomatous inflammation of the conjunctiva in the form of nodules (Fig. 8.57), which resemble follicular conjunctivitis.

- Biopsy of lacrimal glands is positive in 25% of unenlarged and 75% of enlarged glands (Fig. 8.58).

- Biopsy of a superficial lymph node or skin lesion.

3. Serum angiotensin-converting enzyme (ACE) is elevated in patients with active disease but normal during remissions. The normal serum level in adults is 32.1 ± 8.5 IU. In children, the levels tend to be higher and diagnostically less useful. In patients with suspected neurosarcoid, ACE can be measured in the cerebrospinal fluid (CSF).

NB: ACE may also be elevated in other conditions such as tuberculosis, lymphoma and asbestosis.

4. Bronchoalveolar lavage shows a raised proportion of activated T-helper lymphocytes. Sputum examination may also show increased CD4/CD8 ratios.

5. Pulmonary function tests reveal a restrictive lung defect with reduced total lung capacity and are very useful for monitoring disease activity and the need for systemic therapy.

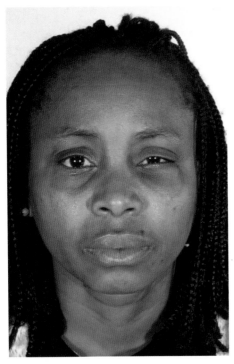

Fig. 8.58 Involvement of the left lacrimal gland in sarcoidosis

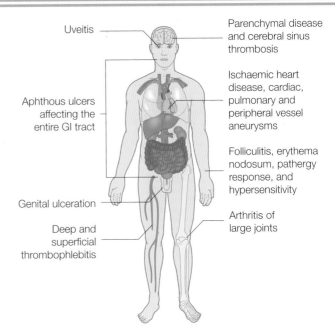

Fig. 8.59 Systemic manifestations of Behçet syndrome

6. **Mantoux test** is negative in most patients. A strongly positive reaction to one tuberculin unit makes the diagnosis of sarcoidosis highly unlikely.

Treatment

Patients with stage 1 and 2 pulmonary disease seldom require treatment, because spontaneous resolution is the rule. Troublesome erythema nodosum, pyrexia and arthralgia may benefit from NSAIDs. Systemic corticosteroids are usually effective in patients with symptomatic stage 3 pulmonary disease or involvement of vital organs. Methotrexate may be used as a steroid-sparing agent.

Ocular features

Uveitis is the most common manifestation, and may be in the form of anterior, posterior or intermediate. Other manifestations include keratoconjunctivitis sicca, conjunctival nodules and optic neuropathy.

Behçet syndrome (BS)

BS is an idiopathic disease characterised by recurrent episodes of orogenital ulceration and vasculitis which may involve small, medium and large veins and arteries (Fig. 8.59). The disease typically affects patients from the eastern Mediterranean region and Japan, and is strongly associated with HLA-B51 in different ethnic groups. However, it is not clear whether the HLA-B51 itself is the pathogenic gene related to BS or some other gene is in linkage disequilibrium with

HLA-B51. The peak age of onset of BS is in the third decade, although rarely it presents in childhood or old age; males are affected more frequently than females.

Diagnostic criteria

1. **Recurrent oral ulceration** characterised by minor aphthous (Fig. 8.60), major aphthous (Fig. 8.61) or herpetiform ulcerative lesions that have recurred at least three times in a 12-month period.

2. **Plus at least two of the following:**

* Recurrent genital ulceration (Fig. 8.62).

* Ocular inflammation.

* Skin lesions include erythema nodosum, folliculitis, acneiform nodules and papulopustular lesions (Fig. 8.63).

* Positive pathergy test, which is characterised by the formation of a pustule at the site of a sterile needle prick after 24–48 hours.

Non-diagnostic manifestations

1. **Major vascular complications**

* Aneurysms of the pulmonary and/or systemic arterial system.

* Venous thrombosis, which may involve superficial veins (Fig. 8.64), deep veins (Fig. 8.65), vena cava (Fig. 8.66), portohepatic vein and cerebral sinuses.

* Coronary artery disease, cardiomyopathy and valvular disease.

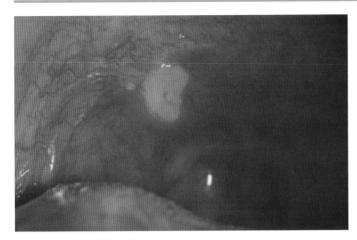

Fig. 8.60 Minor aphthous ulcer

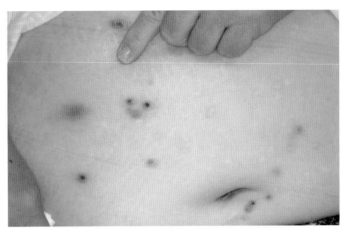

Fig. 8.63 Papulopustular skin lesions (Courtesy of P Saine)

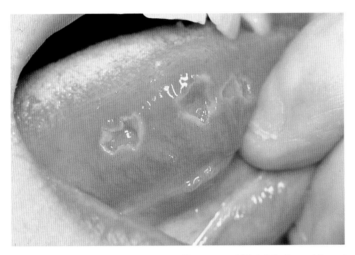

Fig. 8.61 Major aphthous ulceration (Courtesy of M A Mir, from *Atlas of Clinical Diagnosis*, Saunders, 2003)

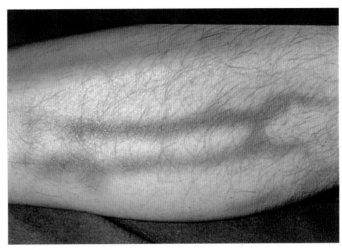

Fig. 8.64 Thrombophlebitis (Courtesy of M A Mir, from *Atlas of Clinical Diagnosis*, Mosby, 2003)

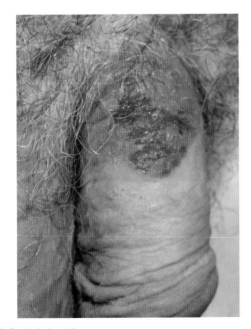

Fig. 8.62 Genital ulceration

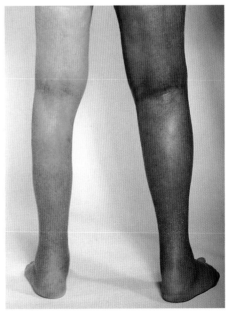

Fig. 8.65 Deep vein thrombosis (Courtesy of M A Mir, from *Atlas of Clinical Diagnosis*, Mosby, 2003)

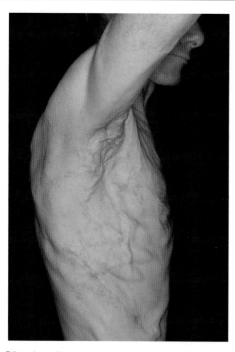

Fig. 8.66 Dilated collateral abdominal veins following vena caval thrombosis

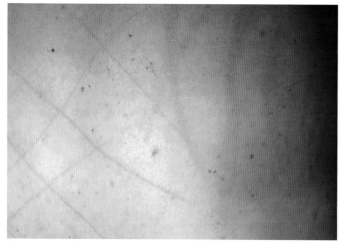

Fig. 8.67 Dermatographia

2. **Arthritis** occurs in 50% of patients. It is typically mild and involves a few large joints, particularly the knees. AS is much less common.

3. **Skin**

- Hypersensitivity demonstrated by the formation of erythematous lines following stroking of the skin (dermatographia) (Fig. 8.67).

- Vasculitis.

4. **Gastrointestinal ulceration** is less common and may involve the oesophagus, stomach or intestines.

5. **Neurological manifestations** occur in 5% of patients and mainly involve the brain stem, although meningo-encephalitis and spinal cord disease may also occur.

6. **Other** uncommon manifestations include glomerulo-nephritis and epididymitis, which is uncommon but very specific.

Treatment

Annoying oral ulceration is treated with steroid mouthwashes or pastes. Systemic disease requires systemic steroids in combination with other immunosuppressive agents.

Ocular features

Panuveitis is common. Other less common manifestations include conjunctivitis, conjunctival ulceration, episcleritis, scleritis, and ophthalmoplegia from neurological involvement.

Vogt–Koyanagi–Harada syndrome (VKH)

VKH syndrome is an idiopathic, autoimmune disease against melanocytes, causing inflammation of melanocyte-containing tissues such as the uvea, ear and meninges.

VKH predominantly affects Hispanics, Japanese and pigmented individuals. In different racial groups, the disease is associated with HLA-DR1 and HLA-DR4, suggesting a common immunogenic predisposition.

In practice, VKH can be subdivided into Vogt–Koyanagi disease, characterised mainly by skin changes and anterior uveitis, and Harada disease, in which neurological features and exudative retinal detachments predominate. Possible trigger factors include cutaneous injury or a viral infection, which may lead to sensitisation of melanocytes.

Phases

1. **Prodromal** phase lasting a few days is characterised by neurological and auditory manifestations.

- Meningitis causing headache and neck stiffness.

- Encephalopathy is less frequent and may manifest as convulsions, paresis and cranial nerve palsies.

- Auditory features include tinnitus, vertigo and deafness.

2. **Acute uveitic** phase follows soon thereafter and is characterised by bilateral non-granulomatous anterior or multifocal posterior uveitis and exudative retinal detachments.

3. **Convalescent** phase follows several weeks later and is characterised by:

- Localised alopecia, poliosis and vitiligo (Fig. 8.68).

- Diffuse depigmentation of the fundus ('sunset-glow' fundus) and depigmented limbal lesions (Sugiura sign).

4. Chronic-recurrent phase is characterised by smouldering granulomatous anterior uveitis with exacerbations.

Diagnostic criteria

These are shown in Table 8.1.

Multiple sclerosis (MS)

MS is a demyelinating disease that typically affects young adults. The characteristic pathologic feature is the presence of focal destruction of myelin sheaths in the CNS accompanied by inflammation (Fig. 8.69).

1. Presentation is with recurrent attacks of focal or multi-focal neurological dysfunction which typically worsen and then remit.

2. Signs

* Spinal cord involvement may cause weakness, stiffness, sphincter disturbance and sensory loss with a 'trouser-like' distribution.

* Brain-stem involvement is characterised by diplopia, nystagmus, dysarthria and dysphasia.

* Cerebral hemisphere disease may cause hemiparesis, hemianopia and dysphasia.

* Psychological disturbance in the form of intellectual decline, depression, euphoria and dementia.

* Visual pathway lesions most frequently involve the optic nerves and result in optic neuritis. Demyelination of the optic chiasm, optic tracts and radiations is uncommon.

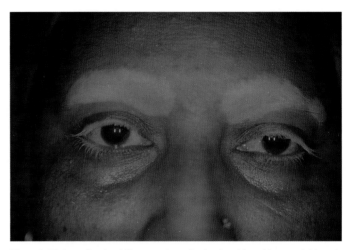

Fig. 8.68 Localised vitiligo and poliosis in Vogt–Koyanagi–Harada syndrome (Courtesy of U Raina)

Table 8.1 Diagnostic criteria for Vogt–Koyanagi–Harada (VKH) syndrome

1. **Absence of a history of penetrating ocular trauma**
2. **Absence of other ocular disease entities**
3. **Bilateral ocular involvement with the following manifestations:**
   a. Early
   (i) Diffuse choroiditis (focal areas of subretinal fluid or bullous serous retinal detachments)
   (ii) With equivocal fundus findings, both of the following must be present:
   * Typical findings on fluorescein angiography (see below)
   * Ultrasonography showing diffuse choroidal thickening, without evidence of posterior scleritis
   b. Late
   (i) History suggestive of prior presence of findings from 3a and either both (ii) and (iii) below, or multiple signs from (iii)
   (ii) Ocular depigmentation in the form of:
   * Sunset glow fundus, or
   * Sugiura sign (perilimbal vitiligo)
   (iii) Other ocular signs:
   * Nummular chorioretinal depigmented scars, or
   * Retinal pigment epithelium clumping and/or migration, or
   * Recurrent or chronic anterior uveitis
4. **Neurological and auditory findings,** which may have resolved by the time of examination:
   * Meningism (malaise, fever, headache, nausea, abdominal pain, stiffness of the neck and back, or a combination of these factors; headache alone is not sufficient to meet the definition of meningism, however), or
   * Tinnitus, or
   * Cerebrospinal fluid pleocytosis
5. **Integumentary findings** (not preceding onset of central nervous system or ocular disease):
   * Alopecia, or
   * Poliosis, or
   * Vitiligo

In complete VKH, criteria 1 to 5 must be present.

In incomplete VKH, criteria 1 to 3 and either 4 or 5 must be present.

In probable VKH (isolated ocular disease), criteria 1 to 3 must be present.

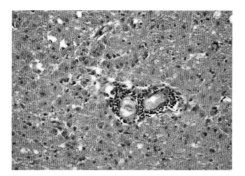

Fig. 8.69 Histology of a demyelinating plaque in multiple sclerosis, showing perivascular cuffing by lymphocytes

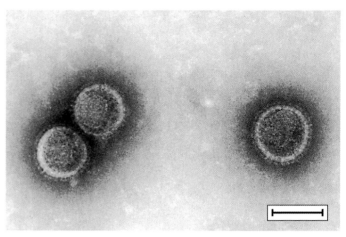

Fig. 8.71 Negative-stain electron micrograph of HIV (Courtesy of Hart and Shears, from *Color Atlas of Medical Microbiology*, Mosby, 2004)

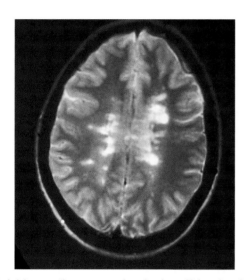

Fig. 8.70 Axial magnetic resonance imaging in multiple sclerosis, showing periventricular plaques

• Brain-stem lesions may result in internuclear ophthalmoplegia, gaze palsies, ocular motor nerve palsies, trigeminal and facial nerve palsy, and nystagmus.

3. Investigations

a. Lumbar puncture shows leucocytosis, IgG level >15% of total protein, and oligoclonal bands on protein electrophoresis.

b. MRI shows ovoid periventricular and corpus callosum plaques of demyelination with their long axes perpendicular to the ventricular margins (Fig. 8.70); acute plaques may be highlighted with gadolinium on T1-weighted scans.

4. Treatment options include systemic steroids and interferon beta-1a.

5. Ocular features: chronic anterior uveitis, intermediate uveitis, retinal periphlebitis and panuveitis.

6. Neuro-ophthalmic features: optic neuritis, internuclear ophthalmoplegia, nystagmus, skew deviation and ocular nerve palsies.

SYSTEMIC INFECTIONS

Acquired immunodeficiency syndrome (AIDS)

Pathogenesis

AIDS is caused by the human immunodeficiency virus (HIV) (Fig. 8.71). On a worldwide basis, heterosexual intercourse is the predominant mode of transmission; in the western world, however, AIDS is commonly transmitted by homosexual contact. Transmission may also occur by contaminated blood or needles, transplacentally or via breast milk. HIV targets CD4 (helper) lymphocytes, which are vital to the initiation of the immune response to pathogens. A steady decline in the absolute number of CD4 lymphocytes therefore occurs, resulting in progressive immune deficiency, particularly cell-mediated immunity. Regular estimation of the CD4 count is therefore a useful measure of disease progression.

Systemic features

1. Progression of HIV infection (Fig. 8.72)

a. Acute seroconversion illness. HIV infection is sometimes followed a few weeks later by constitutional symptoms such as fever, headache, malaise and maculopapular rash associated with generalised lymphadenopathy, soon after which anti-HIV antibodies appear.

b. An asymptomatic phase, often lasting many years, then follows, during which steady depletion of CD4 lymphocytes occurs.

c. Symptomatic HIV infection then follows, characterised by immunosuppression with opportunistic infections, neoplasms and tissue damage directly due to HIV infection.

Fig. 8.72 Virological and immunological progression of HIV infection

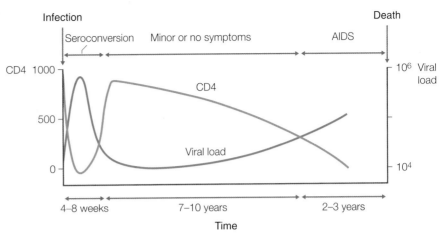

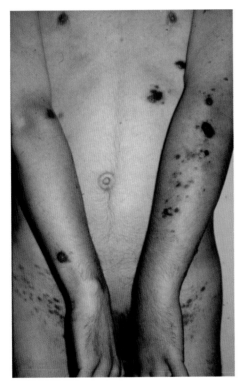

Fig. 8.73 Kaposi sarcoma in AIDS

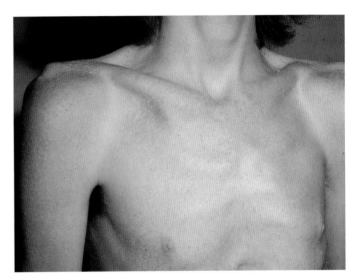

Fig. 8.74 HIV wasting syndrome

3. **Tumours** include Kaposi sarcoma (Fig. 8.73), non-Hodgkin B-cell lymphoma and squamous cell carcinoma of the conjunctiva (in Africa), cervix and anus.

4. **Other manifestations** include HIV wasting syndrome (Fig. 8.74), HIV encephalopathy (Fig. 8.75) and progressive multifocal leucoencephalopathy.

2. Opportunistic infections

a. **Protozoan.** Toxoplasma, cryptosporidium, microsporidium and *Pneumocystis carinii.*

b. **Viral.** Cytomegalovirus, herpes simplex and zoster, molluscum contagiosum and Epstein-Barr.

c. **Fungal.** Cryptococcus, candida and histoplasma.

d. **Bacterial.** *M. tuberculosis, M. avium-intracellulare,* staphylococci, streptococci, *Haemophilus* sp. and *Bartonella henselae.*

Serology

- Serological testing for HIV infection should be performed only with informed consent after proper counselling, due to the profound implications of a positive result. HIV is confirmed most commonly by the demonstration of anti-HIV antibodies in the serum, by enzyme-linked immunosorbent assay (ELISA) and the Western blot test.

- 'Seroconversion' may take 3 months or longer to occur following exposure to the virus, sometimes necessitating serial testing in individuals at high risk.

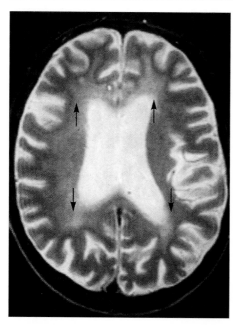

Fig. 8.75 Axial magnetic resonance imaging in advanced HIV encephalopathy, showing cerebral atrophy, widened sulci, ventricular dilatation and white matter abnormalities (Courtesy of Emond, Welsby and Rowland, from *Colour Atlas of Infectious Diseases*, Mosby, 2003)

- Subsequent to the establishment of HIV positivity, CD4 lymphocyte counts are measured every 3 months. A CD4 lymphocyte count <200/mm^3 implies a high risk of HIV-related disease. AIDS is diagnosed when an HIV-positive subject develops one or more of a defined list of indicator diseases.

Treatment

Although there is no cure, the progression of AIDS can be slowed by a number of drugs. The aim of treatment is to reduce the plasma viral load. Ideally, therapy should be commenced before the development of irreversible damage to the immune system.

1. **Indications** for commencement of anti-HIV therapy include:

- Symptomatic HIV disease.
- CD4 lymphocyte count <300/mm^3.
- Rapidly falling CD4 lymphocyte count.
- Viral load >10 000/ml of plasma.

2. **Drug treatment** is with 'highly active antiretroviral therapy' (HAART), which involves two nucleoside reverse transcriptase inhibitors with either a non-nucleoside reverse transcriptase inhibitor or one or two protease inhibitors.

a. **Nucleoside reverse transcriptase inhibitors** include zidovudine, lamivudine and zalcitabine.

b. **Protease inhibitors** include amprenavir, indinavir and nelfinadir.

c. **Non-nucleoside reverse transcriptase inhibitors** include efavirenz and nevirapine.

NB: Antiretroviral therapy is continuously evolving and should therefore be left to a trained physician. Resistance to various drugs is on the rise.

Ocular features

1. **Eyelid:** blepharitis, Kaposi sarcoma, multiple molluscum lesions and severe herpes zoster ophthalmicus.

2. **Orbital:** cellulitis, usually from contiguous sinus infection, and B-cell lymphoma.

3. **Anterior segment**

- Conjunctival Kaposi sarcoma, squamous cell carcinoma and microangiopathy.
- Keratitis due to microsporidium, herpes simplex and herpes zoster.
- Keratoconjunctivitis sicca.
- Anterior uveitis (usually secondary to systemic drug toxicity: rifabutin, cidofovir).

4. **Posterior segment**

- HIV retinopathy.
- Cytomegalovirus retinitis.
- Progressive outer retinal necrosis.
- Toxoplasmosis, frequently atypical.
- Choroidal cryptococcosis.
- Choroidal pneumocystosis.
- B-cell intraocular lymphoma.

Syphilis

Syphilis is caused by the spirochaete *Treponema pallidum*. The organism is thin and has a spiral shape, resulting in corkscrew movements (Fig. 8.76). It is very fragile, does not live in culture, and dies quickly on drying or heat. In adults, the disease is usually sexually acquired when the treponemes enter through abrasions of skin or mucous membranes. Transmission by kissing, blood transfusion and percutaneous injury are rare. Transplacental infection of the foetus can also occur from a mother who has become infected during or shortly before pregnancy. Although the infection is systemic from onset, in some patients clinical manifestations may be minimal or absent. The natural history of untreated syphilis is variable and may remain latent throughout, although overt disease may develop at any time.

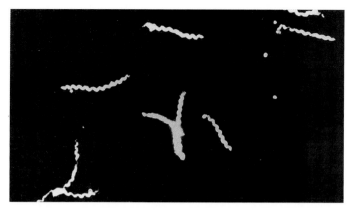

Fig. 8.76 *Treponema pallidum* seen by dark-field microscopy as slightly coiled spirochaetes (Courtesy of Hart and Shears, from *Color Atlas of Medical Microbiology*, Mosby, 2004)

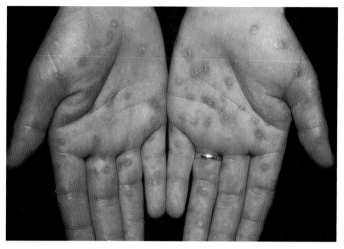

Fig. 8.78 Rash in secondary syphilis

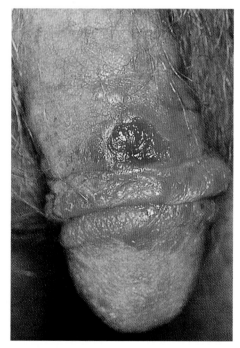

Fig. 8.77 Chancre in primary syphilis (Courtesy of Emond, Welsby and Rowland, from *Colour Atlas of Infectious Diseases*, Mosby, 2003)

Stages

1. **Primary** syphilis occurs after an incubation period commonly lasting 2–4 weeks and is characterised by a painless ulcer (chancre) at the site of infection. The most common site in males is the penis (Fig. 8.77), and in females the vulva. In homosexual men, the anus is a major site. The chancre is associated with discrete, mobile, rubbery enlargement of inguinal lymph nodes. Without treatment, the chancre resolves within 2–6 weeks, leaving an atrophic scar.

2. **Secondary** syphilis usually develops 6–8 weeks after the chancre and is characterised by:

- Generalised lymphadenopathy with mild or absent constitutional symptoms.

- Symmetric maculopapular rash on the trunk, palms (Fig. 8.78) and soles.

- Condylomata lata in the anal region.

- Mucous patches in the mouth, pharynx and genitalia, consisting of painless greyish-white circular erosions ('snail-track ulcers').

- Meningitis, nephritis and hepatitis may occur.

3. **Latent** syphilis follows resolution of secondary syphilis, may last for years, and can be detected only by serological tests.

4. **Tertiary** syphilis occurs in about 40% of untreated cases and is characterised by:

- Cardiovascular manifestations: aortitis with aneurysm formation and aortic regurgitation.

- Neurosyphilis: tabes dorsalis, Charcot joints and general paralysis of the insane.

- Gummata in various organs (Fig. 8.79).

Diagnostic tests

1. **Serological tests** rely on detection of non-specific antibodies (cardiolipin) or specific treponemal antibodies (see 'Investigations' in Ch. 6).

2. **Dark-ground microscopy** of exudate from a mucocutaneous lesion is reliable if positive (see Fig. 8.76).

Treatment

Treatment is with procaine benzylpenicillin (10 days in primary and secondary syphilis; 4 weeks in tertiary syphilis); alternatives in penicillin-allergic patients include doxycycline, tetracycline and erythromycin.

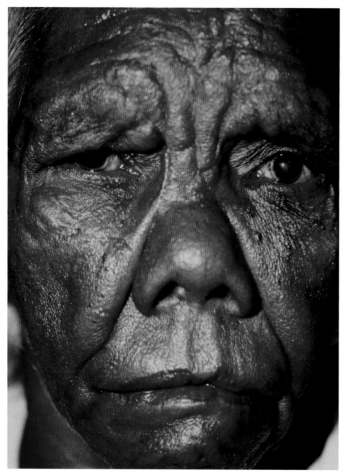

Fig. 8.79 Partial destruction of the nose by gummatous infiltration (Courtesy of C Barry)

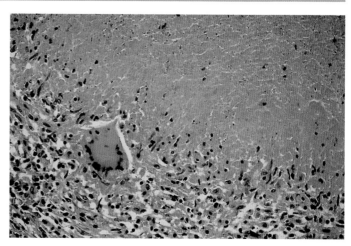

Fig. 8.80 Histology of a tubercule granuloma showing a Langerhans-type multinucleated cell surrounded by a zone of epithelioid cells and an outer shell of lymphocytes (Courtesy of Emond, Welsby and Rowland. from *Colour Atlas of Infectious Diseases*, Mosby, 2003)

Ocular features

These include uveitis, interstitial keratitis, madarosis, optic neuritis, Argyll–Robertson pupils and ocular motor nerve palsies.

Tuberculosis (TB)

TB is a chronic granulomatous infection (Fig. 8.80) caused by the tubercle bacillus that is of the genus *Mycobacterium*, which are non-motile, non-sporing, strictly aerobic rods. The two species responsible for TB in humans are the human strain *M. tuberculosis*, which is acquired by inhaling infected airborne droplets, and the bovine strain *M. bovis*, which is acquired by drinking unpasteurised milk from infected cattle. TB is primarily a pulmonary disease but it may spread by the bloodstream to other sites or form a generalised (miliary) infection. Infection with atypical mycobacteria, *M. avium complex*, may cause disease in immunocompromised individuals.

Stages

1. **Primary TB** usually occurs in children not previously exposed to *M. tuberculosis*. It is characterised by a small subpleural lesion (Ghon focus) and regional lymph-adenopathy (primary complex) which causes few if any symptoms and usually heals spontaneously, often with calcification, within 1–2 months, but the tuberculin test becomes positive.

2. **Latent TB** is characterised by lack of clinical manifestations but a positive tuberculin (Mantoux) skin test or radiological evidence of self-healed TB; the tuberculin test remains positive for many years.

3. **Post-primary (secondary) TB** is the result of reinfection or recrudescence of a primary lesion. Clinical features include erythema nodosum, fibrocaseous pulmonary lesions and lymph node involvement (Fig. 8.81). Miliary (like millet seeds on chest X-ray) TB may involve internal organs, CNS and bones.

Diagnostic tests

1. **Sputum examination** for acid-fast bacilli using Ziehl–Neelsen stain (Fig. 8.82).

2. **Cultures.** Mycobacteria require special media, such as Lowenstein–Jensen, and grow slowly (2–6 weeks) to produce a friable tenacious mass of adherent organisms.

3. **Tuberculin skin tests (Mantoux and Heaf)** involve the intradermal injection of purified protein derivative of *M. tuberculosis* (see 'Investigations' in Ch. 6).

Treatment

Treatment is initially with at least three drugs (isoniazid, rifampicin, pyrazinamide or ethambutol) and then with

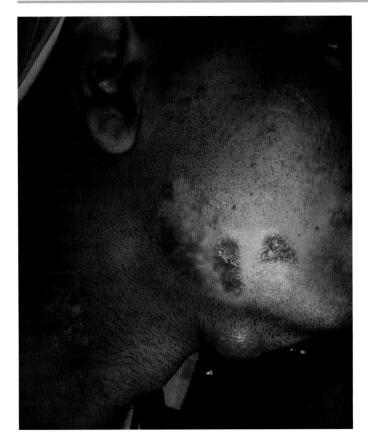

Fig. 8.81 Tuberculous lymphadenitis

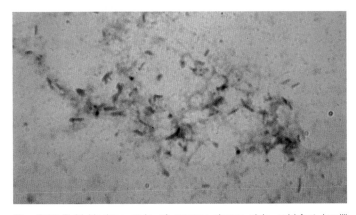

Fig. 8.82 Ziehl–Neelsen stain of sputum shows pink, acid-fast bacilli against a background of pus cells (Courtesy of Hart and Shears, from *Color Atlas of Medical Microbiology*, Mosby, 2004)

isoniazid and rifampicin. Quadruple therapy is sometimes necessary in resistant cases, more frequently seen in highly endemic areas such as India.

Ocular features

The main manifestations are chronic anterior uveitis (often granulomatous), choroiditis and retinal periphlebitis. Other features include solitary choroidal granulomas, scleritis and orbital involvement.

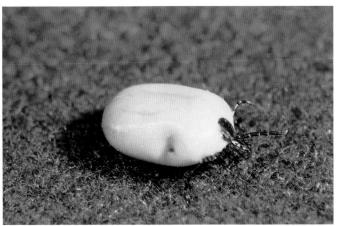

Fig. 8.83 Engorged tick responsible for transmission of Lyme disease (Courtesy of Emond, Welsby and Rowland, from *Colour Atlas of Infectious Diseases*, Mosby, 2003)

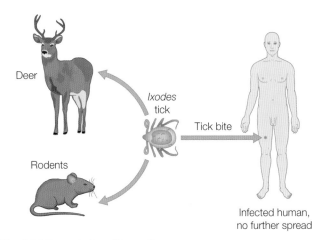

Fig. 8.84 Transmission of Lyme disease

Lyme disease

Lyme disease (borreliosis) is an infection caused by a flagellated spirochaete, *Borrelia burgdorferi*, transmitted through the bite of a hard-shelled tick (Fig. 8.83) of the genus *Ixodes*, which feeds on a variety of large mammals, particularly deer (Fig. 8.84). The disease is endemic in temperate regions of North America, Europe and Asia. It is the commonest vector-borne disease in many areas. Systemic manifestations are complex and are best conceptualised as early and late.

1. **Early stage** presents several days after the bite with a pathognomonic annular expanding skin lesion (erythema chronicum migrans) (Fig. 8.85), which may be accompanied by constitutional symptoms and lymphadenopathy. This may last for several weeks and resolve even without treatment. Complications, both neurological (cranial nerve palsies, meningitis) and cardiac (conduction defects, myocarditis), may follow within 3–4 weeks of the initial manifestations.

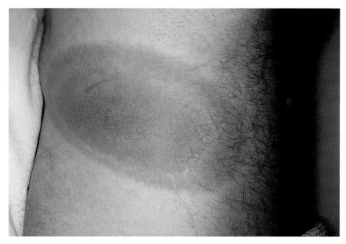

Fig. 8.85 Erythema chronicum migrans in Lyme disease (Courtesy of Emond, Welsby and Rowland, from *Colour Atlas of Infectious Diseases*, Mosby, 2003)

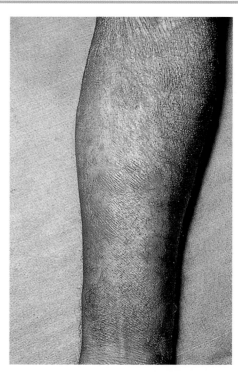

Fig. 8.86 Erythema nodosum leprosum in leprosy (Courtesy of Emond, Welsby and Rowland, from *Colour Atlas of Infectious Diseases*, Mosby, 2003)

2. **Late complications** include chronic arthritis of large joints, polyneuropathy and encephalopathy. Some patients develop a doughy, patchy, skin discoloration, which eventually results in shiny atrophy (acrodermatitis chronica atrophicans).

3. **Investigations:** PCR and ELISA.

4. **Treatment** of acute disease involves oral doxycycline or amoxicillin. Patients with ocular, cardiac, joint or neurological disease require intravenous ceftriaxone 2 g daily for 14–28 days. Prophylaxis with doxycycline should be given within 72 hours of the tick bite.

> **NB:** Protective clothing and insect repellents should be used in tick-infested areas.

5. **Ocular features:** transient follicular conjunctivitis, keratitis, episcleritis, scleritis, uveitis, orbital myositis, optic neuritis, neuroretinitis, ocular motor nerve palsies and reversible Horner syndrome.

Leprosy

Leprosy (Hansen disease) is a chronic granulomatous infection caused by an intracellular acid-fast bacillus, *M. leprae*, which has an affinity for skin, peripheral nerves and the anterior segment of the eye. The exact mode of infection is unknown, although the upper respiratory tract appears the most likely portal of entry.

1. **Lepromatous** leprosy is a generalised, multisystem infection with widespread lesions of skin, peripheral nerves, upper respiratory tract, reticuloendothelial system, eyes, bones and testes. Important signs include:

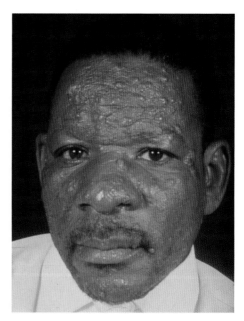

Fig. 8.87 Leonine facies in lepromatous leprosy

• Erythema nodosum leprosum, characterised by multiple painful red nodules (Fig. 8.86).

• Leonine facies, characterised by cutaneous thickening and ridging, nasal widening and thickening of earlobes (Fig. 8.87).

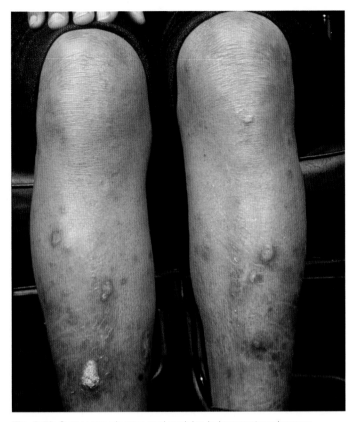

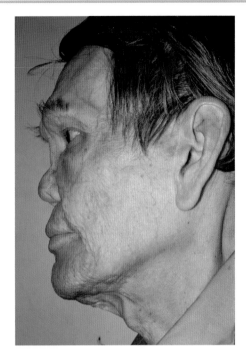

Fig. 8.89 'Saddle-shaped' nasal deformity in lepromatous leprosy

Fig. 8.88 Cutaneous plaques and nodules in lepromatous leprosy

- Peripheral cutaneous plaques and nodules (Fig. 8.88).

- Mucosal thickening and 'saddle-shaped' nasal deformity (Fig. 8.89).

- Sensory peripheral neuropathy facilitates trauma, which may result in shortening and loss of digits (Fig. 8.90).

- Motor neuropathy is exemplified by the 'claw-hand' deformity due to ulnar nerve palsy (Fig. 8.91).

- Autonomic neuropathy leads to dry, cracked, infection-prone skin; often superimposed on this is secondary bacterial infection, with gross tissue destruction.

2. **Tuberculoid** leprosy is restricted to the skin and peripheral nerves.

- Annular, anaesthetic, hypopigmented lesions with raised edges (Fig. 8.92).

- Thickening of cutaneous sensory nerves.

3. **Treatment** is with dapsone, rifampicin and clofazimine.

4. **Ocular features:** anterior uveitis, keratitis, madarosis, trichiasis, conjunctivitis, episcleritis, keratitis and scleritis

Cat-scratch disease

Cat-scratch disease (benign lymphoreticulosis) is a subacute infection caused by *B. henselae*, a Gram-negative rod. The

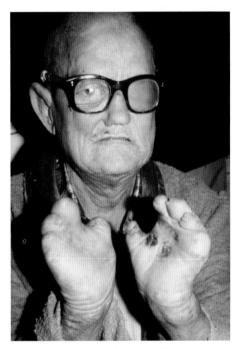

Fig. 8.90 Shortening and loss of fingers due to sensory peripheral neuropathy in lepromatous leprosy

infection is usually transmitted by the scratch or bite of an apparently healthy cat and occasionally by fleas. Ocular involvement occurs in about 6% of cases.

1. **Presentation** is with a red papule or pustule at the site of inoculation, followed by fever, malaise and regional lymphadenopathy (Fig. 8.93). However, general symptoms are

frequently absent or unremarkable and a history of contact with a cat is not always present.

2. **Disseminated** disease is rare but may affect immuno-compromised individuals in the form of endocarditis, encephalopathy, meningitis, splenomegaly, splenic abscess formation and osteomyelitis.

3. **Diagnostic tests** include serology for *B. henselae* and PCR.

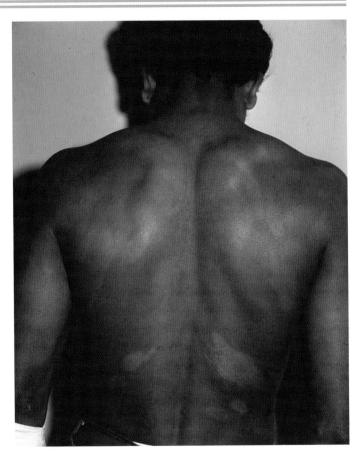

Fig. 8.92 Hypopigmented skin patches in tuberculoid leprosy

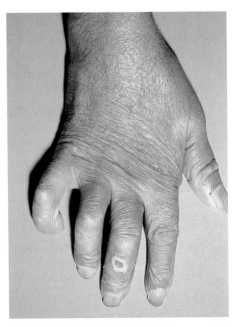

Fig. 8.91 'Claw hand' in lepromatous leprosy (Courtesy of M A Mir, from *Atlas of Clinical Diagnosis*, Saunders, 2003)

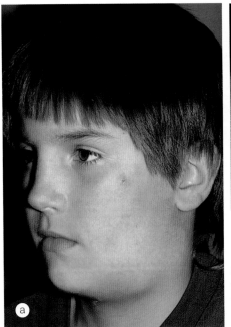

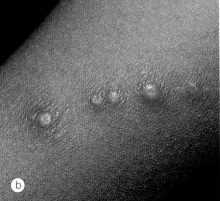

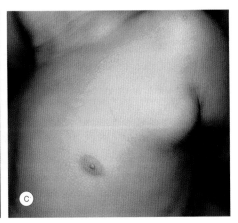

Fig. 8.93 Cat-scratch disease. (a) An ulcerated papule on the cheek caused by the scratch of a cat 2 weeks previously and enlargement of submandibular lymph nodes; (b) a line of papules on the forearm of another patient at the site of a cat scratch 3 weeks previously; (c) marked enlargement of ipsilateral axillary lymph nodes (Courtesy of Zitelli and Davis, from *Atlas of Pediatric Physical Diagnosis*, 4th edition, Mosby, 2002)

Fig. 8.94 Life cycle of *Toxoplasma gondii*

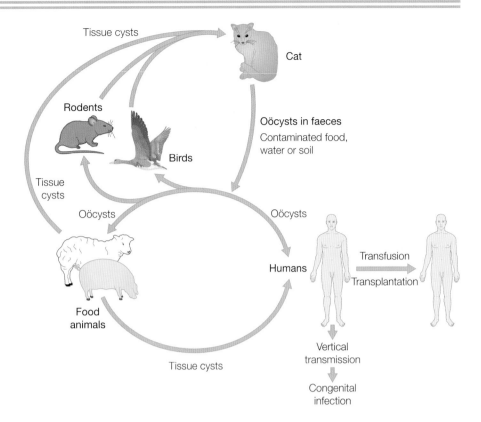

4. **Treatment** is with oral doxycycline or erythromycin, with or without rifampicin; the organism is also sensitive to ciprofloxacin and co-trimoxazole.

5. **Ocular features:** neuroretinitis, Parinaud oculoglandular syndrome, focal choroiditis, intermediate uveitis, exudative maculopathy, retinal vascular occlusion and panuveitis.

Toxoplasmosis

Toxoplasmosis is caused by *Toxoplasma gondii*, an obligate intracellular protozoan. It is estimated to infest at least 10% of adults in northern temperate countries and more than half of adults in Mediterranean and tropical countries. The cat is the definitive host of the parasite, and other beings, such as mice, livestock and humans, are intermediate hosts (Fig. 8.94).

1. **Oocysts** are excreted in cat faeces and spread to intermediate hosts.

2. **Trophozoites** are found in the cytoplasm of cells (Fig. 8.95) and are of two types:

a. **Tachyzoites** are the proliferating active form responsible for tissue destruction and inflammation following rupture of the cell wall (Fig. 8.96).

b. **Bradyzoites** grow very slowly and form tissue cysts which are separated from host tissue by a tough elastic membrane (Fig. 8.97).

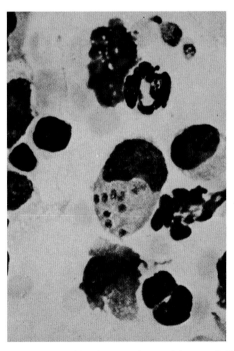

Fig. 8.95 Trophozoites within the cytoplasm of host cell (Courtesy of Emond, Welsby and Rowland, from *Colour Atlas of Infectious Diseases*, Mosby, 2003)

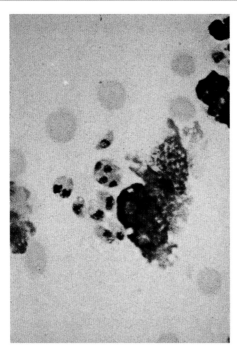

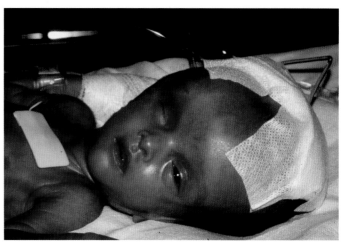

Fig. 8.98 Hydrocephalus in congenital toxoplasmosis; also note left anophthalmos (Courtesy of M Szreter)

Fig. 8.96 Release of trophozoites following rupture of the cell (Courtesy of Emond, Welsby and Rowland, from *Colour Atlas of Infectious Diseases*, Mosby, 2003)

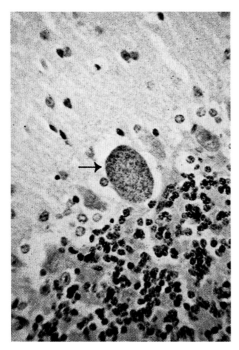

Fig. 8.97 Tissue cyst in the cerebellum (Courtesy of Emond, Welsby and Rowland, from *Colour Atlas of Infectious Diseases*, Mosby, 2003)

3. Mode of human infection

a. *Ingestion of undercooked meat* (lamb, pork, beef) containing bradyzoites of an intermediate host.

b. *Ingestion of sporocysts* following accidental contamination of hands when disposing of cat litter trays and then subsequent transfer onto food. Infants may also become infested by eating dirt (pica) containing sporocysts. It is likely that water contamination plays an important role in the transmission of the disease in rural areas.

c. *Transplacental spread* of the parasite (tachyzoite) can occur if a pregnant woman becomes infected.

4. Serological tests (see 'Investigations' in Ch. 6).

5. Congenital toxoplasmosis

- Toxoplasmosis is transmitted to the foetus through the placenta when a pregnant woman becomes infected. If the mother is infected before pregnancy, the foetus will be unscathed.

- The severity of involvement of the foetus is dependent on the duration of gestation at the time of maternal infection. For example, infection during early pregnancy may result in stillbirth, whereas if it occurs during late pregnancy it may result in convulsions, paralysis, hydrocephalus (Fig. 8.98) and visceral involvement. Intracranial calcification may be seen on CT (Fig. 8.99).

- However, just as in the acquired form, most cases of congenital systemic toxoplasmosis are subclinical. In these children, bilateral healed chorioretinal scars may be discovered later in life, either by chance or when the child is found to have defective vision.

- Infections occurring towards the end of the second trimester usually result in disease that can be detected at birth, such as macular scars, while infections occurring later in the third trimester may result in normal examinations at birth, but with the appearance of ocular or neurological findings in the future.

- The risk of disease later in life can be modified by early recognition of the transmission and long-term therapy.

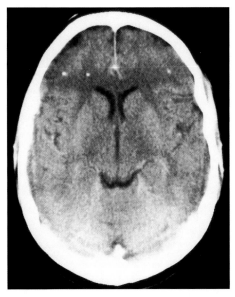

Fig. 8.99 Axial computed tomography showing cerebral calcification in congenital toxoplasmosis

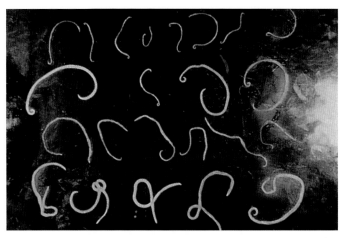

Fig. 8.101 Adult *Toxocara canis* worms from dog faeces (Courtesy of Hart and Shears, from *Color Atlas of Medical Microbiology*, Mosby, 2004)

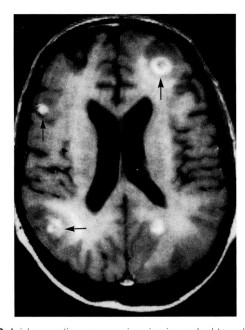

Fig 8.100 Axial magnetic resonance imaging in cerebral toxoplasmosis in AIDS, showing several round lesions resembling abscesses (Courtesy of Emond, Welsby and Rowland, from *Colour Atlas of Infectious Diseases*, Mosby, 2003)

6. **Acquired toxoplasmosis in immunocompetent** patients may take one of the following forms:

a. *Subclinical* is the most frequent.

b. *Lymphadenopathic syndrome*, which is uncommon and self-limiting, is characterised by cervical lymphadenopathy, fever, malaise and pharyngitis.

c. *Meningoencephalitis*, which is characterised by convulsions and altered consciousness, occurs in a minority of patients.

d. *The exanthematous* form, resembling a rickettsial infection, is the rarest.

7. **Acquired toxoplasmosis in immunocompromised** patients may be life threatening. The most common manifestation in AIDS patients is an intracerebral space-occupying lesion which resembles a cerebral abscess on MRI (Fig. 8.100).

8. **Ocular features.** Toxoplasma is the most frequent cause of infectious retinitis in immunocompetent individuals. Although some cases may occur as a result of reactivation of prenatal infestation, the vast majority are acquired postnatally.

Toxocariasis

Toxocariasis is caused by an infestation with a common intestinal ascarid (roundworm) of dogs, called *Toxocara canis* (Fig. 8.101). About 80% of puppies between the ages of 2 and 6 months are infested with this worm. Human infestation is by accidental ingestion of soil or food contaminated with ova shed in dogs' faeces. Very young children who eat dirt (pica) or are in close contact with puppies are at particular risk of acquiring the disease. In the human intestine, the ova develop into larvae that penetrate the intestinal wall and travel to various organs, such as the liver, lungs, skin, brain and eyes (Fig. 8.102). When the larvae die, they disintegrate and cause an inflammatory reaction followed by granulation. Clinically, human infestation can take one of the following forms, which seem to depend on the load of ingested parasites:

1. **Visceral larva migrans** (VLM) is caused by severe systemic infection which usually occurs at about the age of 2 years and is secondary to a large parasitic load. The clinical features, which vary in severity, include a low-grade fever, hepatosplenomegaly, pneumonitis, convulsions and, rarely, death. The blood shows a leucocytosis and marked eosinophilia.

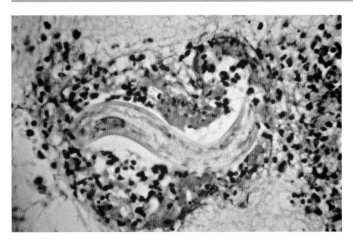

Fig. 8.102 *Toxocara canis* in tissue, with surrounding inflammatory reaction

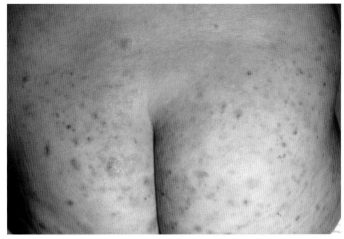

Fig. 8.104 Pruritic papules in acute onchocerciasis

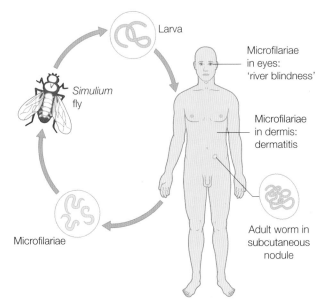

Fig. 8.103 Life cycle of *Onchocerca volvulus*

2. **Ocular toxocariasis** differs markedly from VLM because it involves otherwise healthy individuals who have a normal white cell count with absence of eosinophilia. Parasitic load is very low and no systemic reactions occur. A history of pica is less common, and the average age at presentation is considerably older (7.5 years) compared with VLM (2 years).

Onchocerciasis

Onchocerciasis, or river blindness, is caused by infestation with the parasitic helminth *Onchocerca volvulus*. The normal vector is the black fly of the genus *Simulium*, an obligate intermediate host, which breeds in fast-flowing water. Larvae are transmitted when the fly bites to obtain blood, which then mature into adult worms that produce millions of microfilariae over years (Fig. 8.103). *Wolbachia* (a rickettsia) lives symbiotically in the coat of the microfilaria and

are important for fertility of the female filarial worm. Lipopolysaccharide endotoxins released by the bacteria may be important in the pathogenesis of the disease and the adverse response to treatment in some individuals. Onchocerciasis is endemic in West, Central and East Africa, with small foci in Central and South America, Sudan and Yemen, infecting over 17.7 million people, most of whom are asymptomatic, but with an estimated 270 000 blind and half a million visually impaired. The disease is especially severe in Savannah areas.

1. **Signs**

- Acute skin lesions consist of numerous, small, discrete pruritic papules, usually involving the buttocks (Fig. 8.104) and extremities. Chronic lesions are characterised by thickening and hyperpigmentation, most frequently involving the lower limbs.

- Subcutaneous nodules (onchocercomas) consisting of encapsulated worms develop over bony prominences and the head. A common site for small nodules is just behind the ear. Occasionally, the lymph nodes become grossly enlarged, resulting in chronic lymphatic obstruction and lymphoedema.

2. **Treatment** is with ivermectin 12 mg given as an annual single dose. Although it acts rapidly to reduce the number of skin microfilariae, it depletes them for only a few months, after which they reappear at levels of 20% or more of pretreatment numbers within 1 year, which is sufficient for transmission to continue. New therapies are being developed targeting *Wolbachia*.

3. **Ocular features:** microfilariae in the aqueous, anterior uveitis, keratitis and chorioretinitis.

Cysticercosis

Cysticercosis refers to a parasitic infestation by *Cysticercus cellulosae*, the larval form of the pork tapeworm *Taenia solium* (Fig. 8.105). Pigs are the intermediate hosts and

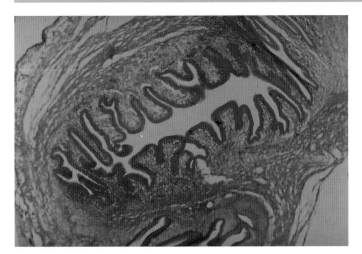

Fig. 8.105 *Taenia solium* (Courtesy of U Raina)

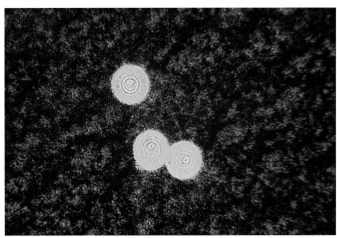

Fig. 8.107 Spores in cerebrospinal fluid in cryptococcal meningitis (Courtesy of Hart and Shears, from *Color Atlas of Medical Microbiology*, Mosby, 2004)

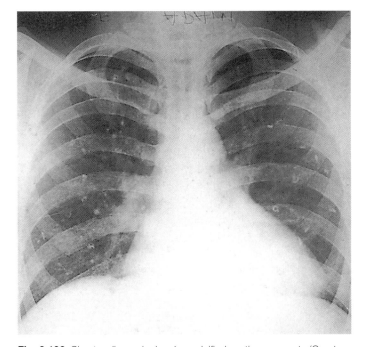

Fig. 8.106 Chest radiograph showing calcified cysticercus cysts (Courtesy of Hart and Shears, from *Color Atlas of Medical Microbiology*, Mosby, 2004)

humans are the definitive hosts, acquiring the disease by ingesting cysts of *T. solium* from contaminated pork or ova from contaminated fingers. The larvae are liberated from ova in the stomach, penetrate the intestinal mucosa and are carried to many parts of the body where they develop and form cysts that contain the head of a young worm (cysticerci).

1. **Systemic disease** often involves the lungs, muscles, brain and subcutaneous tissues.

2. **Investigations** involve radiology of the chest (Fig. 8.106) and muscles to detect calcified cysts.

3. **Ocular disease** primarily involves the vitreous and retina.

Cryptococcosis

Cryptococcus neoformans is a diamorphic yeast that enters the body through inhalation. Infection primarily affects patients with cell-mediated immune deficiency and affects 5–10% of patients with AIDS. Other predisposing factors include lymphoma, active hepatitis with use of prednisone and azathioprine, alcoholism, uraemia, SLE, organ transplantation with immunosuppression, and exposure to pigeons.

1. **Systemic disease** primarily involves the CNS (meningitis, meningoencephalitis and cryptococcoma); it may also cause pneumonia, mucocutaneous lesions, pyelonephritis, endocarditis and hepatitis.

2. **Investigations** involve culture or recognition of spores in CSF (Fig. 8.107), and serological detection of antigen.

3. **Treatment** is with intravenous amphotericin B and oral flucytosine.

4. **Ocular disease**. The most common is papilloedema due to raised intracranial pressure. Choroiditis is present in approximately 6% of patients with cryptococcal meningitis.

Nocardia

Nocardia asteroides, a Gram-positive, aerobic bacterium, is a cause of opportunistic infections in immunocompromised patients, particularly those with lymphomas, long-term pulmonary disease or receiving long-term systemic steroid therapy. The organism is usually acquired by inhalation.

1. **Systemic disease** has a predilection for the brain and soft tissues, with suppurative necrosis and abscess formation.

2. **Ocular disease** is characterised by keratitis, choroidal abscess and endophthalmitis.

Congenital rubella

Rubella (German measles) is usually a benign febrile exanthema. Congenital rubella results from transplacental transmission of virus to the foetus from an infected mother, usually during the first trimester of pregnancy. This may lead to serious chronic foetal infection and malformations. It appears that the risk to the foetus is closely related to the stage of gestation at the time of maternal infection.

1. **Fetal infection** is about 50% during the first 8 weeks, 33% between weeks 9 and 12, and about 10% between weeks 13 and 24. Each of the various organs affected has its own period of susceptibility to the infection, after which no gross malformations are produced.

2. **Systemic complications** of maternal rubella include spontaneous abortion, stillbirth, congenital heart malformations, deafness, microcephaly, mental handicap, hypotonia, hepatosplenomegaly, thrombocytopenic purpura, pneumonitis, myocarditis and metaphyseal bone lesions.

3. **Ocular features:** cataract, microphthalmos, glaucoma, retinopathy, keratitis, anterior uveitis and iris atrophy, extreme refractive errors, pendular nystagmus and strabismus secondary to poor vision.

Whipple disease

Whipple disease (intestinal lipodystrophy) is a rare, chronic, bacterial infection with *Tropheryma whippelii* that primarily involves the gastrointestinal tract and its lymphatic drainage. It occurs mostly in white middle-aged men. The disease is fatal if untreated.

1. **Presentation** is with weight loss, arthralgia, diarrhoea and abdominal pain.

2. **Extraintestinal manifestations** include primarily the CNS, lungs, heart, joints and eyes.

3. **Diagnostic tests.** Jejunal biopsy shows infiltration of small intestinal mucosa by 'foamy' macrophages that stain with periodic acid–Schiff. Electron microscopy shows small rod-shaped bacilli within the macrophages.

4. **Treatment** is with trimethoprim–sulfamethoxazole; the organism is also usually sensitive to tetracycline, erythromycin, penicillin, streptomycin and chloramphenicol.

5. **Ocular features** may be secondary to CNS involvement or caused by various types of intraocular inflammation.

BLISTERING MUCOCUTANEOUS DISEASES

Mucous membrane pemphigoid

Mucous membrane pemphigoid is a mucocutaneous blistering disease that may affect the mouth, nose, pharynx,

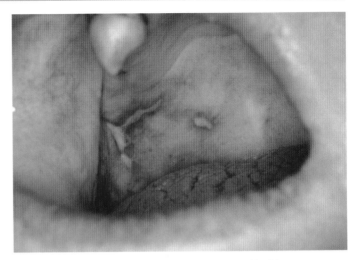
Fig. 8.108 Oral blisters in mucous membrane pemphigoid

trachea, genitalia and anus. The condition affects women more commonly than men (2 : 1), with a mean age of onset in the sixth decade. Conjunctival disease (ocular cicatricial pemphigoid – OCP) is seen in 75% of cases with oral involvement but in only 25% of those with skin lesions; occasionally, it occurs in isolation. OCP is always bilateral, but frequently asymmetric with regard to time of onset, severity and rate of progression.

Systemic features

1. **Mucosal** subepidermal blisters, most frequently oral (Fig. 8.108), rupture within a day or two, leaving erosions and ulcers that heal without significant scarring. Ulcers in other sites typically heal with scarring that may result in stricture formation. Stricture of the oesophagus (Fig. 8.109) can result in potentially lethal inhalation of food. Laryngeal or tracheal stenosis is a medical emergency.

2. **Skin** lesions are less common and present as tense blisters and erosions. They are common on the head and neck, the groins and extremities (Fig. 8.110); generalised involvement is uncommon (Fig. 8.111).

Stevens–Johnson syndrome and toxic epidermal necrolysis

Stevens–Johnson syndrome and toxic epidermal necrolysis (Lyell disease) reflect different severity of the same mucocutaneous blistering disease process. Both are uncommon but potentially lethal conditions that may be associated with severe ocular complications. They have the same clinical signs, treatment and prognosis, although ocular changes are much less common in toxic epidermal necrolysis. Males are affected more often than females, with a mean age of onset of 25 years.

Fig. 8.109 Barium meal showing an oesophageal stricture in mucous membrane pemphigoid

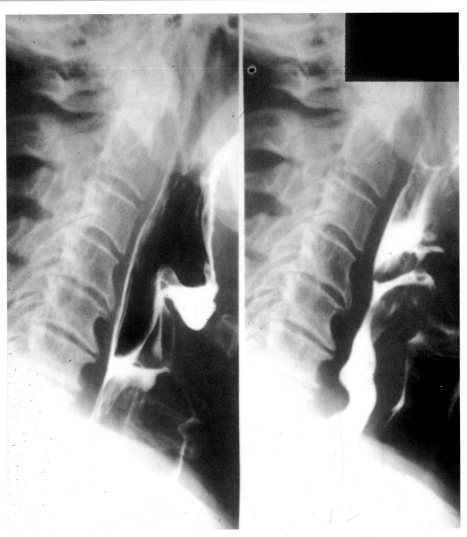

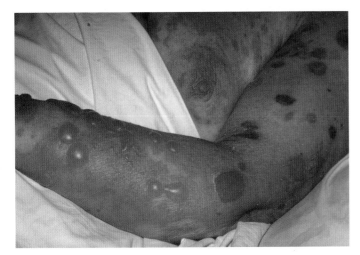

Fig. 8.110 Cutaneous blisters in mucous membrane pemphigoid

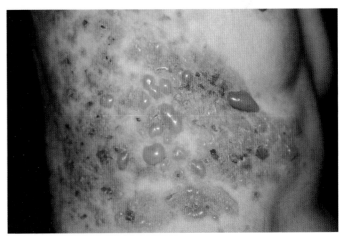

Fig. 8.111 Generalised mucous membrane pemphigoid

Systemic features

1. **Presentation** is fever, malaise, sore throat and possibly cough and arthralgia, which may last up to 14 days before the appearance of mucocutaneous lesions. In many cases, the patient is very ill and requires hospitalisation.

2. **Signs**

- Mucosal blisters of the mouth and nose, which rupture, forming erosions.

- Haemorrhagic crusting of the lips is characteristic (Fig. 8.112); genital involvement is less common (Fig. 8.113).

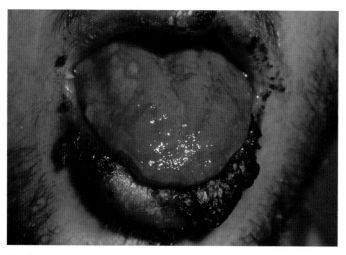

Fig. 8.112 Involvement of the mouth and haemorrhagic crusting of the lips in Stevens–Johnson syndrome

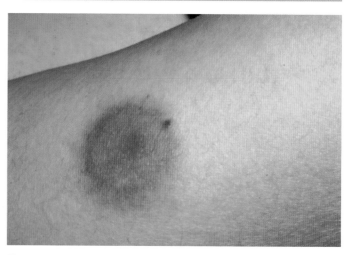

Fig. 8.115 Target lesion in Stevens–Johnson syndrome

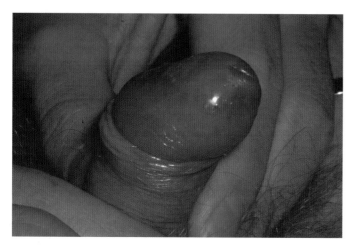

Fig. 8.113 Involvement of the glans penis in Stevens–Johnson syndrome

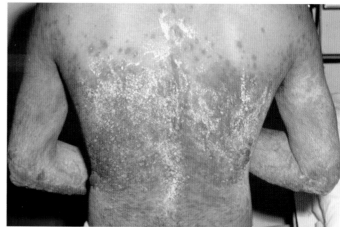

Fig. 8.116 Widespread haemorrhagic blisters in Stevens–Johnson syndrome

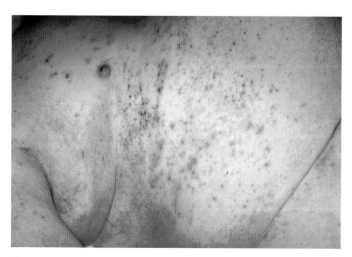

Fig. 8.114 Generalised papular rash in Stevens–Johnson syndrome

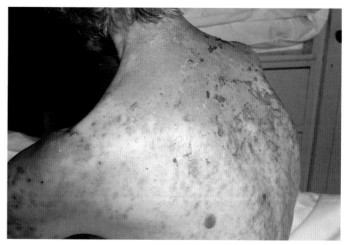

Fig. 8.117 Toxic epidermal necrolysis

- A generalised erythematous papular skin rash (Fig. 8.114), which evolves into 'target' lesions, consisting of erythematous centres surrounded by pale areas, in turn encircled by erythematous rings (Fig. 8.115).

- Blisters are usually transient but may be widespread and associated with haemorrhage and necrosis (Fig. 8.116).

Healing occurs within 1–4 weeks, usually leaving a pigmented scar.

- In toxic epidermal necrolysis, there may be widespread sloughing of the epidermis (Fig. 8.117).

Index